The Making of British Oral and Maxillofacial Surgery

Voices of Pioneers and Witnesses to its Evolution from Hospital Dentistry

Andrew Sadler

With the voices of:

Ordered by date of their first professional qualification

Professor Sir Paul Bramley (1944), Gordon Fordyce (1946), Michael Awty (1953), Laurence Oldham (1955), Russell Hopkins (1956), Khursheed Moos (1957), John Bradley (1958), Michael Bromige (1958), John Williams (1961), Professor John Langdon (1964), Andrew Brown (1968), John Cawood (1969), David Vaughan (1969), Adrian Sugar (1970), Brian Avery (1971), Richard Thornton (1971), Tony Markus (1972), Robert Hensher (1972), Michael Davidson (1976), Ian Martin (1979), Mark Cutler (1984)

The Making of British Oral and Maxillofacial Surgery Voices of Pioneers and Witnesses to its Evolution from Hospital Dentistry

© Andrew Sadler

ISBN: 978-1-9993612-4-2

Library of Congress Control Number: 2021909589

BROKESLEY HOUSE   2021

******

Cover Images:

Top Row. Left & centre: *A skin graft on gutta percha for an epithelial inlay.*
Right: *Silver cap splints.*

Centre Row. Left & centre: *A chrome-cobalt sub-periosteal implant for lower denture stabilisation.*
Right: *A plaster of Paris headcap supporting a maxillary fracture.*

Bottom Row. Left: *A fractured mandible fixed with external pins* **Centre:** *Intermaxillary fixation with arch bars.* **Right**: *Lateral oblique X-ray images.*

Contents

Prologue... *v*

1. *Why Become a Dentist?* *1*

2. *Getting into University*.. *8*

3. *Dental School 1939 to 1975*... *14*

4. *Surgery at Dental School*.. *25*

5. *Dental Students Gave Anaesthetics* *33*

6. *Early Hospital Experience* *40*

7. *Inspiration to Oral and Maxillofacial Surgery*........................... *62*

8. *Medical Training: Why and How?* *69*

9. *Medical Training: Paying For It* *85*

10. *Medical and Surgical Experience*.. *92*

11. *Applying for Jobs and Reminiscences of Prof. Homer Killey*....... *108*

12. *Higher Training* *121*

13. *Kaduna and Elsewhere Overseas* *148*

14. *Becoming a Consultant*.. *166*

15. *The Battle for Cancer* *188*

16. *Liverpool - The First Super Unit* *209*

17. *Facial Trauma* *221*

18. *Orthognathic Surgery* *232*

19. *Dento-alveolar Surgery* *254*

20. *Cleft Lip and Palate Surgery* *260*

21. Pre-prosthetic Surgery and Implantology *270*

22. Temporomandibular Joint Disorders *278*

23. Becoming a Medical Specialty and the Influence of Europe *285*

24. The Name *293*

25. Maxillofacial Fellowship of the Royal College of Surgeons of Edinburgh *297*

26. Professional Relationships, Co-operation and Antagonism *305*

27. The Early Greats, Terence Ward and Norman Rowe *321*

28. The Influence of the British Association of Oral and Maxillofacial Surgeons. *335*

29. Brian Conroy and the Evolution of Maxillofacial Technology *339*

Appendix 1 The Interviewees *353*

Appendix 2 Some Hospitals Mentioned in the Text *368*

Appendix 3 Timeline *374*

The John McLean Archive *382*

Acknowledgements *382*

Also by Andrew Sadler *382*

Prologue

The story told here starts in the 1940s before the start of the National Health Service and finishes in the 1990s when the specialty of oral and maxillofacial surgery was universally recognised both within the hospitals of the United Kingdom and the wider medical community, and as a medical specialty by the regulatory authority, the General Medical Council.

I started my career journey into what was then called oral surgery as a house surgeon in July 1975 in a northern teaching hospital. I had been in post for only a few days when, on my first ever evening on-call, I was summoned to the casualty department to see a patient with a broken jaw. I was shown by a nurse to a curtained cubicle across the corridor from the office where a handful of nurses and junior doctors were sitting, drinking tea, joking and flirting. The department was quiet in the early evening.

I was standing looking at the lateral oblique X-ray images of the mandible, when a fresh-faced young humourist put his head around the curtain and said, 'Excuse me, did a dentist do that?' There was laughter from the office behind. That was the first sign to me that the 'dentals', as we were known, were regarded, at least among the junior doctors at the Infirmary, to be a laughing stock. The perspective afforded by the passage of time confirms to me that this reputation was somewhat deserved, but at the time I felt demoralised.

Some years later I started work as a consultant oral and maxillofacial surgeon. On arrival I found the clinical repertoire similar to my house surgeon days. There were two operating lists a week, all wisdom teeth and dental clearances, with the occasional apicectomy.

I performed my first cancer operation three weeks later. It was simple stuff, a radical neck dissection, floor of mouth resection and reconstruction with a pectoralis major flap. The operation went well, but it took a good while. It was the first I had done from beginning to end entirely myself, apart from my three month elective in Sri Lanka earlier in the year.

Three days later when I went to the theatre I was told that the surgical director had been looking for me. A few minutes later, I had found him in his office and introduced myself. He explained that there had been something in the way of a complaint from an anaesthetist. 'You overran your operating time, and the dentist has operated on a neck and has a patient in intensive care; we've never had a dental case in intensive care before.'

I must have looked somewhat alarmed, but before I could open my mouth to make my case he quickly reassured me. 'Don't worry, I told him to piss off, now are you planning to do any more of these cases? Then you had better take my afternoon operating list so you can combine it with yours to have an all-day list.' Clearly someone expected the new dentist to do more than just extractions.

How did this expectation come about? How was it that the hospital dentist evolved into the oral and maxillofacial surgeon? I decided to investigate by becoming trained in oral history and interviewing some of the pioneers and witnesses to the process.

I chose people to interview who I knew were surgical big hitters by reputation or who I personally knew to be so. Some of the later ones were people who were mentioned in earlier interviews. Most were pioneers who really advanced the specialty either by introducing new techniques to our discipline or who inspired trainees, some of whom became pioneers themselves. They produced others who became disciples, like myself, who were not innovators but who took what they had learned or been inspired to do. The decision of whom to interview was mine; a couple declined. Some I asked because they had worked as juniors to pioneers, and in all these cases they advanced the specialty themselves, such was the inspiration that can be driven by enthusiasm and charisma.

I was interested in the politics, of course, but mostly in the social history because most of the advance was made at the 'coal face' in the clinics and operating theatres of the land. Several of my subjects had made substantial contributions to advancing our specialty through medical or dental politics and had become Presidents of our British Association of Oral and Maxillofacial Surgeons. But this was not my reason for asking them, they were asked because of their contribution to clinical oral and maxillofacial surgery, inspiration and training. Eight of my subjects have been awarded the Down Surgical Prize of the British Association of Oral and Maxillofacial Surgeons, for making 'a major contribution to oral and maxillofacial surgery in its widest sense'.

And of course it wasn't all completely wonderful. Besides the pioneers, witnesses and disciples there were others who made no such contribution but carried on just removing wisdom teeth or more often delegating it to juniors. They won't be mentioned again.

The recordings quoted in this book were made between 2012 and 2020, as part of the British Dental Association John McLean history archive, mostly, but not exclusively, in the subjects homes. The recordings were made on broadcast quality equipment in a lossless format and were transcribed literally, i.e. exactly as spoken. The copyright of the original recordings is held by the British Dental Association.

I have edited the 450,000 words of transcript into a readable text. The resulting text was sent to the subjects for them to check and modify as they thought appropriate.

In reading the text of peoples' memories, please consider that oral history is the recollection, opinion or interpretation of individuals. I have included some contrary opinions, and all opinions expressed are those of the speaker and not necessarily my own. I have attempted to keep my introductions to the quotations to a minimum; where it is not obvious what time they are talking about, I have added the years in [square brackets].

In reading the text please consider:

'Even where there is no malice, imagination will still be active. People believe or disbelieve, repeat or suppress, according to their own inclinations.'

James Anthony Froude (English historian 1818-1894)

Or put more succinctly:

'It ain't necessarily so.'

Ira Gershwin (1935)

Or more recently:

'Recollections may vary.'

Queen Elizabeth II (2021)

Andrew Sadler

July 2021

Chapter 1
Why Become a Dentist?

'Most of the college wanted to go into medicine'

In the middle of the 20th century, a career in medicine conferred a higher social standing and income than dentistry. Those who could afford the long training were therefore more likely to be drawn into medicine. During the Second World War, entry to the dental schools had fallen by 30% whereas medical recruitment had held up.[1]

All of my interview subjects went to dental school before undertaking any medical training, but what was their motivation? Although intelligent high achievers, just like dental school applicants today they were often naïve and only superficially informed about their intended career. Perhaps unlike many of today's applicants sometimes they lacked self-confidence; but just like today's recruits, they were often inspired by dentists who had treated them.

Paul Bramley was 16 when he applied for dental school, but he wanted a medical degree as well! [1939].

> *I did two years in the science sixth, and most of the college wanted to go into medicine. I felt well, I'll go into dentistry. It was partly because my mother took me to the dentist regularly, a very distinguished practice where both partners were doubly qualified. One of my contacts was a young dentist which I had quite a lot to do with socially, so I thought 'well that's a good life, that's what I'll do'.*

> *It was also something to do with your hands, it's to do with people, it has medical overtones and expressions of service and that sort of thing. It became clear to me that I would get qualified in dentistry and practise dentistry, but with a medical qualification.*

Gordon Fordyce applied for Dental School during WWII [1942].

> *I think it was because I had a good, attractive, young male dentist and I think he was the one who influenced me to go towards dentistry. I thought about doing medicine but I thought no, I would do dentistry because it was a subject which I thought I could see round and that it*

---

1 The Teviot Report-Recruitment and the Dental Schools. Wilkinson F C. British Dental Journal 1946 Vol 80 (7) 215-219

was possible to know as much as was available about it. Whereas medicine I thought it would have so many side-lines that I couldn't concentrate on. I saw dentistry as my future.

Mike Awty was also influenced by being a patient. It was soon after World War II [1948].

I really was interested in medicine, but that was not a burning desire. Just before the Health Service came in I went to a dentist who had just come down from Guy's, who diagnosed an unlined silicate filling in my canine, which was slowing dying and giving me terrible grief. He performed a root treatment, and I was very impressed, as he drew diagrams of what was going on and made it all very interesting, which sounded much more fun than I thought filling teeth was.

So I talked more and more to him as he put my mouth in order and I thought, well, this sounds rather fun. I'm quite good with my hands and I thought I could cope with the academic side. That was why, a considerate and interesting dentist had talked to me at an impressionable period of my early life.

Status was much more important than now and although there had been university degrees in dentistry from 1904, it was not until after the Dentists Act of 1956 that a degree became the prominent qualification; before that it was the LDS diploma from one of the royal colleges, most usually the Royal College of Surgeons of England.

In 1923, two years after the Dentist Act of 1921, which established the register, only 40% of registrants had any form of qualification. It was therefore no wonder dentistry was considered of lower status and that many dentists wanted the approbation of a medical qualification and many considered medicine first.[2]

Laurence Oldham had applied to study medicine but ended up doing dentistry in Birmingham. He explains why [1949].

I applied to medical school because that was my first love, but I came out of the secondary education at a time, 1949-50, when a lot of ex-forces people were in the market for university places, and they seemed very much more mature. I think the interview panel in medicine realised that here was a relatively insignificant newcomer straight

---

2 125 years of development in dentistry 1880-2005 Part 5: Dental education, training and qualifications Gelbier, S. British Dental Journal 2005. Vol 199 (10) 685-688.

from school who wasn't really up to the medical course.

My parents took my younger sister to Birmingham Dental Hospital so she could have orthodontic treatment. I can remember going with the family up the stairs to the orthodontic department and I had one of those rare flashes of insight which said to me, this is what you want to do.

Russell Hopkins entered Dental School in 1951. His route was complicated, he wanted to study medicine but failed his Higher School Certificate[3] so he applied for dentistry. He subsequently turned down an offer of a medical place.

The results of my Higher School Certificate were of no surprise to me, I got a distinction in biology, passed physics but failed my subsidiary pure maths and chemistry. I then left boarding school, went to the local grammar school, spent a year working hard, and then took the first A levels. Chemistry, Physics, and Biology, and I passed sufficiently to satisfy the requirements for the dental school, which I then accepted. Then I was rung up by the medical school and they said they had a place for me because I'd reached the standard to get into medicine. I mulled about what to do, and I thought oh bugger this, what am I going to do? I became a dental student.

The dental schools took a lot of people who'd failed to reach the standard required for medicine. That subsequently I reached the standard to get into medicine, was something that caused me a lot of anxiety and I turned it down, which may well have been a mistake, but anyway, I went to dental school.

The shock of failing that exam caused a major depression during that summer afterwards and it took me some time to recover from my loss of confidence. I never failed another exam as an undergraduate in medicine or dentistry, or my fellowship or primary, or anything else. I made damn certain I never failed another exam. So, it was a lesson, but it was a lesson hard learnt.

Khursheed Moos wanted to do medicine but went to Guy's as a dental student [1953].

When I was at school, I was quite interested in the medical side of

---

3 The Higher School Certificate was taken two years after the School Certificate usually at age 18. It was replaced in 1951 by A-levels. Russell took both because he had failed the 'Higher'.

things and was advised to apply to Oxford for a scholarship to get in to do medicine. I hadn't really thought much about dentistry and I applied for medicine but unfortunately did not get the scholarship and there was only one. I was offered a place but my father could not afford to pay for me to go to Oxford and so I applied then for dentistry in London University because I had had some experience in dentistry as an orthodontic patient.

Mike Bromige considered medicine [1954].

The thought process was something like well a doctor would be all right but they get called out at night therefore perhaps dentistry would be better.

John Bradley wanted to be a dentist like his father [1954].

I was always interested in healthcare. I was good with my hands, so I wanted to do something practical and I wanted to work with people. So I decided that I would do dentistry, I had an insight into it from my father who was a dentist.

John Williams was influenced by a physiologist who taught at Guy's. [1956].

At school on a Saturday when I was working towards A-Levels, we had a person who came and taught physiology who was actually a professor of physiology for dentistry at Guy's. He really was the person instrumental in first introducing me to the concept of doing dentistry. I thought it was a good idea.

I had two compatriots who wanted to do medicine, and I was perceived as possibly not being as bright as they were, and it was questioned whether I would be able to do medicine.

John Langdon. [1960].

My hobbies were all based on manual dexterity, building models and the usual, and my grandmother had been a dentist in Shoreditch, so I thought that dentistry might suit me.

However, David Vaughan was in Ireland where it was easier to secure a place in medicine than dentistry. He went to University College Cork in 1962. Why dentistry?

Most of my family are in the medical profession and I thought I'd be slightly different, so I applied for dentistry.

In those days, 1962, I think the reason dentistry was competitive in

Ireland was because it was well known that you can make a lot of money as a dentist. Pre-registration house officers in medicine weren't even paid, they got their board and lodgings, and that was it; and they worked 120 hours a week. Whereas if you did five years of dentistry you were out and you could make money; and quite a few people made very big money doing dentistry.

In those days, we had a general pre-med/pre-dental science class and the dental school I was applying for had a place for 15 dental students. When we did the exam, 20 of us passed and the five with the lowest marks went on and did medicine; the first 15 did dentistry.

There was a chap in the first dental year who developed an osteogenic sarcoma of his leg and died and so we were down to 14 in the year. And the chap who was 16th in the exam results, who was now doing medicine, applied to the senate of the university to change from medicine to dentistry, and they wouldn't allow him, so we ended up with a class of 14 people.

By the 1960s, the status of the Dental Profession had improved. Andy Brown went to Guy's [1963].

I had poor dental health, so I spent quite a lot of time in the dental chair in my early teens. The dentist used to run two surgeries. He'd put the local anaesthetic in and leave you cooking, and while I was waiting for the anaesthetic to work I used to fiddle and play with all the knobs on his dental machines and his kit, and pick up instruments and look at them. And I started to think to myself, because I enjoyed the biological sciences, perhaps I'd like to get into this.

John Cawood [1963].

It was very much a spur-of-the-moment decision, prompted in my final year at school when our careers master confronted our class and went round each individual saying, 'What would you like to do when you leave school?' I was on the back foot because, really, I hadn't given it very much thought.

I was sitting beside Graham Wood, who you know was an oral and maxillofacial surgeon first in north Wales and then latterly in Glasgow. Graham and I were great friends and as soon as he was asked he said, 'I want to be a dentist,' I thought that's an interesting prospect. So without further thought I said, I think I'd like to do dentistry. That's about as much thought as I could muster at the time.

Also by the 1960s is was known that a good income could be earned by dentists, a reason for going to dental school which was supplied by Brian Avery [1965].

I think my father influenced me, mostly. He said to me that dentistry appeared to be a good well-paid job and I should consider taking that up. And when I heard that it was a good well-paid job, ears pricked up, and I thought, right, okay, I'll apply.

Tony Markus went to Newcastle [1967].

I did my sciences at school and I thoroughly enjoyed it. I had some wonderful teachers but I didn't work terribly hard. There were six of us who were going to go do medicine. Anyway, I didn't do terribly well so I didn't get into medical school as I was hoping to and follow my two brothers; so I was advised to apply for dentistry.

Mike Davidson [1972].

It was an accident. I'd wanted to read medicine and my A-level grades were not up to scratch, and the headmaster said, 'Oh, well, why don't you go off and do dentistry? A friend of mine who was at my college, is now the Dean at the London Hospital dental school and they're always after people in clearing and you're just the sort of chap I'm sure they'd look at.'

Adrian Sugar [1965].

I only ever really wanted to do dentistry or medicine and I couldn't decide which. And I applied for medical and dental school and I didn't like the interviews I had for medical school, especially one I remember in particular; it put me off a bit. So I eventually ended up doing dentistry at Leeds.

When Ian Martin was a sixth former, he was sent by his school to various places to get inspiration for a career choice [1974].

One place they sent us was the dental school in Manchester. I think it was an open day or something that we were all enrolled to go along. They had lots of these big plaster teeth and they gave you a go at drilling them and that sort of thing. And a chap came up over my shoulder and he said, 'Oh, that's jolly good. Had you thought of doing dentistry?' 'Well, no.' He said, 'Well, I think you should think about it.'

And, of course, I looked around. I was from a borderline of working/lower middle class background, and in the town that I lived, which was Chorlton-cum-Hardy, all I really knew about medicine was the GP lived in a semi, round the corner from us and had a Rover and the dentist lived in the biggest house in the town and had a Mercedes and a Bentley. Well, hmm, that sounds fun.

Chapter 2

Getting into University

'If I'd got one D, I might have got into Medicine'

Getting into dental school was not difficult; before the start of the National Health Service in 1948, there was inadequate recruitment into the dental profession. Prior to WWII the average intake into dental schools was 375 a year, and it was anticipated that doubling that number would not lead to an overcrowded profession.[4] In 1943 the Minister of Health had set up the Teviot Committee to report on dentistry, education, research, legislation and a state dental service. The committee submitted a final report in 1946 and suggested that 20,000 dentists might be needed in the UK within 20 years.[5] This was the start of expansion in dental training.[6]

Gordon Fordyce [1941].

It wasn't difficult to get into. The war was on; they wanted people to go in. I was only seventeen when I started. So I was still a young lad.

Mike Awty was in a hurry to get a place before National Service. Conscription into the armed forces started at the beginning of WWII and continued until 1957 for young males. After 1948 they had to do 18 months in active service and remain on the reserve list for four years. But going in with a professional qualification meant the possibility of being an officer [1948].

National Service was a big threat because I thought if I could get to university I could postpone that for a bit and then perhaps have a more interesting time in the Services once I'd qualified in something.

So I did one year in the science sixth and then applied to Guy's for a pre-med entry. I did the chemistry, physics and biology at Guy's in a year course. The hurry was that I was rather afraid that I'd be taken for my National Service if I didn't get a university place quickly.

---

4 British Dental Journal. Leading article August 3rd 1945 74-75.
5 Final Report of The Inter Departmental Committee on Dentistry. HSMO, February 1946.
6 For a summary of the important changes in dental training see: Milestones in Dental Education. David Mason. Dental Historian 1999 35; 4-14.

An essential part of the selection process for Dental School was the interview. Mike:

The headmaster at the grammar school where I had matriculated wrote a testimonial. It seemed to do the trick. I had made quite a lot of models, which had been appreciated, and this seemed to impress the chairman of the interviewing committee, which was Fred Warner.[7] He was a very imposing figure, sitting across the table, big shoulders, big man with a   double-breasted black jacket; he could have been Al Capone. Very intimidating, but I evidently passed muster, and I was accepted. I ended up being his house surgeon later.

Laurence Oldham was applying to Birmingham [1949].

We had a manual dexterity test, as well as an interview, and I remember we had to do the professor's initials in bending wire. We had to bend it to JO, John Osborne, who seemed to be in charge of the interviews. And then we had to carve from a cube of wax, I think it was an incisor, and when I finished the manual dexterity test with about 25 others, we looked around and some of them had done beautifully artistic wire bending for JO and very authentic carving for teeth. Mine were rather mediocre. The offer was unconditional, providing I'd got through A levels. I did chemistry, physics, biology and subsidiary maths, and I passed all of those and was accepted straight away.

Mike Bromige, also Birmingham [1954].

I wrote to Birmingham and got myself an interview and met Professor Osborne. I had an interview and there was a practical test. We had to bend some wire into a circle and carve some wax into a pyramid and mount six anterior teeth on a wax strip in the correct order. Then I went back and saw Prof. Osborne and he said, 'You're in.' I went home with a university place in my pocket. Oh, I think it was conditional on getting my A-Level biology, because I must have had chemistry and physics at A-Level already.

The years 1951-1955 saw a fall in the already inadequate number of recruits into the dental profession. The McNair committee was set up to recommend how recruitment could be increased. The report recommended that 1000 training places were required each year. Not only was there a shortage of dentists, many were older and the shortage

---

7 Dean of the Guy's Hospital Dental School.

was forecast to get worse. This meant that potential recruits to dentistry had little difficulty in gaining a training place.[8][9]

Khursheed Moos had been offered a place for medicine at Oxford. However, he had failed to get a scholarship; his father could not afford to pay for Oxford [1953].

The closing date there had passed for medicine and therefore I applied to Guy's Hospital for a studentship in dentistry. I applied to Guy's for no special reason except I must have been given some advice, and I don't know by whom, that I should apply for that. To some extent, I had drifted into dentistry.

When I went to Guy's in 1953, at my interview I was told that there was a dual degree course in medicine and dentistry and that it would be possible for me to join that later. Originally I had expected I would do dentistry and then go on to do medicine as it was implied at the interview that was likely.

John Bradley [1954].

I didn't seem to have any difficulty getting a place at all. Everybody seemed to want me, which is rather nice. I think it was because I was the son of a dentist. We were interviewed properly and I think they got a sense of what the prospective students were like as people. I remember my interview well with the Dean, who was FS Warner. They asked quite a few pointed questions why I wanted to do it, and we were tested for manual dexterity.

John Williams [1956].

When I went for an interview at Guy's I was greeted on the doorstep by Declan Anderson.[10] I think he'd primed the Committee, and I had a very sensible interview. We had to do our three A-Levels, but because I was doing the scholarship as well, I had to do an additional bit.

John Langdon [1960].

I applied to dental school, was summoned to the London, where I was interviewed by Harry May, who was the Dean of the medical school, on his own in his study. We chatted for ten minutes, he said,

---

8 McNair Report (1956) Report of the Committee on Recruitment to the Dental Profession. Cmnd 9861, HMSO.
9 The Dental Service. Office of Health Economics Publication. February 1969.
10 Declan Anderson the Professor of Physiology who had taught him at school.

'Okay, you can start in September.' So I ended up going to dental school.

John Cawood [1964]

I planned to go to Glasgow University but I had a very unpleasant interview with Professor Aitchison who was then the Dean and that prompted me to think again so I applied for the University of St Andrews and I had a totally different experience with Professor Hitchen, he was very friendly and welcoming. On that experience alone I decided to accept an offer from St Andrews and turn down an offer to go to Glasgow. The St Andrews the dental school is actually in Dundee and was part of Queen's College.

Andy Brown [1963].

I dipped one of my A Levels and although I had a place at Guy's I had to start on what was called the first MB, or the first BDS course to re-sit physics, which paradoxically was the one A Level which all my schoolmasters told me I would sail through!

At no stage in any of my interviews for dental school was I asked to perform any form of manual dexterity test. They just assumed, I presume, that you could train anybody to use their hands, which is rather strange.

By 1967 there were still only 14980 dentists in the UK.[11] The McNair report of 1956 had given impetus to new buildings for dental schools and one new school, which had increased the number of places available for training to 800 a year. But still there was difficulty in recruiting into the schools. Prospective students found it easy to get a place.[12]

Brian Avery [1965].

I applied in the last year before they introduced the UCCA, the University Central Council for Admissions.[13] I could apply to four dental schools. And because my home was in London, I applied to four of the five London dental schools.

---

11 Dental Services Office of Health Service Economics 1969.

12 .Dental Recruitment H Colin Davis 1968 British Dental Journal 125(5) 206-211.

13 UCCA administered university applications, replacing individual applications to Universities, from 1961. the London medical and dental schools did not join the scheme until 1967. In 1993 it merged with the Polytechnics Central Admissions System to form UCAS (University and Colleges Admissions Service).

I got a place at Royal Dental first and then at University College Hospital (UCH) and then at the London, and UCH wanted me to accept within a certain date. And I'd heard that Guy's was the best dental school, so I was about to accept UCH, and I suddenly got a letter offering me an interview at Guy's a couple of weeks ahead. My father realised that I'd miss the chance to go to Guy's if I accepted UCH and met the deadline, so he rang up Guy's and said, 'Look, my son's got three places already how about interviewing him quickly?' So they interviewed me the next day.

It was a very interesting interview. I met Fred Warner who was the Dean, and I forget who else. I went in to them and they said to me, 'We understand you've already got three places?' and I said, 'Yes.' 'But you'd like to come here?' I said, 'Yes, I would.' So they said, 'Okay,' and they interviewed me. Then they said, 'Would you like to go outside and take a seat. We've got a little bell here on the desk and we'll ring it and you can come back in and we'll tell you if you've got a place?' So I went outside, and I was just squatting to sit and the bell rang; I hadn't even sat down. Fred Warner called me back in and they offered me a place. So I accepted.

Tony Markus [1967].

I got two Es in history and English and I got three Es in my sciences. So I got five Es. They gave me an unconditional offer. I think if I'd got one D, I might have got in to medicine.

Tony had an interview at Newcastle [1967].

I got in my Morris Minor and the big end broke down just south of Darlington on my way to interview and I couldn't go any further. Having got my hands covered in black oil, I had to ditch the car and get up to Newcastle for the interview dishevelled. They asked me about my manual dexterity and I said I play the piano and they said that's very good, 'And what else do you do, do you fix cars?' I said, 'No, I just had a problem today.' Anyway, they offered me a place there and then. Newcastle was very easy-going; this was 1967. I was very grateful to be given an unconditional place. I knew little about Northumberland, but I knew that there were some very good rivers there and I could indulge in fishing.

Mike Davidson [1972].

When clearing started, I was invited down to the London; it wasn't The Royal London in those days; it was the London Hospital Dental school, for an interview with Roy Duckworth who was Dean and a friend of my headmaster. It was just me and him in a room and I got offered a place in dentistry.

Ian Martin [1975].

I hadn't done biology because it looked like too much hard work; I'd done physics and chemistry. So because it was a small school they were very helpful they said, well if you want to do dentistry you really ought to get some sort of biology, the easiest one to do is human biology. And so they organised, in the summer holidays, for the biology teacher to give me a bit of private tuition, all free, and I took the O level in the November sitting, and that made me eligible to apply for dentistry.

I went to visit King's, and there was something about it, it was really nice; they made you feel welcome; they made you feel you were somebody special. I was shown round, and it seemed quite modern. And unlike most of the other places where you had to wear little tunicky things or half size white coats, at King's they all wore long coats like proper doctors and proper dentists. So I quite liked it there, and they offered me a C and two Ds, so I'm like: ah, that's the place for me.

Chapter 3
Dental School 1939 to 1975

'I can remember the smell of burnt dentine to this day'

Paul Bramley was an undergraduate at Birmingham in wartime [1940-44].

> *It was the beginning of the Second World War and I was then of course in a reserved occupation.[14] I lived in the old VD[15] ward in the General Hospital, which was in Steelhouse Lane in the absolutely the centre of Birmingham, next door to all the industrial installations; it was a pretty dangerous place. We fire watched there for one shilling a night, and had bed-and-breakfast and an evening meal in the General Hospital.*

> *When there were air raids and incendiary bombs we had to get up on the roof and deal with them, which we did on several nights, and that was pretty scary because the firemen were coming up with their hosepipes, not seeing you on the roof and this great jet came round.*

> *The way that dental hospitals were run before the advent of full-time academic teachers, was the honorary consultant system. That meant they gave their services to Guy's, Barts, the London Hospital, etc., for free, but they got the student contact for future referrals, they got the kudos of working at a great teaching hospital. They also had their private practices in Wimpole Street or Harley Street or thereabouts, which flourished under this and financed their largesse in teaching in a dental hospital.*

> *In Birmingham the teachers were distinguished local people who came into the dental hospital perhaps once a week, twice a week or something like that, and retired back to their own practices. But the same thing happened in the way of kudos.*

Gordon Fordyce was still only 17 years old when he started Dental School, St Andrew's [1942].

---

14 An occupation considered important enough for the holder to be exempt from being conscripted into the armed services and forbidden from enlisting e.g. medicine or the police.
15 Venereal disease.

The main things we did were done in the laboratory. Most of what we learned about dentistry was from a very old and very capable dental technician. He taught us more than almost anyone else.

After the second year-- we were four years-- we were treating patients. It was a busy, small dental school. I don't think there were over nine students in my year. We had a schedule of quite extensive filling work and we'd make crowns and inlays in the laboratory and we were allowed, in our second clinical year, to do crowns and a bridge or two on patients. Not many because only in the last six months of my time in dental school did we have an electric engine to use. There were two electric engines in the dental hospital and in our final six months we were allowed a week or two to use them, when they were working, otherwise it was all done with a treadle engine. I think I made somewhere like twenty to twenty-five dentures.

When I qualified, I went into general practice for a few months until my call-up papers came and I was off to the army.

In the late 1940s and early 1950s, many went to University after their National Service, so school leavers were mixed with mature students. Mike Awty started soon after WWII at Guy's, at that stage many of the undergraduates were ex-service [1948].

Oh, they were nearly all ex-Service. I mean I was one of five, four boys and a girl, in my dental year who were not, the rest were ex-Service. They'd all been killing people for years. You see, they were grown up, comparatively we were like children in short trousers.

In those days you had to do 18 months in the prosthetics department. There was a great deal of technical mechanical work, metalwork, gold work, porcelain work, so your manual dexterity was quite taxed. I suppose that in later life stood me in good stead, because we had a very hard grounding in all those disciplines. Towards the end of that course, we had our patients for full and partial dentures. There were a lot of edentulous people around in the early 1950s in London.

After the 18 months in prosthetics we did a period of working on a phantom head and carving up teeth, more and more manual dexterity training. Having done all the standard cavity styles in the phantom head room, you moved to the conservation room and started doing simple restorations on patients.

Laurence Oldham was at Birmingham [1949].

For the first year we were a combined medical, dental course, and we had lectures on physiology and anatomy and then we separated into discrete lectures for dental students, which were taken by a surgical registrar called Bevan. He was very clever at drawing on the blackboard; it was all done with a blackboard and chalk. So the first year was basic science with the medical students and we joined in the lab work with them, with the frog's legs muscles, action potentials for nerves, we did all the basic physiology for the medical course, the same.

In the second year we then went to the dental laboratory course which was again in the medical school on the second floor, where we each had our own station where we worked to do our prosthetic mock-ups. It was all to do with prosthetics, how to mix plaster, how to flask a denture, how to wax up a denture, how to get the right teeth, mould, shape, size, bite blocks, how to register a bite, flasking, burning out the wax, casting the acrylic, compressing the acrylic, waiting for it to set.

In the third year we left the medical school and went down into the centre of town to Great Charles Street, and a prefab building for the Op. Tech. course. We had phantom heads and treadle drills. Each student had a station with a treadle drill rather like a Singer sewing machine worked by the foot, with a series of arms and cords, and on the end you could put an old-fashioned hand piece. And then we had phantom heads which you had teeth set into plaster and we had to do cavities on these teeth and I remember it was quite hazardous because of the dentine dust; we were not given any protective masks or anything to wear, and we must have all inhaled this dentine and enamel dust over quite a protracted period of time.

When we got through the Op. Tech. course and R.J. Smith felt we were able to go, we went up to room six in the Birmingham Dental Hospital. Room six had about 25 to 30 chairs in several rows. We were given a list of patients which we called in, so that's when we started our conservative work on patients.

Almost half of the students were ex-forces, we had people from the army, navy and from the air force, and they seemed to us very mature and they knew how to study.

One such student was my uncle who had stayed in the army in north Africa after the war, he was in the same year as Laurence who described how they met.

16

I'm not proud of this incident, but with all these ex forces graduates among the undergraduates in the year, I was led astray on a pub crawl to Stratford-on-Avon. In those days, 1950, we all drove. I wasn't a driver, but I joined a group, four of us in a Ford Popular, and a whole convoy of cars drove from Birmingham to Stratford stopping at various pubs, however we did it I don't know.

By the time we got to Stratford we were all practically oiled and I remember entering The Swan at Stratford and tripping on a ledge on the floor halfway down the corridor just after purchasing a pint of beer and that Dennis Sadler was sitting on the ground with his legs out in front of him, just smiling benignly. As I tripped, I emptied the whole pint on the top of his bald pate and I can't remember him showing any displeasure or irritation or anything at all. I was very apologetic because it hadn't been intentional, but Dennis seemed to take it as a matter of routine.

Alas, this acquaintance was short-lived, my uncle Dennis continued his beer drinking, failed his second year exams and was chucked out.[16]

Many took the LDS examinations of the Royal College of Surgeons as well as BDS from their own university, Laurence:

I went to London as an external candidate to the LDS.RCS because I thought that would be valuable in coming up to qualification from Birmingham and I was very well versed in the basic science, medicine and anatomy, so I got through the LDS.RCS part one straight away, which was quite thrilling. I came back to Birmingham and then sat the BDS later. The LDS.RCS part one was the written work, and then for the second part we were examined with a viva in London. I don't remember any clinical work; I was asked to delineate the tumours from the alimentary tract starting from the mouth, through to the anus which I was able to do. And the examiner seemed quite happy with that.

1950s

Russell Hopkins was at Newcastle [1951].

A significant number of the students were ex national service people and there were still odd people around who'd been in aircrew and other things like that. We had two or three people who'd been bomber crew who'd stayed in the RAF for a time after the war.

---

16 He qualified in dentistry from a better university a few years later.

The first year and second year was anatomy, physiology etc. Bradlaw insisted, any lecture we went to, we wore undergraduate gowns.[17] Dental students had to be on a par with anybody in terms of dress and behaviour. I think he was seeking to get dentistry regarded as an equal with medicine.

The third year was a waste of time because we then did dental mechanics and also dental pharmacology. The dental mechanics bored the pants off just about anybody, but we could all do set ups, cast gold inlays, and did all the stuff the mechanics did and we learnt how to make dentures from the beginning, and put wax on and take impressions, and then put teeth on, and set them up and all the rest of it. Not for patients; they were all done for models, and there was a senior technician training us, and I think everybody was bored to death.

We had phantom head, started carving bits of chalk and then cut cavities in chalk teeth, and then cut cavities in extracted teeth. So we used to go skiving around and nicking teeth from extractions so we could have the teeth to set up do gold inlays in and things like that. We went through this rigmarole in phantom head of doing some really rather lovely work, supervised etc., and all the angles had to be right, no sharp edges and everything had to be bevelled and so on. It was good training, useful. And so when we went into the fourth year, we had three years of clinical training; we were already able to do the limited clinical work that we had to do in conservation.

We used to get points. You got one point for a single surface filling, two points for a two surface filling, three points for three surface and gold inlays you got bigger points. And for dentures you got points; everything was pointed, and I used to work faster than a lot of the people, and I was second in the table of point scorers. I established a reputation of being good at cons,[18] and in those days of course we were good at extractions, because we were taking a lot of teeth out. I must have taken roots out and done some simple stuff, I don't think I had much training in surgical procedures at that stage.

Most of us played sport on a Wednesday afternoon, and the fifth year used to do conservation work in the dental hospital on a

---

17 Sir Robert Bradlaw was Dean of the Newcastle Dental School. We will hear more about him later.
18 Conservative dentistry

Wednesday afternoon; the other two years we had the afternoon off to play sport.

John Bradley went to Guy's; he wanted to be a dentist like his father [1954].

When we got there, we had one or two ex-servicemen in the year. We started off with lectures in anatomy, physiology, biochemistry and dental anatomy and, with that, comparative dental anatomy as well. Also, we did anatomical dissections of the head and neck region, didn't stray much beyond that. We could go to the post-mortem rooms as well, we were told it would be good experience for us to see that.

The second year was essentially in prosthetics, where we did all the clinical work and did all the laboratory work as well. We had great fun doing that; we cast our own chrome cobalt frames for partial dentures and we did all the set-ups for the teeth and made the acrylic dentures ourselves and we had a marvellous professor Herbert Fenn, a consummate craftsman.

Mike Bromige, Birmingham [1954].

The dental school was based in the medical school in Edgbaston, and in fact the dental school was one corridor in the medical school building. We did a lot of the preliminary work, physiology and biochemistry and that kind of thing with the medics, branched off as I recall for the practicals but lectures were all of us, medics and all the dental students together.

We did an awful lot of comparative dental anatomy so I knew an awful lot about alligator teeth and baboon teeth and it was sheer paddy. We did an awful lot of dissection, there were eight of us to a body and we dissected most days for a year and a term, doing meticulous dissections of head and neck, thorax, abdomen, one limb and a brain 'spotter'.

We did a junior op course, which was an extraordinary experience. It was on the top floor of an ex-factory in a couple of streets away from the dental hospital. The dental hospital was still in Great Charles Street. That was a bit of a caper and we were all on treadle machines to begin with and then there was this wonderful time when we walked in and it had been equipped with hanging electric motors and flexible drives.

I can remember the smell of burnt dentine to this day with about 35 people all busy drilling dead teeth set up in phantom heads. We started off with amalgam fillings. Amalgam was processed in a finger stall by dropping in bare mercury and amalgam powder and then mixing it between finger and thumb, squeezing the rubber finger stall and then tipping it out and then using it. Then we went on to capsules as I recall and the amalgamating machine, but you still loaded that to begin with mercury from the dropper bottle, and later on they came preloaded.

We walked in one day, and suddenly there was an air rotor in the clinic. In Great Charles Street, the dental hospital there, like many up and down the country, you walked into a vast room and there were dental chairs and spittoons and bracket tables as far as the eye could see. But there were adjacent single cubicles that had been built, and suddenly an air rotor appeared in one of these. They were used by David Shovelton and Ivor Whitehead who were the lecturers, and slowly we could use it very occasionally. But if you ask if I was taught on an air rotor, the answer is no. And the moment I did some work in practice, of course there were air rotors as they were taken up by practices very quickly.

I can't tell you exactly how many amalgam fillings I did, other than it was well over 500 to 600. Gloomy people in the year did the LDS. They did it as a safeguard and to make sure they got a qualification so they could practise. And the other advantage of course was that it was taken six months before the BDS and therefore they could actually go out and earn some cash by working in the evenings whilst they were completing the final six months of the university course.

1960s

John Langdon was dyslexic and had failed five out of eight 'O' levels at his first attempt at school, but he thrived at the London Hospital Dental School [1960].

I loved the dental course. In those days it was fairly old-fashioned. The first year was basic science, which included materials science. Then the second year we did phantom head and prosthetic laboratory work and then went onto patients. And I was one of these curious undergraduates; with no real effort I ended up winning all the prizes except the oral surgery prize. So I won the London prize for prosthetic dentistry, children's dentistry, which was an honorary membership of the American Academy of Dentistry of Children, the Harold Fink Prize, which was for restorative dentistry, and so it went on. I really enjoyed dentistry.

Andy Brown went to Guy's [1963].

In those days there was a full pre-clinical course, which were the standard subjects, anatomy and physiology. We spent a lot of time cutting up bodies in the dissection room and time in the physiology lab and the biochemistry lab for three terms. And then they integrated into that pathology and some other clinical subjects related to dentistry. You didn't go on to the conservation room until the following third year of a four-year and one term course. Local anaesthesia and drilling holes in teeth and restoring teeth was at the beginning of year three.

In the prosthetic dentistry year you worked in the laboratory and you made dentures for a whole year, and you did all the laboratory work yourself and saw patients and treated them. You had to make quite a lot of dentures, I can't remember exactly how many, but partial dentures and full dentures. It was very good technical training in a way. I remember that you spent all of your time either in the clinic or at the laboratory bench. Dental prosthetics was important in that there were a lot more edentulous patients then, and also I think it was their way of teaching manual dexterity and learning, if you were going to work with a dental lab, how you could interact with them.

When I was a dental student, Pat O'Driscoll was appointed as a new consultant at Guy's. He was actually the first consultant appointed with the title of Consultant Oral Surgeon, or at least adopted that title. Until then all the senior consultants were called Consultant Dental Surgeons and that's exactly what they were. Most of them had Harley Street practices, and they came over to Guy's as part-time consultants the two days a week or so they were scheduled to attend. The rest of the week many of them were doing general dentistry in west end practices. They were like the old consultants pre-1948, they were descendants of the 'honoraries'.

John Cawood trained at St Andrews Dental School in Dundee [1964].

The first two pre-clinical years we did with the medics. In the clinical years it was mostly small group tutorials. We had to spend an extra 10 weeks in the summer between third and fourth years working in the dental hospital mainly doing dental mechanics. It was fairly intensive 5 year course.

There was a lot of personal interaction between lecturers and students. The people who I found most interesting were the oral surgery faculty.

Tony Markus went to Newcastle [1967].

I did laboratory work, taught by a wonderful chap called Dr Naru who was a doctor as well as a dentist. And he was a terrifically gifted artist and musician and a part time GP, part-time general dental practitioner and a part-time gynaecologist. He taught me how to carve teeth in wax.

I attempted to make a denture and got into terrible trouble. For one lady I put the wax set up into her mouth to try it in and it was all perfect, so then I discharged her. And she rang up and spoke to Professor Storer, who was the Professor of Prosthetics. Very, very angry because she'd gone down to the railway station in Newcastle, had a quick cup of tea before getting on the train and guess what? 'Are my teeth supposed to come out in my mouth?' So the whole setup had melted. I got into frightful trouble, I almost thought I was going to get thrown out. He accused me of doing it on purpose. I didn't, purely forgetful! So that was prosthetics. I think that was the only one I ever made, the only one I was ever allowed to make.

I remember doing one crown and one inlay. I don't know how many fillings, probably not very many. I'm sure I did a few. I think I did a root filling probably, one. I don't think I was awfully good at it; I didn't put my mind to very much. It may have been that we had quotas, but they certainly weren't very stressful quotas and we had plenty of time for drunken lunches.

It was very pleasant I'm not sure that it was intellectually stimulating, but there were some nice things that went on in Newcastle. There was some good music, there was a good concert hall, there were good theatres. There were plenty of opportunities to learn about tying flies for fishing, which was pretty intellectually stimulating. It was a very pleasant time. I thoroughly enjoyed myself.

Adrian Sugar was at Leeds [1965].

I got involved in student union politics. I sat on the Student Union Council and Senate Staff Student committee; I spent most of my spare time at the student union in my first year or two. Also, in the medical school I played bridge in the breaks and lunchtimes; I enjoyed that very much.

I don't think any particular individual inspired me but there were several people I respected and I learnt from, and often they were registrars. When I went back to Leeds later as a registrar in '76 I was quite influenced by the senior registrars there; we did a lot of work together.

1970s

Mike Davidson at the London Hospital [1972].

I had a good time. Socially, it was great and academically it was challenging. When I got to the dental school, my academic drive and enthusiasm seemed to just click back in again, and I found it interesting. I really loved the academic challenge, the learning of new material. We were very lucky there were some very talented teachers, very interesting people, some of whom were slightly eccentric, and I would say, not run-of-the-mill. particularly people like Aubrey Sheiham and Jack Lozdan.

In the oral medicine and perio there were some really good minds, people like Roy Duckworth and Roger Sutton. And in what was then termed the oral surgery department, there were people like Gordon Seward and David McGowan, they were the academics, and they were good value. One of my teachers was a guy called Ian Millward, he was a dentist who'd gone back to read medicine but was teaching us oral surgery. I was very impressed by this; he was very influential on me; he was very kind and took me under his wing a bit. But also in my year there were a lot of students who were academically quite gifted and some of them very good technically as well, so you had to keep alert to keep up with the rest of them, so it was very good in that sense.

I really enjoyed my time at the London doing dentistry because it was such a good group of teachers who were enthusiastic. There was also some deadwood there, but then that's true of all dental schools.

Ian, Martin King's [1975].

The first bit you did in an ordinary university, so it wasn't all just in dental school. So I started off in King's on the Strand in 1975, where we did our preclinical. And we used to pop into the Royal College of Surgeons and see all these odd exhibits in the dental anatomy section of the Hunterian collection and stuff. And it was right in the centre of town, I had a lovely time there. The National Theatre was opposite, and I quite liked theatre and music.

The only problem was because it was a proper university rather than a dental school, you did biochemistry with people who were doing proper biochemistry as opposed to dental school Mickey Mouse biochemistry; and physiology with physiologists, and so forth. So the failure rate in those days at second BDS at King's was about twenty, twenty-five per cent. And most of the people who failed, failed biochemistry. There was a particularly aggressive professor of biochemistry, and he didn't particularly like the medical and dental undergraduates. He felt they were all a bit dodgy. So quite a lot of people either got booted out completely or got put back a year. For some reason, I scraped through unscathed.

At King's dental school, you all wore long coats and were distinguished by the colour of your badge. First years (very dangerous) orange badge, green was the middle eighteen months, and then in your final year you got a red badge.

As an orange badge you did the phantom head room initially, but you were also introduced, fairly quickly, to giving local anaesthetics, doing local extractions, on the clinics. And I was in a firm of five blokes, and I was quite lucky in that on the local anaesthetic clinic I was with Phil Rood, who was a senior lecturer then. And you started off supposedly doing simple extractions. But this was south London and a big West Indian population, and they had really thick bone and a lot of their teeth were quite difficult to take out.

King's was good you had the set pieces you had to do like cons on Monday and perio on Tuesday, or whatever, but there was quite a lot of spare time where you could opt to do things you wanted to do.

Chapter 4
Surgery at Dental School
'We did take out an awful lot of teeth'

I have heard much criticism of the level of practical experience dental undergraduates have in minor oral surgery. In previous generations there was significantly more advanced dental disease. But how much experience had these previous generations of dental students had in surgical procedures, including lifting muco-periosteal flaps and removing bone?

Paul Bramley was at Birmingham and can remember a lot of extractions under general anaesthetic [1940-44].

As an undergraduate dental student, you went into the general anaesthetic department and you did half the anaesthetics or half the extractions that morning until 11 o'clock. From nine to eleven you were at it all the time.

Gordon Fordyce, St Andrew's (Dundee) [1943-45].

There were a lot of dental extractions. The clinics started at nine in the morning and there'd be a queue of people coming to have their teeth out. We might have had to lift a flap to get a root out, but I can't recall doing it.

Laurence Oldham was at Birmingham Dental School [1950-55].

We just did straightforward extractions, I don't think I did any surgicals at all. We were taught by Mr Brown, Father Brown he was known, and he took us one at a time in a single room with a patient and he would always loosen the tooth with a straight elevator before we were allowed to extract the tooth, we never approached a virgin tooth with a view to extracting it unless he'd loosened it with an elevator; always under local anaesthesia and he would guide us in the technique; it was one-to-one with a succession of patients.

Mike Bromige was a little later at Birmingham, and can remember doing surgery [1954-58].

I did a lot of oral surgery early on, certainly I raised flaps and removed bone, I did minor impactions. For third molars that could've been elevated we raised the flap and took some bone and then elevated it, fairly straightforward simple things.

We had two fortnight periods in the gas room. And although there was somebody standing by, you did the majority of the work and you'd probably get through something like 20 patients in a session, taking out single teeth and occasionally doing a clearance; pretty horrific.

It's quite extraordinary how lax things were because you could do a locum house job in the General Hospital. There was a notice on the dental hospital gates that said, 'After 5 o'clock go to the General Hospital for treatment,' and that resulted in anything, up to 20, 30 patients attending in the evening which had to be seen by the housemen, there were two housemen. But if you were locuming as a student then it was your job and if teeth needed to be removed we were allowed to remove them and did, under local anaesthetic, totally unsupervised.

I think it was a very good training. I do think we benefited from our general surgery and general medicine training, which was taken very seriously by the medics who undertook the tuition. We did ward rounds, had lectures and case examination of patients; they took it fairly seriously, and we did as well.

John Bradley was at Guy's at the same time. He did one surgical procedure in his final exam! [1954-58].

I did quite a lot of extractions. We didn't actually do any clearances. You might do four or five teeth maximum at a time. This was with the patients sat in a chair, upright with the anaesthetist there. You had to put a gag in, put a throat packing down the back, which was really an oral pack, and then you took the teeth out. Practical surgical experience was very spasmodic, it was really the luck of the draw whether you actually got a patient who needed a flap reflecting to take out a root.

The final examination was three hours long, and I had done my inlay in two. There was an hour left. They gave me a patient who had a root to take out. I needed to cut and reflect a flap and drill it out, and that was the first one I'd ever done in my life, and it was under exam conditions.

Some students at Guy's had much better experience, especially if they had been appointed as an assistant house surgeon. Mike Awty explained [1948-53].

In the final six months, I was an assistant house surgeon. And in fact, I got my real interest stimulated in surgery by working when John McLean was supervising.[19] He was a registrar, and he much preferred to sit on the window sill carving crowns and experimenting with impression materials than surgery. And once he realised I was quite interested and quite good at it, he said, 'Well, you carry on, you do it all and I'll just be nominally here to be responsible.' The assistant house surgeon was a sort of halfway house. I imagine it was the better students, as they became near the end, were given more responsibility. In fact, probably grooming them for a house job, to see how they shaped up.

John Cawood [1964- 1969].

At Dundee we did a lot of extractions. We didn't raise any flaps, but we watched a lot of oral surgery. We were attached to the Dundee Royal Infirmary, so went to theatre quite frequently to see oral surgery being carried out by Peter Brown and at Ashludie Hospital by Derek Henderson.

Derek Henderson was the consultant, and he made a very big impression, not least because there was a very nasty car accident involving a dental student, two dental nurses and one of their husbands. Sadly, one died and the other three were very badly injured, it being in the pre-seat belt and laminated windscreen days. Some of them sustained very bad maxillofacial injuries, which Derek Henderson managed. He gave us a lecture, not about the individuals, but about his specialty, and that really fired me up. So oral surgery in general, and Derek Henderson in particular, made a big impression at dental school.

Brian Avery, Guy's [1965-70].

Towards the end of my training, I put myself about a lot to make sure that I got as much training as I could. So when I was in my last year they'd created a post, I think they called it assistant house surgeon, this was before you were qualified, and I got one of these posts in oral surgery so I was taking out wisdom teeth as an undergraduate, largely unsupervised. A wild rough estimate might be 20 or 30 cases of surgical removal of wisdom teeth. We took out an

---

19 John McLean became an eminent restorative dentist and material scientist who taught part time at Guy's.

awful lot of teeth. We had the gas room at the dental hospital and if you went to a session, there you could easily take out 20 or 30 teeth at a session and I took out hundreds as a student.

Andy Brown, Guy's [1963-69].

In your final six months of training you could apply to be attached to a 'firm' of a consultant and a registrar and a house surgeon. So for three to six months, I can't remember the exact time, I was an assistant house surgeon to one of the consultants. And, although we had been overseen in taking out buried roots and apicectomies and things like that, that's really when I did quite a lot of minor oral surgery, by today's standards.

John Williams, Guy's [1956-61].

We had firms that you were attached to and I did my general anaesthetic experience with Alan Thompson, who was the consultant in charge. Alan Thompson did a lot of minor oral surgery, removal of 8s, apicectomies, under a general anaesthetic. So I learnt a lot of oral surgery quite early on . It triggered my interest and made me determined that his was the house job I wanted to do if I could get the chance of doing it.

Khursheed Moos had his horizons lifted higher at Guy's [1953-57].

I came to Guy's in 1953, I much enjoyed my time there and especially doing and being involved with surgery. I seemed to manage that quite well and do most things that were needed. My interest in surgery was partly related to a Guy's consultant who was a doubly qualified and took us off to New Cross Hospital where he did orthognathic surgery.

As a student I was an assistant house surgeon for Mr Mansie, I believe it was for 3 months. It was delightful. I liked working for him and we got on very well. As assistant house surgeon at Guy's, you did some assisting and preparing the cases for Mr Mansie. I believe the full-time house surgeons did much more. I don't think I did many surgical extractions and things like that. I was keen to do some but then there was little opportunity, there was not a lot of minor surgery for students to do, that I remember.

John Langdon was at the London Hospital [1960-64].

We had requirements we had to do. I think it was twenty extractions and ten surgical procedures, roots and wisdom teeth, which I did and enjoyed doing. And of course we were also trained in general anaesthesia, intubation, outpatient anaesthesia and inpatient. Most of the practical clinical teaching was done by the registrars and senior registrars. I can't remember there being a lecturer in oral surgery, if there was, I can't remember who it was.

Adrian Sugar, Leeds [1965-70].

In oral surgery I took a lot of teeth out but I can't honestly remember being taught one-to-one how to remove a tooth surgically, but I think I must have done because when I was a house officer, I spent most of my time doing that with students. But it was unlike some schools, for example in Manchester where I worked as a locum senior registrar for a short period. There it was didactic one-to-one teaching of surgical removal of teeth; every student had to do that, the teaching was much more formalised. It was more informal in Leeds. Ninety per cent of the time of a first-year house office in that dental school was spent supervising students doing dental extractions. And there were hundreds of patients a day and lots of broken teeth. There were a lot of oro-antral communications, we house officers would close them stat. I must have done dozens.

Mike Davidson, the London Hospital [1972-76].

In the oral surgery department you had attachments at varying times throughout your career, but most years you had a regular weekly commitment and that was mainly in the extractions department. We would also go to the 'emergency clinic' seeing people who turned up at the door. They would take the first thirty people in the queue, and after that children came through and adults were told to come back in the afternoon, or the next morning as appropriate. You saw a vast amount of off-the-street pain and this emergency clinic was run by the oral surgery department.

You did a lot of diagnosis and you saw a lot of cases and very quickly you learnt how to take a history, make a decision and investigate appropriately, and that was good fun. There were people keeping an eye on you when you would take teeth out, and then if you snapped them, normally either one of the residents or one of the qualified staff would come and do the surgical, but you would assist. That was the deal, you had to assist, and then if you got more experienced, you could do the surgical under supervision. In amongst that, you had to do a certain amount of half days and be signed up by the person in charge of whatever clinic you were doing in oral surgery, that you had been satisfactory during that time.

You got a massive grounding in what I would describe as basics and you saw trauma coming through the door. But also you would see some more complex operations coming back, the osteotomies, the trauma and some malignancy. When you were doing oral surgery at the London, you got attached to the resident team. It was usually only a couple of days, but that was also on-call, but had to go to a few inpatient theatre sessions, and you had to write up a case report on one case that you had seen both in clinic, on the ward, in theatres and post-op. So, you got the idea that there was something beyond dental extractions.

You were expected to have done some surgical procedure, lifting flaps and drilling bone to extract difficult teeth, but I don't think there was a formal number. When you went in on Saturdays, you were expected to get yourself out of trouble, with support admittedly. So, I've probably done twenty to thirty surgicals at a guess. Also, I did quite a few periodontal flaps when I was a student and a couple of apicectomies when I was doing restorative dentistry.

Ian Martin, King's [1975-79].

So in week one on local anaesthetics in the first year you gave the local and then a houseman came along and took the tooth out. Week two, you put the local in and you had to take the tooth out.

So in week two, all five of us at the same time snapped the incisors off at the root. And Phil Rood[20] came along, and they had these big paper towels over the sink, and he pulled one of these big paper towels down and he said, 'Right, you lot gather round.' And he drew on it, 'Here's the teeth, here's the gums, right? The mental nerve is there. So you're going to cut with a knife round the neck of these teeth, right? You go down into the socket there, mind the nerve, scrape it back with this thing. It's called a periosteal elevator', he said, 'When you've done that you're going to get the drill, you're going to drill away the bone until you see the root, it's a slightly yellower colour, and then you're going to stick this thing in,' which was a Coupland's, 'And turn it, and you'll find that the root comes out.' And he says, 'If you get stuck, the nurse knows what to do, all right?' So, in our first week

---

20 Senior Lecturer in oral surgery, later Professor in Manchester and subsequently back at King's.

taking out teeth, we were doing minor oral surgery.

And, of course, you did it in your bare hands; you didn't have any gloves or anything like that. So you got quite adept at being able to use elevators and get teeth out, whatever. And basically, the rule was if you snapped it; you had to get it out. So I really quite liked that.

And then you also did general anaesthetics in the first year as well. So you had to do partly giving general anaesthetics and partly taking teeth out under general anaesthetic. And I was on a Friday morning, and on a Friday morning the anaesthetist was a very laid back chap called Dennis Potter, and the surgeon in charge was Malcolm Harris, who was, at the time, a senior lecturer at King's. And unlike on the other days of the week where they were all taking kids' teeth out, Malcolm Harris always put things like wisdom teeth onto this outpatient general anaesthetic list.

So my first experience of the general anaesthetic room was with Malcolm Harris, and the first case that he got me to do was a wisdom tooth. So this is literally a few weeks into clinical dentistry. And he said, 'Right, you cut the flap like this,' 'Scrape it back, yeah, yeah, go on.' And he's there assisting me. 'All right, scrape it back, scrape it back, yeah, right, now you get the chisel, because of course, we didn't use drills then. He said, 'Right, bevel back, put a stop cut there. Knock this thing off, grab the bone out, put that in there, turn that out. Yeah, very good, very good, scrape it clean and then stitch it up,' black silk, of course. And so I did that. Loved it. And Malcolm Harris came up to me at the end of this and he said, 'Well my boy, did you enjoy that?' 'Ooh, yes, Mr Harris, thank you.' So from day one, almost, in dental school, we were encouraged to do minor oral surgery.

And one of the big things we could do, there was an open invitation to go to ward rounds in the morning, so there was a group of us that were interested in the surgical side. Whenever we could, we'd go up to do the ward rounds with Geoff Forman, Malcolm Harris, or with Phil Rood, John Sowray, very occasionally. We got to see stuff on the wards and were also invited to go to the operating theatre whenever we wanted to as well. So we started to see quite a lot of surgery.

At the same time, you were actually getting quite a lot of hands on experience doing minor surgery. And that was absolutely encouraged. So I fairly rapidly decided that that was the bit that I found the most interesting, much more interesting than drilling holes in teeth and doing crowns and scraping people's perio and stuff. And so I spent a lot of time going to ward rounds, going to the theatre, and a lot of time in minor oral surgery taking teeth out. By the time I qualified I would have taken out well over 100 wisdom teeth and done loads of apicectomies, and god knows how many biopsies and stuff, as a dental undergraduate.

I had a great time at King's. It was a great place, everybody was made to feel like they were an important somebody. You were treated like a professional, so loved it.

Chapter 5
Dental Students Gave Anaesthetics

'I used to give anaesthetics for the ENT list'

It was only in the late 20th century that dentists stopped giving general anaesthetics themselves. Practical anaesthetic instruction and experience used to be part of the undergraduate training.

Paul Bramley, Birmingham [1940-44].

> *As an undergraduate dental student, you went into the general anaesthetic department and you did half the anaesthetics or half the extractions that morning until 11 o'clock. From nine to eleven, you were at it all the time. So you had a huge soaking in nitrous oxide and oxygen. There wasn't any Trilene then, it was during wartime.*

After he qualified from the Birmingham Dental School, Paul Bramley became the dental house surgeon at the Queen Elizabeth Hospital in Birmingham [1945].

> *I used to give anaesthetics for the ENT list in the Queen Elizabeth Hospital as the dental house surgeon, and that was Schimmelbusch mask and pour on the ether for all their quickies. Why I was doing it and the department of anaesthetics not doing it, I really don't know. It all happened like this; it was very casual.*

He also gave anaesthetics when he was a medical student [1948-52].

> *When I was a medical student I was appointed as an honorary anaesthetist to Monyhull Colony.[21] I had worked for Harold Round,[22] and his partner in his Birmingham practice was a woman called Jessie Rowbotham who was a foil for the great man. She used to have to do the dental extractions at this Monyhull Colony and somehow or other she asked me to give her anaesthetics. So without being appointed and so on, I used to turn up regularly to her clinics and I did the dental anaesthesia. So it was all very informal. It was plain, straightforward nitrous oxide and plenty of oxygen, a lot of skill and occasional squirts*

21 The Monyhull Colony was a mental hospital at King's Norton near Birmingham. It was a self-sufficient community with the patients working the farmland to supply their own needs.
22 More of him in chapter 6 and 7. Harold Round was also one of the two first U.K. dentists to qualify with a degree, at Birmingham University in 1904.

of ethyl chloride when people got really stroppy. I put it onto a pack. It seemed to work. It wasn't ether; it was ethyl chloride.

When I started dental practice myself during medical qualification, there were two cylinders on the floor, one of nitrous oxide and one of oxygen, and you stood on them and turned the taps on and off with your foot and gave the anaesthetic through a nose mask and that was straight forward nitrous oxide/oxygen. So by the time I came to Monyhull Colony I was pretty experienced in dental anaesthesia and did a far better job of it than the general practitioners who used to give anaesthetics for dentists.

Once I frightened myself stiff by giving a general anaesthetic and doing an extraction at the same time, and the chap stopped breathing. But we got him round in the end.

Mike Awty, Guy's [1948-53].

At dental school we had minimal instruction on how to give general anaesthetics, nitrous oxide and oxygen; I think we might well have used ethyl chloride too, for children, but you had to be much more careful with that. There was a consultant anaesthetist there, usually sitting on the window sill with his newspaper, but I'm sure that they had 'antennae'. They knew exactly what was going on. But you felt responsible because they were not actually doing it and of course actually doing things is the way to learn.

Russell Hopkins, Newcastle [1951-56].

You had to do twenty or more to be signed up, and part of your exam always included problems related to general anaesthesia. I was actually quite a competent dental anaesthetist. We were trained, in the early days on gas, nitrous oxide, oxygen and Trilene. We induced patients to a degree of cyanosis before turning rapidly to oxygen mixes to get them through the stage of cerebral excitement as quickly as we could. It was hairy stuff, but we were much better trained than most medical practitioners, who at that time were the anaesthetists for general dental practitioners.

After he qualified, he worked in General Dental Practice [1956].

The first job I'd got was a temporary job in a practice in west Hartlepool. Every morning I gave up to about eight to ten general anaesthetics whilst they whipped out the teeth. They picked me as the most junior person in the place because I'd just come out of dental school and knew more about general anaesthesia than anybody else there. So I became the anaesthetist to the practice.

And then later, as a Senior House Officer in Nottingham [1958-59].

I actually became the anaesthetist for casualty, I used to give them two anaesthetic lists a week to do breast abscesses and Colles fractures and this, that and the other. I gave them gas, oxygen and Trilene. They could never get anaesthetists in time so it became my anaesthetic list. It was unofficial, everything was unofficial, no one gave approval for this, it was just done. The nurses used to pull the Colles fractures back and put the back slabs on, and I gave the anaesthetic.

Mike Bromige, Birmingham [1954-58].

We had two fortnight periods in the gas room and you alternated day by day giving an anaesthetic or extracting teeth. Although there was somebody standing by, you did the majority of the work and you'd probably get through something like 20 patients in a session, taking out single teeth and occasionally doing a clearance. Thinking back, it was pretty horrific.

Brian Avery, Guy's [1965-70].

The gas sessions, as they used to be called, were very exciting because initially the patients were anaesthetised by inhaling nitrous oxide and oxygen and the patients got very excited as they went under. Some patients had to be strapped to the chair with big leather belts because if they were big aggressive men they could injure people if they jumped up when they were being induced. I can remember a docker from the London port who got so excited that he put his feet on the ground and stood up with the heavy old dental chair attached to him via a big leather belt. They were quite exciting sessions, but they taught you a lot.

Mike Davidson, the London Hospital [1972-76].

We had to do about twenty dental extraction sessions, ten general anaesthetic sessions where you were taking the teeth out, and about ten where you actually gave the anaesthetic. You gave general anaesthetics to children, and it was very much smash-and-grab, it was almost anoxia technique, it was pretty rudimentary.

Ian Martin, King's [1975-79].

You did general anaesthetics in the first clinical year. So you had to do partly giving general anaesthetics and partly taking teeth out under general anaesthetic.

It wasn't always dental cases that dental students gave anaesthetics for. Paul Bramley as a dental student gave anaesthetics in the Birmingham General Hospital casualty department during the war [1940-45].

It used to be the biggest casualty outpatients in Europe. There was a huge turnover in central Birmingham, particularly in wartime. I was the one dental student, the other 10 or 11 people, were medical students. We used to man casualty in the evenings if we'd got nothing better to do. So we bailed out of our wards into casualty and I got all the anaesthetics to do because, unlike the medical students, I had some knowledge of the problems. So I got a lot of practical hands-on things there. Anaesthetics were just part of dentistry.

Laurence Oldham was a student in Birmingham. He gave anaesthetics in casualty [1950-55].

In year four we were surgical dressers and rotated down to the hospital in Steelhouse Lane, Birmingham General Hospital and we were required as dressers to give anaesthesia for general surgical problems like breast abscesses or paraphymoses, under supervision, while the medical students did the surgery. I found it was the most exciting thing I'd ever done. I look back on those dresser days, rotating out to the General Hospital with great satisfaction, interest and enjoyment.

Mike Bromige agreed.

I'm sure I'm right in recollecting that the dental students used to give anaesthetics for minor ops in A&E, not minor ops dental, but minor ops generally.

Tony Markus was a registrar ay Guy's [1975].

There was a lovely chap who ran the dental emergency unit and also taught me how to take out teeth properly under general anaesthetic and we used to have these quick general anaesthetic sessions. There was a wonderful anaesthetist called Halliwell, and he used to get the patients blue. He said, 'There you are, dear boy, you've got until they get red.' And you tussled with these big brutes of chaps who'd come in for extractions.

My friend and colleague Richard Thornton was an anaesthetist for oral and maxillofacial surgery and general dentistry. He qualified in medicine from St Thomas' in 1971.

We got two weeks of anaesthetics. And within those two weeks we were actually expected to anaesthetise patients and did so. One can't imagine we were on our own, but it felt like it because the anaesthetist wasn't in the room. So that was the first sort of experience I ever had of doing anything medical at all. I suppose it stays with you, actually doing something for once, and also anaesthetists seemed to be nice people, I thought.

Richard described the usual technique for dental anaesthesia.

My training in dental anaesthetic was in the '70s and the techniques were the same as had been used when I was a child on me. It was sitting the patient in the chair sitting upright, using a gas induction with nitrous oxide, in various concentrations. I don't think at that stage we were using an anoxic technique, but we were certainly using hypoxic. You would use a nitrous oxide concentration of between 80 and 85 per cent for induction. You would then possibly add something else, like halothane. But halothane was unnecessary if it was just for one or two extractions, you'd just keep going on nitrous oxide. If the dentist needed more time, you would add halothane from a Goldman vaporiser. Usually, as the last tooth was about to be extracted, you turned everything off and just turned oxygen on.

The airway was maintained with a jaw thrust, and the anaesthetic was delivered via a nasal mask. The dentist would put a pack at the back of the throat, but obviously not right in the pharynx, usually just under the soft palate. This would be enough to maintain an airway and stop too much air breathing through the mouth. The dentists were usually very experienced at this and just knew how to pack a mouth properly so you didn't get mouth breathing.

I never had any disasters with that technique. But because the patient wasn't ever so deep and if an extraction proved difficult, then it might become impossible to complete the extraction. So it wasn't the ideal technique for getting the job done.

It was a very good and safe technique because it was such a light anaesthetic; the patients weren't properly anaesthetised. It was slightly hypoxic. Having got the induction done, you didn't maintain sort of 85 per cent nitrous oxide, you would then go onto about 75 per cent nitrous. So at that stage they weren't really breathing a hypoxic mixture. If there was any obstruction to respiration, they quickly became very hypoxic with that amount of nitrous on-board.

One issue that we have in modern times is with efficiency of production. How many patients would you have done on an afternoon list at the dental hospital or in the community clinic for extractions?

Well, definitely a dozen, maybe more. The most I ever did was sort of 18, something like that, less than 20. But let's say you did a dozen patients, you would expect to do those in about an hour and a half, not that long per patient. The patient was in and out of the surgery within 15, 20 minutes.

It was more difficult to induce an adult with gas, so that in the '70s adults coming into the clinic usually had an intravenous induction, which was with methohexitone. That may or may not have been a cannula placed, it wasn't absolutely always the case. You'd sometimes just put in an ordinary needle and pull it out after the induction.

One improvement has been monitoring. Of all the monitors, the one that's made a huge difference has been the pulse oximeter. And of course it's one of the simplest to put on. It tells you exactly, at the time, what the oxygen saturation is within the blood and will alert you to changes before the eye can detect cyanosis. You'll see cyanosis with the saturation of say 85 per cent, in a patient with normal haemoglobin. With pulse oximeter, you can see that the saturation has maybe changed from 98 per cent to 95 per cent. Now that may mean nothing, but it will alert you to the fact that there's a downward trend.

When I was starting anaesthetics, hardly a case went by without the surgeon at some stage saying the blood looks a bit blue here. The surgeon would have spotted it within the theatre lighting before the anaesthetist would have seen it, say, in the lips or the face. You never hear that now. Hypoxemia during an anaesthetic is never something that is suddenly discovered to have happened. People always know it's about to happen or something is going wrong before it becomes apparent clinically.

Do you think we're looking back at what were the good old days, or the bad old days?

The old-fashioned dental anaesthetic was really safe; probably safer than hospital anaesthesia. But if anything did go wrong, it was hopeless to try to resuscitate; and the monitoring was very poor, and it was seen as an absolute disaster, and something that shouldn't have happened, whereas if something goes wrong in a hospital, people feel it's obviously a disaster, but they'll feel more that everything has been done that should have been done. So if you asked me, would I go back and give an old-fashioned anaesthetic again in a surgery, the answer's emphatically no.

Eventually the idea of dentists giving anaesthetics became an affront to the anaesthetic community but when Paul Bramley became professor at the Sheffield dental school anaesthesia was still on the undergraduate dental curriculum but the professor of anaesthetics had different ideas. [1969-88].

I really had my trouble later on as professor of oral surgery. The General Dental Council specified what you had to do about dentists and giving general anaesthetics and what practical work they had to do. The professor of anaesthetics had a very different view, and I had an absolute stand up row in which he became livid and lost his temper and I finished by trembling myself. It got to that pitch. I had a duty to do and was bloody well going to do it and he felt he had a duty to mankind. It was all in the early days of the intravenous stuff with Drummond Jackson, so that stirred up the anaesthetic community.[23]

I had to teach it, so it was a very uncomfortable time with the professor. I think he really wanted a tube down for every one of them, which is ridiculous.

---

23 Stanley Drummond Jackson was a dentist from Sheffield who in the 1960s formed the Society for the Advancement of Anaesthesia in Dentistry which ran week-end courses for dentists teaching them to give anaesthetics using intra-venous methohexitone. An article was published in the British Medical Journal saying this technique was potentially dangerous and Drummond Jackson sued. This lead to one of the longest ever libel cases in British legal history which was never concluded as both sides ran out of money. See: Physiological responses to intermittent methohexitone for conservative dentistry. Wise C, Robinson J, Heath M, Tomlin, P. British Medical Journal 1969 2; 540–543.

Chapter 6
Early Hospital Experience

'Anything complex was passed on, usually to ENT'

Paul Bramley qualified in 1944.

I did a year's service as a resident dental house surgeon at the Queen Elizabeth Hospital in Birmingham to a great man of the past, Harold Round. That was a marvellous year. I was a proper old-fashioned resident, £72 a year, all meals, all accommodation, all laundry and being looked after as a proper doctor. And I looked after my patients as a proper doctor. I wasn't medically qualified, but I was interested in that, and I put up the drips and all that sort of thing.

The work in the hospital was mostly what the consultant dental surgeon did at the beginning of the Health Service. It was dento-alveolar stuff, mandibular fractures, infections and a lot of impacted wisdom teeth; also dentistry under anaesthesia, for those who couldn't tolerate it otherwise.

Joe Sankey the plastic surgeon did the major stuff, but Harold Round applied the dental expertise. He had a superb mechanic who worked for him and did the facial prostheses; he was doing a lot. Monyhull Colony was a sort of mental institution that housed a plastic surgery unit which Harold frequently went out to; and which I went out to with him when I was his house surgeon.

When Harold Round visited the hospital, I always used to meet him on the steps. I had his itinerary worked out for him with all the consultations which he'd got to do on the various wards, who we were bringing down to the clinic and so on. That was twice a week, but he operated twice a week too. With all his hospital appointments, he would be probably doing half the week on a quasi-voluntary basis. I say quasi because I don't know whether any money passed hands in those days. I don't think it did. If he was doing at least two days' work a week for no payment, so he must have been doing quite well in his practice. And then, of course, I earned a bit more by assisting him in the nursing home jobs he did.

Voluntary hospitals had an elite number of dentists who were recognised by their fellows as being worthy of a position of consultant, a handful of these in every place. They were the people who were issued with honorary FDSs soon after that, that was in '48.[24]

The patients adored Harold Round. He would go on over time in the outpatients department with me in the morning, and arrive at about three o'clock in the afternoon in his practice in Birmingham, and walk through the waiting room where his first patient was supposed to have been at one o'clock. He was so charming it was a privilege for them to wait for him. I don't know how he did it. He treated everybody exactly the same, so he gave the 'poor' in the hospital just the same amount of time and the same care that he was going to give in the afternoon in his practice, and they waited for him.

Gordon Fordyce qualified and went into Dental Practice and subsequently got his first surgical experience in the army [1946].

It was a few months until my call-up papers came, and then I was off to the army. The first place I went to was a unit in Carlisle for a few months, and then Chester for some more months. The patients were recruits who were not suitable to go straight into the army because they were underfed, as quite a lot of them were, or were way overweight, or needed some more education. Their English wasn't good enough.

Then I was posted to Austria where I did in a clinic in Klagenfurt and then after six months or thereabouts I was posted to the 31st British General Hospital as a number two dentist. And then number one finished, and I was made the senior dental officer there, and that's when I was responsible for any trauma that came in to this area of the British Authority.

I had such a wonderful time; I was skiing in the winter, and in the summer sailing yachts and doing all the things I loved doing. I came out of the army when my number came up; we had age in service release numbers; it was before we were on a fixed time contract. So my number came up, and I went back to St Andrews, went to see Professor Dow and he said, 'All right, Gordon, if you take my advice you had better do what the doctors do, and that is come back to the anatomy department and do six months as a demonstrator in the dissecting rooms.' So I set to and did this and read my physiology at night and worked in the anatomy department.

---

24 The Diploma of Fellow in Dental Surgery started in 1948 at the English Royal College of Surgeons and the following year at Edinburgh.

David Dow, the anatomy man, had told me that the way ahead was do your anatomy and get on with your fellowship, which had then started; the Edinburgh Fellowship in Dental Surgery. If I remember correctly, the examination was in two parts, a primary and a second part. And the primary bit was anatomy, physiology, pathology. And once you'd passed that you could do the second part, which was clinical dentistry and oral surgery.

So I set to and worked on that and passed the primary, and by that time I was ready to apply for a job. I was told that because I'd been in a hospital in the army and I had some experience I didn't have to do a house job.

So I looked at the journals and there came a job to go to be a registrar in dental surgery at Hill End Hospital. So I put an application in and was called to meet Ben Fickling, Paul Toller and Alexander MacGregor, who were the consultants. And I was successful and was taken on to start as soon as I could. There was an Irishman, whose name I have forgotten, who was the senior registrar, full time, and I'd be the full-time registrar and I could get enough experience to sit the second part of the fellowship.

Mike Awty's interest in surgery was stimulated as an undergraduate. After he qualified, he got a house job at Guy's [1953].

I was house surgeon to Warner, who was the Dean, and a chap called Holland, and they didn't get on, so that was my first lessons in professional diplomacy. Warner would look at the operating list and see that Holland had more interesting things on his, and I would be summoned to the Dean's office to explain why Holland had this patient and he didn't. So I learned to tread the line very early on.

I had to organise both of their clinics, take notes and then put people on the waiting list or on the operating list. I organised the operating list and liaised with the anaesthetist. The operating lists were usually late in the afternoons because they'd been working either in their clinics or up in the West End until they came back.

To begin with, you scrubbed with them and then once they realised you were okay you did half and after that you were off and did it while they were there; they were nearly always there, which justified their position. We did wisdom teeth and apicectomies; we had very limited horizons in those days. I had looked in on an ENT list and thought, there's more to this than pulling out teeth.

In 1954, Mike was then appointed as house surgeon at East Grinstead.

I was paid £350 a year the first year and then I think it went up by £50. Mind, I lived on £5 a week all the way through student time. I was very poor. I used to send my washing home, at Grinstead I got my laundry done and I was fed well.

I shared a hut with Sir Archibald's[25] chief assistant, who was a very experienced Canadian plastic surgeon, but he had problems with barbiturates. We had this Nissen hut, and we had a room each with a bathroom and a great big coke stove in the middle to keep us warm. There was enough heat to have a shower. In those days, Sir Archibald's chief assistant did some general surgery at the cottage hospital as it was and he would be called at night and he'd bring up his Tuinal[26] and do it. And if it was cold, he'd scream at me, 'Michael, go and orgasm that stove, will you?' He was a very colourful character. It was full of colourful characters in those days. You worked 24/7 I think I had Saturday afternoons and Sunday off on alternate weeks.

Laurence Oldham graduated in 1954.

The first job I got was house surgeon at the Birmingham Dental Hospital for six months. We used to rotate round from the examination room, that is diagnostic and treatment planning, through to the local and general anaesthetic departments. We did periodontal attachments under supervision of a chap called Dr Fox; we seemed to rotate around most of the departments except orthodontics. I was paid 540 pounds for a year; considering I'd earned nothing for all my life until then, I thought this was a jolly good start, because the value of 540 was quite good in 1955.

Then I did the second house surgeon's job, which was split between the dental hospital and the general hospital. We were on duty every night of the week, there were two of us in this split job. There was a room in casualty, with no chair, just an operating bench, and we did all our extractions and dressings there. We used to use carbolised resin for toothache, because we didn't want to extract every tooth that came in because we'd get 50 or 60 people at a weekend. The demand was enormous. The second house job was far more formative as we worked

---

25 Sir Archibald McIndoe the plastic surgeon who was in charge.
26 Tuinal, now discontinued, was a combination of barbiturates secobarbital and amobarbital.

in theatre with a consultant on his operating lists. So here I was in the environment which I wanted to be in.

The chief at the general hospital was RWH Tavenner, who was doubly qualified, a very nice chap who was a single man. He used to make us laugh because he said, 'I've got to go away for the weekend to see my aunt, could you look after the shop?' that was one of his statements, and the other one was, 'Oldham, keep a sticky eye on that,' meaning be very careful with what you were doing.

The work wasn't terribly adventurous; I mean I never even did a malar. All the surgery was cysts, odontomas, extractions, a bit of pre-prosthetic surgery like removing tuberosities if they were stopping a denture, basic oral surgery really, nothing very exotic. If there was a malignant case, that was a big deal, a very big deal, and we got the plastic surgeons.

Russell Hopkins qualified from Newcastle in 1956. He spent two years in dental practice in Hartlepool, Cambridge and Rhodesia. After that he became senior house officer in Nottingham. Tom Battersby was the consultant [1958].

I loved living in; in those days you lived in the hospital, it was your home. You were on-call 24 hours a day, but you could go out to the cinema or the pub.

I took over all the facial lacerations, I could sew them up much more tidily than the others, and so I became the accepted sewer of all facial lacerations. Tom taught me to cut skin and to lift the cheek bone. I didn't pull the upper jaws back at that stage, but he was the guy that introduced me to facial trauma. And there was a lot around because this was before seat belts and crash helmets, so people went through windscreens daily. It was an absolutely wonderful experience.

In casualty, I used to give anaesthetics, and the nurses used to pull the Colles fractures back and put the back slabs on. Sister Postlethwaite had been in the Army and seen and done everything in the kitchen sink. So the nurses were good, they were practical; they did a lot of the stuff; the housemen used to come out and the nurses would teach them, because they'd done it.

There was a wonderful mess at Nottingham, so we had our own doctor's dining room, and we had monthly lunches where consultants came and gave us a speech and we met and talked. And we had dine-ins and then had a dance afterwards. The nurses used to come, and they knew it was going to be a fairly alcoholic do. You worked hard, played hard, and they looked after you. We had our own proper accommodation and proper dining room. It was a wonderful year.

John Bradley had intended to qualify and go into general practice with his father and godfather in Wimborne [1958].

In those days, we still had to do national service, and I was one of the last tranche of people liable for this. Six months before my army medical, which was in August of '58, I suffered a tension pneumothorax of my right lung, which meant that I was rejected for military service.[27] So I thought I would do something similar in the hospital service. I would learn a lot, it would stand me in very good stead for general practice, they didn't pay you very much, but that didn't matter.

As a houseman, you had your own list, once a week on a Friday in basement theatres at 5:30, for taking out teeth, clearances basically.

John's first operating list was in his first week, the only surgical dental extraction he had done before was in in final LDS examination.

The list started at 5:30 and I'd finish around about seven. The first time I only had three patients. There were two dental clearances and one lady who had only five lower anterior teeth to come out, that was all. The two clearances were very easy because they had suffered from advanced periodontal disease and the teeth fell out. I taught myself to stitch that evening at the operating table but I had put a few stitches in in my finals exam.

The clearances went off fine but the third case was this lady with only five lower anteriors to come out; that was a real challenge because it was the glass in concrete syndrome and I had to reflect a flap, remove buccal bone and managed to prise these things out. It took a while and Sister Fessy was in charge of the theatres and she realised I'd got a difficult one, so she came and scrubbed up and assisted me. She was very experienced, was Sister Fessy. I think she must have seen just about everything. And she told me what to do, so it was fine.

My learning curve was almost vertical at Thomas'. I was given

---

27 Conscription into the armed services started in 1939 and ended gradually between 1957 and 1960.

tremendous challenges; there was very little supervision because the staff comprised of the consultant John Hovell, the houseman, me, a senior registrar, who was called Donald Winstock, who was a very well-known chap in the end, and we had one technician, Mr Dark. We had a part-time staff nurse in the outpatient department, so it was a very small department. But it was John Hovell that fired my interest; he did a mid-facial osteotomy after I'd been there about four months.

I was at St Thomas' for six months. At the end of the six months I could take out teeth pretty well, I could stitch up anything inside the mouth, and Donald Winstock taught me how to take out impacted third molars, so I was reasonably confident at that.

We saw a little oral medicine; we didn't see very much cancer. One thing we did see was syphilis of the mouth, we saw quite a lot of that. The first syphilitic I saw, I'd only been in the job ten days, was this classic snail track ulcer on this man's tongue. I recognised it from an illustration in a book.

After six months as house surgeon at St Thomas', John moved to the Westminster [1959].

There was a senior house officer job going there for 12 months but there was a gap of three months, so I did some general practice down in New Cross. I got paid a vast amount more money , compared with the hospital.

The consultant at Westminster was Rupert Sutton Taylor . He was an eccentric; he was a bit of a Lancelot Spratt,[28] actually; he was very much a military man, and he ran his unit like a military unit. So when I asked John Hovell to act as a referee, his immediate reaction was, 'What on earth do you want to work for Mad Rupert for?' He was known as Mad Rupert. He wasn't mad at all.

So I started there but if I wanted to ask Rupert Taylor a question, the question was put to the registrar and put to the senior registrar, to put to the senior hospital dental officer, who put it to the boss and the answer came down the line again. Well, I put up with this for about a couple of weeks and I thought this is daft. I'm not going to learn anything from Taylor if I have to communicate in this way, so I told him so. Nobody, I was told immediately afterwards, had ever spoken to Mr Taylor like that. I wasn't rude, but I was to the point and I told

---

28 Fictional character in books written by Richard Gordon.

him I thought it was a poor show if I couldn't talk to him directly about this, that and the other. He threw, best described as a fit, and wouldn't speak to me for the next two weeks. After those two weeks elapsed, I was taken into his room, where I thought I would be given the sack. Quite the opposite happened. He said, 'Bradley, I've been thinking about what you said. You're quite correct.' And from that point on, he was instrumental in my career.

Khursheed Moos was denied the opportunity to the double degree course or get a house surgeon job at Guy's in spite of his academic record, so went to Brighton as a house surgeon [1958].

I enjoyed my house surgeon post at Brighton working for Paul Gillett, who was a most unusual man. He left you to do things once he saw that you could do it, for example, taking out wisdom teeth and similar minor surgery. Although you were very much left to yourself, you could always ring up and speak to him.

We used to go to Cuckfield Hospital[29] once a fortnight, and the anaesthetist, surgeon and myself would go for a drink at the local pub after finishing the morning list. In those days it was always a gin and (French) vermouth or rather several. It started with a double from the surgeon and then a double from the anaesthetist and then a single all round. I hadn't had time for breakfast so I used to go up to the station in Haywards Heath to return to Brighton, 'feeling my way' because I knew I had had too much and it was somewhat uncomfortable and I usually promptly fell off to sleep when I got back to the hospital. Surprisingly, I always got back each time.

I enjoyed that first house job. I also had the opportunity of going to see other medical and surgical conditions, and I took an interest in what was going on in the hospital in general, especially in the casualty department. I often used to help or carry out procedures with the casualty officers, apart from doing just oral surgery. From there I went to do medicine.

Mike Bromige got a job at Selly Oak Hospital, Birmingham [1958].

There were a lot of hospitals with dental departments in and around what is now the West Midlands. So there were lots of house

---

29 Cuckfield Hospital was located in an old Victorian workhouse which had been commandeered as a hospital for the war injured in WWII. Like many such establishments it remained as a hospital after the war. It was closed in 1991.

jobs going, even if you didn't move out of the Birmingham area. I felt that I wanted more experience, surgery attracted me and so I signed up for a house job. It was down to a personal approach to the consultant who was Mr Hoggins.

Most of the consultants were part time and also ran a practice in Birmingham somewhere. Often they had been appointed pre-war and had been honorary appointments, and then they became official salaried appointments after the war. Hoggins wasn't one of those because he was ex-Army. Other ones were taken on as jobs were created. They were called consultant dental surgeons, and when fellowship[30] became available, they took it.

I was the only member of junior staff and there was one senior hospital dental officer. This was a time when all the dental staff in a hospital were paid less than their equivalent medical grades, significantly, for consultants as well. Then within a year or two the salaries were aligned, and this was immediately evident because every consultant went out and bought themselves a new car. So I was resident for six months, then I got married and we lived out, but I was still on call and I did that for a full year.

The duties of the house surgeon were to admit patients for two lists a week, but that was always done out of hours after the day's clinic was over. I attended clinic each day, if the boss wasn't in I did dentures, because there was a large elderly population in Selly Oak, in the geriatric wards. So there was a lot of denture work, quite a bit of cons,[31] often for mentally and physically disabled patients, and a few deformity patients.

I treated an awful lot of acute ulcerative gingivitis, trench mouth, which seemed to appear with astonishing regularity. The treatment was chromic acid and hydrogen peroxide, which was a fairly technicolour procedure that instantly relieved pain, whatever else it did. We also got an awful lot of abscesses, so that incision and drainage of abscess was another thing I did a large amount of, both extraoral and intraoral.

John Williams qualified in 1961 from Guy's and initially had a house job

---

30 Fellowship: The Diploma of Fellow in Dental Surgery of the Royal College of Surgeons of England. FDSRCS. The first examination was in 1948.
31 Conservative dentistry.

there.

I became house surgeon to Alan Thompson.[32] He was into precision attachments and I was interested in this.

After six months, I went to Plymouth as a senior house officer with Paul Bramley. Paul's job was known about. It was a job where you got a lot of hands-on experience; it was a busy job and there was a lot happening. It was out of London, right away from the teaching hospitals, and I thought this would be a tremendous opportunity to see what I wanted to do, and see what the environment was outside.

The way Paul Bramley practised oral surgery was as much as a specialty of medicine as it was of dentistry. The breadth of trauma we got and experience was huge. My wife Jill will say I spent every night in casualty sewing up faces because it was toughened windscreens, masses of glass in the face. The problem of getting all those pieces out and restoring somebody, who was almost always a girl because they were in the suicide seat with no seatbelts, was a challenge and a challenge that I liked. I liked the concept of trying to restore somebody to normality again.

John Langdon became a registrar at the London Hospital after a senior house officer job at the Eastman [1967-68].

It was a joint job in restorative and oral surgery, so it was half and half. When an opportunity came up, I transferred to oral surgery full-time. It was twelve months resident at Honey Lane in Waltham Abbey, which was the regional inpatient unit, and twelve months up in Whitechapel. We were doing outpatient clinics, emergency clinics, the regular review clinics, inpatient activity and all the trauma.

There was only one emergency theatre kept open at night. So the team would go out into the Whitechapel high street and go to the pub opposite, the Blind Beggar, and would drink and have typically sausages and ratatouille that they served from the bar. But quite often the Kray twins would be in there. And it was patently obvious if you came from the hospital, you were better dressed and you spoke differently to the rest of the East End crowd. So you would walk into the Blind Beggar, and one of the gang drinking in the bar or one of their hangers on, would turn round, and say, 'Ah, have a drink on us,

---

32 Consultant at Guy's who taught him minor oral surgery as a student.

doc.' And they would buy a round of drinks for us.

The East End in those days was a very interesting place. If you were clearly from the hospital, whether you were a nurse or a doctor, or a dentist, same thing, you could walk around at any time of the day and night and nobody would touch you. And any shop you went into would say, 'Oh, you're from the hospital, aren't you, doc.' And they just automatically knocked 10% off the price of anything you were buying. It was quite remarkable. At Easter time and Christmas time there would be a queue of locals, usually Jewish, offering their services to help on the wards or whatever so that the regular staff could have time off. And the Jewish community would send in food every Friday for the doctors' mess. And it was fillet steak and smoked salmon, every single Friday. It was a wonderful time to be there.

Trips to the pub often included a consultant.

Terry English was an affable Irishman and at the end of a clinic he'd always want you to go off to the pub and have a drink with him. But he would always touch you for a tenner. He never had his wallet with him.

When John was at the Honey Lane Hospital, Waltham Abbey end of his job he had to do an operating list at Bishop's Stortford on a Friday morning.

It was an operating theatre with two tables in it, and I would operate on one table using drills and things and producing dust clouds of burnt dentine and bacteria. And in the adjacent table there was a female eye surgeon doing eye surgery. Those were the happy days of cross infection control.

John Cawood went back to his hometown of Glasgow after dental school [1969].

I was in general dental practice for about a year and was quite disillusioned, it was not very stimulating. I was restless and so after a year, in 1971, my wife and myself went to Cape Town and I worked in a very good practice. Compared with anything I'd experienced in Scotland, it was progressive. It allowed me to practise dentistry at a level which I couldn't achieve within the confines of the health service in Scotland. We did quite a bit of dento-alveolar surgery, so I really enjoyed the overall experience. But I realised that the idea of being a hands-on dentist was not going to be my career choice. I arrived back in the UK and got a senior house officer job in Southend, working with a consultant called Ted Wisely; it was 1972.

I was the only member of staff other than the consultant, Ted Wisely, so I got a solid training in the basics of oral surgery and medicine and quite lot of exposure to trauma. I enjoyed the year in Southend. It was quite low key; we did mainly dento-alveolar surgery, fractures using inter-maxillary fixation, elevation of fractured zygomas, and some dental cysts, and quite a lot of what now falls into the realms of oral medicine. Any other surgery would be referred, usually up to the Royal London.

While I was there I was able to attend the primary course for the fellowship at the College of Surgeons.

After a year John then became a registrar in Edinburgh where the consultant was Dr (later Professor) W D MacLennan [1973-1977].

It was an annual rotation between the Royal Infirmary in Edinburgh and the Plastic and Jaw Surgery Unit at Bangour which was, more or less, half way between Edinburgh and Glasgow.

There were cordial relations with the plastic surgeons. We got very involved with quite major surgery and we also worked closely with the neurosurgeons who were based in the Royal Infirmary in Edinburgh. I suppose our practice was dominated by maxillofacial injuries being a pre-seatbelt era, and this famous road between Glasgow and Edinburgh, the old A8 which was an experimental three-lane road; it produced horrendous injuries. So a lot of my experience in Edinburgh was related to the management of facial injuries. Edinburgh covered the east coast of Scotland virtually up to Dundee and down to the borders so we registrars used to go out on calls to other hospitals in the region and if patients couldn't be transferred we do operating, mainly for trauma cases.

MacLennan was a very good teacher. He had a very logical way of assessing facial injuries and treating them. His ward rounds were quite legendary. Even if you'd been operating all night he would insist you attended the ward round after which he would say, 'right go and get some sleep and I'll pick you up at lunch time and we'll go for a slap up lunch'. He nurtured us very well.

In terms of elective surgery, again a lot of dento-alveolar surgery, not so much orthognathic surgery, no malignant surgery, although we got involved with some management of those cases which was largely done by the plastic surgeons out at Bangour. But I got exposed, either directly through the oral surgery department or our close associations with plastic surgery and neurosurgery; so I saw the full range.

Andy Brown [1969].

I qualified and was appointed as one of the two resident dental house surgeons at Guy's Hospital. And that's when I first got more interested in surgery per se, besides the overall treatment of the pathology of the oral cavity which was what the consultant dental surgeons used to run their clinics to do. They did everything from oral medicine through to the wisdom tooth assessment.

Brian Avery had done 2nd MB at Guy's after 2nd BDS with a view to becoming doubly qualified. After qualifying in dentistry, he did a dental house job [1970].

I remember a character called Bret Day who was half French, half English. He was a man with great charisma who used to do oral surgery, and another one called James Mansie who I worked for. After qualifying I did the resident house surgeon post which was an incredibly busy job, I was technically the house surgeon of James Mansie.

The job was for six months. It was a prime job if you wanted a career in oral and maxillofacial surgery because you did the on call. We were resident, and we had a huge volume of work, not of trauma but of people coming into A&E with toothache. At the time I wasn't too pleased about it but I realise the huge experience it gave me. It was not at all unusual for the two resident dental house surgeons, over a bank holiday weekend, which would be three or four days, to see 300 or 400 patients in A&E and treat them as well. There was a dental surgery there. Literally we had queues all the way up the corridor waiting to see us. We were there dealing with abscesses and occasionally organising general anaesthetic sessions for kids, and that was very busy but invaluable experience.

After the job I had a gap between July and September and I went off and did a locum in dental practice in Middlesex to earn some money. Then I went back and started medicine in September of '71.

Adrian Sugar qualified from Leeds dental school in 1970.

I did a year as a house surgeon in four specialties, cons (which I suppose would be restorative now), perio, something else that I can't remember and oral surgery. The junior house officer was not on call, so I didn't get to see trauma; trauma was just something that I heard the registrars and the consultants talking about in the background.

After the house job I went into practice for a short while largely because a guy I vaguely knew had to go into hospital to have surgery; he needed somebody to run his single-handed practice for six months. It was an interesting experience, partly because he was one of the last of a dying breed of dentist-anaesthetists who would give general anaesthetics and take teeth out at the same time. But boy, was he slick at doing it. I made it clear to him that I would not be doing that. I was in dental practice for just six months. Then I went off to do a course in London at the College[33] and then came back, did another period in practice while I was looking for jobs in oral and maxillofacial surgery.

Eventually I went up to Teesside as a very young, inexperienced registrar. I never did a senior house officer job; my senior house officer job was, I suppose, my first year as a registrar. They had a senior house officer there, and she knew a lot more than me as she constantly reminded me, and I couldn't argue with that. But I was there for a few years, and it didn't take me too long to get up to speed. And it was a unit that had two consultants and both of them singly qualified, and they had a lot of trauma, sometimes double figures a week in terms of fractures.

I was thrown in at the deep-end, and I remember the first mandibular fracture that I personally treated, and wired her jaws together. She had been beaten up by her husband who'd kicked her in the face when she was on the ground, and that shocked me and I wondered where I'd got myself to.

Tony Markus qualified from Newcastle in 1972.

I did my first job in Newcastle as a house officer. I remember Walkergate Hospital[34] because that's when I was taught to scrub up by a fierce theatre sister who made me put on six pairs of gloves until I got it absolutely right for the first time I went into theatre. Walkergate Hospital, was one of these very old Nissen hut type hospitals. I can't even remember where it was. It wasn't very stressful. I certainly didn't work the hours I put in at Barts which was my next job. I had six

---

33 Primary Fellowship course at the Royal College of Surgeons of England.
34 Walkergate Hospital closed in 2011

months there, a very nice time. We did some trauma, but it was nothing compared to what we do now. For many reasons, technology hadn't advanced then and also I don't think we were doing things that our specialty expects to do now.

Tony became a senior house officer at Barts [1973].

Barts, was wonderful. David Glendinning was the registrar, but it wasn't very advanced stuff. There was Theo Schofield, Frank Coffin, Donald Winstock and Markum, who was a very nice chap. They all had their interests around London in different hospitals and they were all part time, as was the custom then. Donald Winstock was at the Middlesex and Edgware and he had to be given a different colour surgical skin prep for each hospital. For Barts it was green, Middlesex was orange, and so presumably it was iodine based, and somewhere else was pink, chlorhexidine.

They used to breeze in. Donald always tried to get a discussion going about some hot topic. He was very unhappy if he didn't have one, so we always made sure he was made happy. A clinical topic, but sometimes something slightly different, but mainly clinical. Frank was difficult to work for, he hated the smell of curry, so David and I would always have the curry on Sunday night prior to his Monday morning alternate week list, just to annoy him. Then he'd be using his hammer and chisel and he'd say, 'Tap, tap,' and we would hit his knuckle instead of the end of the chisel. And after a few knuckle hits he'd look at us and say, 'You've b-b-b-been eating c-c-c-curry, g-g-g-get out.' And so David and I had the morning off and left him to the beautiful Barts nurses.

But we learnt a lot from him. There were lots of interesting things going on and it was good old-fashioned early oral and maxillofacial surgery. There was some trauma and lots of dento-alveolar, quite a lot of working with the ENT doing maxillectomies, and Frankie always did the obturators. We saw quite a few people with trismus who were always given lots of elastic bands to chew; they had to be of a certain thickness and colour red.

The highlight in my year there were the two big bomb blasts, one at the Old Bailey and one at Moorfields Station, the IRA. Both were very close, especially the Old Bailey. I remember going to do a ward round somewhere else in the hospital with the senior registrar. We came back into the big waiting hall in Barts and it was totally empty. The outpatients sister told us there'd been this huge blast.

Then the place filled with severely traumatised people with global injuries, including pan-facial injuries. And we didn't have major accident plans in those days. The waiting hall full of people working in the city with minor ailments who didn't have time to go to their GP or didn't want to go to their GP were all just thrown out and the whole place was cleared, and we got on with it, on both occasions. I can't remember the details, but I just remember there was lots and lots of trauma, and that was my first exposure to severe cranial facial trauma and working as a team to sort these people out.

The mess was a terrific place at Barts but food was horrendous and so we would go up to the Angel Market on a Saturday morning, buy in some really lovely food, go over to Charterhouse Square to get the wines and we would gourmandise all weekend, unless we were asked to do some work. And then on the Sunday night before Frankie's list, David and I would always go out for a curry. We drank quite a lot, and the mess was above casualty, and when we were needed, sister would come up and remove the glass from our hand, take us downstairs. If we needed sobering up, she would give us black coffee and peppermints, and then she'd take us round to see the patients.

We didn't do any restorative dentistry, but I remember Theo Schofield coming in one day with two wonderful patients: one was a porter at Smithfield Market, and he came in with a white bloodstained coat on, and he sat down in the chair. Theo just walked out and there was this silence. I talked to the patient for a moment or two, and then I went out to see what was going on. And I found him in the lab where he was sitting talking, and I said, 'Shall I get on and do something?' He said, 'Yes, tell him to go away and get a clean coat because I won't see him until he does.' He did, he went away and got himself a clean coat.

Another one was the management of sore, painful dentures. This lady came in with a painful denture which she might have had made there for some reason. So he took it from her, took it to the lab, found a tiny little piece of plaster a couple of millimetres roughly in diameter, popped it into the fitting surface of the denture and gave it back to her and asked her if it was any better. And she said no. So he took it away back to the lab, took the little piece out, gave it a rinse out and gave the denture back to her and said, 'Is it better now?' 'Yes, thank you very much, sir.' It took about 20 minutes each time he was in the lab. And I said to him, 'Why did you do that?' He said, 'bench rest dear boy, bench rest.'

There was lots of oral medicine, lots of people with trismus and I'm not sure why they had trismus, whether it was a post infection, whether it was ankylosis, and I think we did a few ankyloses there but I can't remember in detail. And so we had a jolly good time. We were on call phenomenal hours because we would only get paid overtime for over 80 hours. How we occupied those hours was another matter.

When I left Barts I decided I was going to do the primary FDS and I got a job working part time as a locum in a dental practice. It was a dental factory just behind the Bank of England and I think there were about ten surgeries in there. And we used to just go in and do fillings. And it was great because I could earn a bit of money whilst I was studying for the primary.

Tony went on the primary FDS course at the College of Surgeons [1974].

There was David Israel teaching pathology, frothing away at the mouth and sitting cross-legged on the bench at the front of the lecture theatre, disappearing now and then whilst we were furiously writing notes, which we didn't need to do because all he was doing was from memory reading out the content of his book.[35] And every now and again you'd look up, and he wasn't there. He was out in the corridor snorting, removing the mucous from his nasal passages.

And then another pathologist was a chap called Reece, who had just brought out a rival little book.[36] It was the better, because it was all there very quickly and it was great. He always turned up in his three-piece suit. He had a bowler hat and umbrella always, even in summer. He was very good. And we had immunology, it was really early days for immunology. I didn't understand a word.

I got the primary in 1974 and passed the final FDS in that very hot summer, June 1976. It was horrendous because we were in Queen's Square Examination Hall. And we were all downstairs in the basement cloakrooms, it was wicked really; the chap came to read out the numbers. I don't know how many people were there, 60, 70 people perhaps. And I can still remember this, he read out, '14,' and I thought oh this is nonsense, I haven't got a chance in hell, cat in hell's chance. So I was just making for the door and then he said, '56,' and I thought

---

35 Walter and Israel. General Pathology.
36 AJM Reese. Principals of Pathology.

well that's it. And then I heard 57, and that was my number. I stopped, and he had to say it again. I'd passed. And there were only three people who passed that day.[37]

Adrian Sugar had been the course at couple of years earlier.

I realised afterwards how fortunate I had been to do it. Prof Slome lectured on physiology and painted graphic images of physiological concepts such as the alveoli of the lung spread out would occupy the area of the tennis courts in Lincoln's Inn Fields. And all of this was said in his South African accent with a glass of water in his hand because he had Sjogrens syndrome. He was a fantastic lecturer as was Prof. Last, the anatomist, who also lived in as warden of the Nuffield College.[38] As a student I noticed that all our anatomy demonstrators used his book – they were working for primary FRCS– and so did I. We had lectures on immunology by Prof Turk. This was a whole new world to me and all of us.

Mike Davidson qualified in Dentistry from the London in 1976.

When I graduated, I then applied for the oral surgery resident job, which I did, and that was on call one-in-two resident at the London. And my main base was the hospital and the emergency department, but I also did some sessions in the dental school, in the oral surgery department, predominantly in the extraction area.

Occasionally you would do the general anaesthetic children, almost smash-and-grab session, you would occasionally do that on a Saturday. You did some clinics but your main duties were the inpatients and the A&E within the main hospital, so you were mixing very much with the medics, you were part of the residents.

I did that for six months and I worked for Prof. Seward, Patrick James, Terry English, and Hugh Cannell who had had just become a consultant. And that was for six months on a one-in-two on call. And

---

37 The Examination Hall at 8-11 Queen's Square was where generations of medical students went for their 'conjoint' finals examinations and doctors and dentists for their Fellowship and Membership examinations. The building was originally owned jointly by the Royal College of Surgeons and the Royal College of Physicians and latterly just by the surgeons. On the afternoon of the last day of the examination candidates gathered in the basement cloakroom next to the toilets to hear their result after the examiners meeting. The numbers of the successful candidates were read out.
38 The Nuffield College was the residence for the Royal College of Surgeons in the adjacent building.

the clinical work was pretty good because you began to do trauma, you got to do zygomas, again under supervision, so it was elevation in those days. I didn't fix anything, there were no bone plates being used. Fractures were wired and put into inter-maxillary fixation and went back to the ward with wire cutters pinned to their theatre gown, and you had to, as the house officer, draw a diagram of the wires in case the nurse had to cut them, and that diagram was pinned above the patient's bed while the patient was on the ward.

Though by then it was becoming increasingly clear if you wanted a career in oral surgery you were going to have to do medicine. They still called it Oral Surgery, although some more enthusiastic registrars called it the Oral and Maxillofacial Department, but most of the consultants called it Oral Surgery Department and to be honest, the bulk of the work, that's what it was, it was oral surgery, if you look at the sheer volume that was going through.

Although Mike qualified at the London Hospital and became a house surgeon there, and very much enjoyed it, he was not enthusiastic about staying.

By the time I started being a houseman and became more competent I realised that all dental schools have quite a bit of deadwood and are static, and very insular institutions. When I moved to other dental schools, I realised that the London in many ways was one of the better ones. But I found some were academically static, they had not moved on at all; they were teaching the same things, and they weren't really pushing, and that was particularly true in oral surgery at the London at the time, I thought.

Gordon Seward, obviously well-known and had done a lot of good work and had pushed things forward, but he didn't really have the support around him to take things further. I think a lot of these guys got involved in the politics of the College[39] and all sorts of other things. It was a unit that I just didn't think was going anywhere.

To be honest, you were there as a workhorse; they weren't really interested in you going off and being a supernumerary at any other clinics where you weren't needed, because if you were in a clinic, you were there to take impressions; you were there to fetch and carry. So, as a resident, you would go to the boss's clinic, but you were there very

---

39 The Royal College of Surgeons of England.

much as his handmaiden.

In Patrick James' case it involved doing the clinic 'til he arrived from the Golden Nugget[40] somewhere, and in another thing you'd take a patient off and take them elsewhere in the hospital to make sure they got there, you would chase up results, you would go down and lean on X-ray to get something done quickly. You might go off and do a biopsy, you would be there to take sutures out, you would be there to remove wires or cap splints, or whatever. So, you were very much the boss's supernumerary.

Patrick James described you as his right-hand man, so in theatres you physically had to be on his right hand because that's where you stood. And I remember once being with him in a list, and a new registrar said, 'Oh, you don't need to scrub, you can go across there,' and sort of pushed me out and made sure I couldn't get anywhere near. Patrick just turned to him and said, 'No, no, my right hand-man stands there and that's not you.' Because he would ask things that as the resident you knew, he was very good actually in the sense of giving you some chance to see what was going on.

The National Health Service consultants had their strengths but were very much visitors at the London. Their base was then Honey Lane Hospital at Waltham Abbey and that department later on moved to Epping, that was their power base. Patrick James was an interesting surgeon and did a moderate range, some rather strange temporo-mandibular joint procedures, but that's beside the point. His main interest was private practice. Terry English again was an often under-estimated surgeon. I think he did some good work, but again was quite distracted by private practice and the London wasn't really his base, it was much more Honey Lane. And we, as students or as house-surgeons, didn't get to see that side of things because the National Health Service practice was about fifteen/twenty miles away. So, I never wanted to stay at the London. Whether I would have wanted to come back later in my career is perhaps a different question, but that never arose, but I don't think I would have done, because by then I was very suspicious of dental schools and teaching hospitals in general.

He then became a senior house officer in Brighton [1978].

---

40 Euphemism for private hospital.

Richard Juniper was the only consultant. Very much a Guy's man and very much an East Grinstead man. There were two of us, resident housemen, so you're on call one-in-two. If your colleague was away, you were on a one-in-one; it was internal cover, and that was part of your contract, that was the deal; and if a colleague was ill, that was also part of the deal.

There was a lot of dento-alveolar work. Richard Juniper was just beginning to get into his temporo-mandibular joint work. He'd been doing some research into which muscles were effective around the temporomandibular joint at Brighton University with one of the chaps there, and he was beginning to do some temporo-mandibular joint surgery, but that didn't really kick off until after I'd left. So, there was a lot of dento-alveolar surgery, there was a little bit of trauma, not a vast amount but there was some, there was a little bit of salivary gland work in the way of submandibular glands. The cancer work was minimal, anything complex was passed on, usually to ENT.

You did a lot of clinics and minor oral surgery by yourself in a room in A&E, separate from everywhere, and you would have three or four cases on that and a nurse who would lug all the kit up there. So, it was a bit of a hand-to-mouth existence in that sense. Poor old Richard who was a single consultant, very small beer around the hospital because he didn't have the muscle of a large department.

Ian Martin qualified in Dentistry in 1979.

So, until the time I was due to do house jobs, there had been a fairly traditional pattern of two six-month house jobs which was the norm. And if you wanted to do oral max-fax surgery, or oral surgery, as it would have been then, you needed to get one of the resident oral surgery house jobs. The year I needed a house job, in 1980, they changed things. They made them twelve month posts split into three sections which I wasn't very happy about because it meant you had to do more of other stuff. I wanted the resident oral surgery post, but I also had to do four months of prosthetics and four months kids. Although I hadn't really been particularly keen on doing the prosthetics job, it turned out to be actually quite useful because I was making really complicated dentures for people who'd had commando operations done by the ENT surgeons.

So after that I did a senior house officer job, and that was at the time when Bob Ord was there, and then David Vaughan came. And it was a transformational time, I think for the specialty because this was the time, or certainly in King's, when you had people who had double degrees, were looking to expand things, weren't afraid to do new stuff that was uncharted territory, and they were supported to do it by John Sowray.[41]

---

41 Professor of oral surgery.

Chapter 7
Inspiration to Oral and Maxillofacial Surgery

'I thought this was wonderful'

Most of my interviewees had been primed towards an interest in oral surgery as undergraduate dental students but decided to pursue a career in it when they had more experience as junior hospital staff. Some of them had been lucky enough to have been exposed to inspirational surgeons early in their careers, and some had made the decision when they were still students.

Paul Bramley was inspired by Harold Round [1944].

Harold Round got an MDS in about 1910 on his method of wiring a fractured jaw.[42] He was a distinguished general practitioner who had honorary sessions at the Queen's in Birmingham and then eventually after that at the Queen Elizabeth. And because he had a powerful mind and because he was a good man, he seems to have created a lot of opposition and he was excluded from the dental hospital, but he practised in the two general hospitals and he had a following and I was one of those following whilst I was an undergraduate in the dental school.

Much to their disgust, I attended his clinics, and I thought I want to be like this chap. I wanted to do what he, Harold Round, did and he was at the time in advance of most other people.

Russell Hopkins spent a couple of years in dental practice after qualifying [1956].

I'd had this feeling gradually dawning on me, I woke up one day and I thought, I can't fill teeth for the rest of my life. And I'd had two years of filling teeth and dental practice, and I thought, this is the most boring bloody job I've ever come across. And I couldn't cope with it.

He became senior house officer in Nottingham where he was inspired by

---

42 Harold Round was also one of the two first U.K. dentists to qualify with a degree, at Birmingham University in 1904. Previously the only qualification was the LDSRCS examination. See: 125 years of developments in dentistry, 1880-2005. Part 5 Dental education and qualifications. S Gelbier. British Dental Journal. 2005; 199: 685-688.

Tom Battersby, the consultant [1958].

I loved it from day one, and Tom Battersby had been a Dental Officer in the war, had been involved in the treatment of facial injuries and Tom was one of the first three to sit the FDS, (Norman Rowe and Killey were the other two).[43] Tom cut skin and lifted cheek bones, and treated mandibular fractures, and I thought this was wonderful.

There were several things attracted me, one I enjoyed the atmosphere of working in a hospital. I enjoyed cutting skin; I enjoyed doing things which I thought were important, relative to teeth. I'd gone off teeth, and I got more pleasure out of spending three or four hours pulling glass out of a patient, in the middle of the night, than I ever did from filling a tooth and getting a decent result from a filling. So, I enjoyed the work. I was in my element and it goes back to the days as a dental student. I always enjoyed the medical things of the dental course, rather than the dental things, even though I was pretty competent at doing dental things. My enjoyment and pleasure came from medicine.

John Bradley expected to become a dental practitioner like his father. But on qualification he turned to the British Dental Journal to look for a job [1958].

There was an advert in the British Dental Journal wanting a house surgeon at St Thomas' Hospital so I applied. I went to have an interview with a man called John Hovell. He was a consultant orthodontist at the Royal Dental Hospital, north of the river, and if he couldn't do it with springs and wires he shipped them south of the river to St Thomas', where he corrected the deformity surgically.

He fired my interest; he opened my eyes. This bouncing man, who was a bit of a flash Harry, quite a character, bounced around the place and he was doing all these quite incredible things and I'd had no idea this is what oral surgery was about. So he enthused me.

John moved to a senior house officer job at the Westminster Hospital where he worked for Rupert Sutton Taylor.

He was instrumental in my career. He was my mentor; he was my

---

43 In fact there were 7 candidates, those mentioned are the ones who passed. The first final FDS exam was in April 1948 3 weeks before the NHS started. See: The Faculty of Dental Surgery of the Royal College of Surgeons of England: An overview of the first 70 years of achievements. Stephens C. Dental Historian 2017; 62(1) 24 - 32.

encourager, and I wouldn't be here if it wasn't for Rupert Taylor, It was Rupert that encouraged me to do oral surgery because he said, 'Look Bradley, you've got to get the fellowship. You've got extremely good hands, Bradley, you've got to do this,' and he really encouraged me to aim for oral surgery and forget about general dental practice.

John Williams was inspired towards oral surgery as a student and house surgeon at Guy's from where he qualified in 1961. Subsequently, he worked as a senior house officer for Paul Bramley in Plymouth [1962].

I'd developed an interest in the latter part of my student time. When I saw the difference between the type of routine conservative work done by the people I knew at Guy's against what Alan Thompson was doing, I realised there was a lot more. I became house surgeon to Alan Thompson, because of his particular interests from the surgical point of view.

He then went to Plymouth as senior house officer.

Paul Bramley insisted that his senior house officer was able to do a tracheostomy, could do cardiopulmonary resuscitation and could manage head injuries; so much so that when I went back ultimately and did medicine and became a house surgeon in ENT, I personally had done more tracheostomies than the senior registrar. Those three things he insisted on, and that was the measure of the type of work that was going on. Paul Bramley was the dynamic lead. Paul was a mover and shaker, and he always came over that way.

I worked there for just over 12 months. At that time I decided that I wanted to do max-fax.

John Langdon qualified from the London in 1965.

But then of course it came to house jobs afterwards. And I was very much influenced by a senior registrar in oral surgery, Colin Parker. Who was a bigger than life character, very laid back and very skilful; he was singly qualified. So I did an oral surgery house job. I then did a six months house job at the Royal Dental Hospital covering inpatient duties at Tooting Hospital.

After that I was a bit lost; I didn't really know what I was going to end up doing. And somebody suggested I ought to go and see Robert Bradlaw, who was the Dean at the Eastman Dental Hospital. So I phoned up his secretary, and got an appointment to see Sir Robert.

He asked me a few questions, and he said, 'What you're going to do is come here as a senior house officer in oral surgery. You will sit the primary FDS. and we'll take it from there.' And without asking if that's what I wanted to do, he picked up the phone, spoke to Professor Killey and said, 'I've got a young man here. I'm sending him round to you. He's starting in a month.'

At what stage did Andy Brown take an interest in surgery as a career? [1968].

I didn't want to go into general dental practice (although that was my initial interest) because I didn't fancy the rest of my life locked in a room with a 17-year-old school leaver and not working in an environment where I could interact with other people. Now that was a very naïve assessment of dental practice, but that was my assessment!

When Pat O'Driscoll arrived at Guy's he was the first person who really impressed me as an oral surgeon. He had been better trained I suspect than the more senior guys. He had worked at East Grinstead as a senior registrar and he had a very good pair of hands. I think that was just another link in the chain that confirmed to me that this is something that I want to do. He was the one who really started to steer me to oral surgery.

I went to Roehampton Hospital in my final medical year for a medical elective period. I sat in with Norman Rowe at Roehampton. Again, that convinced me that oral surgery was something I wanted to get back into because I could see just what they were doing at Roehampton. It was one of the major units.

For David Vaughan it was at a lecture in a pub in Cork where he was a student that decided him to be a cancer surgeon [1969].

Gordon Russell was the professor of oral surgery; he had trained in Newcastle and had befriended a plastic surgeon there, J S P. Wilson.[44]

In my final year of dentistry, Professor Russell called us all together and said, 'Would you like to hear a lecture from a very famous plastic surgeon who is on holiday in Kinsale?' So we said yes, and armed with two projectors we descended to Acton's Hotel, where we met the great J S P. Wilson, who was actually on his honeymoon; it was his second

---

44 We will meet JSP (Tiger) Wilson again in chapters 12 and 26.

marriage, and he was obviously rather bored, so he decided to give a lecture.

So in the bar of Acton's Hotel, we set up the projectors, put the screens up, and I sat there with an untouched pint of Guinness, looking at what he was showing and saying 'You cannot do that to humans.' Wilson was the great man for reconstructing defects of the head and neck, and I think really that was what implanted the idea that that's what I wanted to be

Adrian Sugar qualified from Leeds dental school in 1970.

I did a year as a house surgeon. That was when I really had something of a revelation. It was when I was doing the oral surgery house job that I just realised that that was for me, that I enjoyed every minute, and I knew that that's what I wanted to do. Whether I even had any idea what maxillofacial surgery was then I very much doubt because I never really got to see any.

Brian Avery qualified in dentistry at Guy's. He had decided in his first year at Dental School that he wanted to become an oral and maxillofacial surgeon [1971].

I don't really know why; I twigged that that's what I needed to do. I'd realised that it was a more interesting career than a dentist. There are several people who had inspired me. I remember in oral medicine there was Professor Cawson and Professor Lehner who were good teachers. Then there were the oral surgeons; Pat O'Driscoll used to do a few osteotomies and I can remember him doing what was probably the first sagittal split osteotomy at Guy's at the end of my training, which would be in about 1969. I was in theatres at the time and there was a huge crowd of people there.

Rob Hensher was inclined towards oral and maxillofacial surgery as an undergraduate at Liverpool [1971].

In the final year you could steer yourself into more exposure of oral and maxillofacial surgery if you wanted to. So, I was given the opportunity to get a flavour of that. Simple extractions, a bit of periodontal surgery, raising flaps, you could do that under supervision.

You could rotate into the hospital general anaesthetic lists at the Royal Infirmary where the oral and maxillofacial docs were doing more difficult or more extensive surgical extractions and watch and sometimes hold a retractor in bigger things. Towards the end of the course, when the more mature aspects of medicine, surgery and oral and maxillofacial surgery were introduced, I began to get really quite interested in it. My mentor at this time was Lawrence Finch, who was a consultant there, and I had some chats with him about it.

What was attractive about oral surgery, or oral maxillofacial surgery was the broader aspect of treating patients, and treating people. When we were given medicine and surgery tuition, I began to realise that there is a whole interesting world there. I thought I can still do the dental stuff, but it will be broader. And we had Mr Finch as an example, and his juniors. That opened up my outlook, really.

Tony Markus had no idea when he qualified in 1972 what he wanted to do in his career.

I did my first job in Newcastle as a house officer and was influenced by Jack Murgatroyd, who was a wonderful oral and maxillofacial surgeon, doubly qualified, a terrific Yorkshire man and inspirational. A balanced good surgeon, lots of good advice, and he told me what I should do with my career.

John Cawood had been inspired by Derek Henderson when he was at Dental School [1969].

I enjoyed oral surgery at dental school. I think that was the subject that was most interesting and I realised that this was a fascinating field and I wanted to pursue it.

Derek Henderson presented a very impressive lecture on what could be done to repair very serious facial injuries. This was a seminal lecture and I also remember a lecture I went to at the College[45] by Hugo Obwegeser. The first slide was a very disfigured young patient. Obwegeser's remark was 'this is how God made this patient'. He clicked on the second slide, after his reconstruction, and said 'this is what I did for this child'. It was an inspirational lecture and I was amazed at what could be achieved in terms of reconstruction using bone grafts.

But for me, it was my experience in Edinburgh that really fired me up because I was lucky to work as a registrar under Professor MacLennan, or Dr MacLennan as he was in those days.

---

45 Royal College of Surgeons of England.

Mike Davidson qualified in Dentistry in 1976 and had to decide what to do.

At the London they had a rather good system, as long as you had completed all the number of dentures, fillings, etc., you could apply to what they called a student internship. You were allowed a maximum of three, so I did oral surgery, oral medicine and oral pathology, and you did it for two months and you had a certain number of sessions you had to turn up to and you did clinics, a one-on-one with a senior person in the relevant department. I really enjoyed it and I thought, this is what I want to do.

But I couldn't decide, would it be oral pathology, would it be oral medicine? Because oral medicine was Roy Duckworth and Roger Sutton, both of whom I respected tremendously, both clinically and academically, and it was an area that did interest me, but I also quite liked the surgery.

He became an oral surgery house surgeon.

It was hard work, but it was interesting work, and I enjoyed it. It made me think I wouldn't mind taking this a step further and see how far I could go.

Ian Martin had performed a lot of minor oral surgery (over 100 cases of third molar removal) and had been encouraged to go to ward rounds and theatres by Malcolm Harris, Geoff Forman and Phil Rood at King's [1979].

I rapidly became bored and disinterested with stoppings, crowns, and bridges, and perio, and stuff. I made my mind up fairly early on that I'd like to do surgery. I thought, well I'll just see how far I can go, and if they stop me, well fine, I'll be a dentist and do that. But as it happened nobody ever did stop me, I just carried on.

So after I did this year's house job, I got a senior house officer job in oral max-fax surgery. In fact, I was also offered a lecturer's post in restorative dentistry by Ivan Curzon, who was the professor of restorative dentistry, which was very flattering, but thankfully I was sensible enough not to accept it because I would have been bored rigid.

Chapter 8

Medical Training: Why and How?

'You're only a bloody dentist'

Before the National Health Service, many dental surgeons who had hospital appointments had a dual medical and dental degree. Often they had studied a shortened combined course which possibly would not have been well rounded in the general management of medical or surgical conditions.

John Cawood was a registrar in Edinburgh. His chief WD MacLennan was medically qualified.

He had a medical degree. They had what was called the Triple in his day. They went to dental school and then they could do an extra year at the conclusion of dentistry and convert to a medical qualification.

I don't know if he ever went on the Medical Register, but he certainly got the Triple qualification and he got an honorary FRCS.[46] But he was very much an oral surgeon in his outlook, and he didn't step beyond his own boundaries He concentrated on what he could do, politically, safely, and well.

When the issue of a medical degree came up I felt that people were taking medicine, more or less, for the sake of it. It didn't lead on to general surgical training and they just continued in maxillofacial surgery as before I didn't see the value of it. That is until later when we saw what David Vaughan and Ian Martin did in obtaining general surgery training as well.

This was more to do with status and the presiding culture of the time than having the skills to provide comprehensive patient management which was one issue in 1981 when the British Association of Oral Surgeons decided that from 1991 a medical qualification would be necessary for a consultant appointment.[47]

---

46 The diploma of Fellow of the Royal College of Surgeons.
47 British Association of Oral Surgeons Working Party Report.- Medicine as a second degree for dental surgeons practising oral surgery and oral medicine (1979).

In 1948, when National Health Service consultant dental surgeon posts were established, it was not necessary to have a medical qualification. The Faculty of Dental Surgery of the Royal College of Surgeons of England was also established in 1948, and it was considered that passing the examinations to become a Fellow in Dental Surgery of the College was sufficient to demonstrate the skills needed to become a consultant.

Throughout the 1960s and 70s there was much debate and disagreement about whether a medical qualification was necessary for consultants in dental surgery, or oral surgery as they were starting to call themselves. In 1966, the British Association of Oral Surgeons council appear to be prevaricating when they stated:

> 'Council were unanimously of the opinion that in the future development of oral surgery a registered medical qualification will tend to come to be regarded as desirable for the holder of a consultant appointment in dental surgery who aspires to have full medical charge of beds'.

The Fellows of the Association (who at that time were all consultants) had voted in a questionnaire. For medical qualification: 81, against 41, reply not analysable: 7, not replied: 34.[48]

Nevertheless, some aspiring oral surgeons sought to gain a medical degree and others not. Why? Paul Bramley wanted to be doubly qualified because he was inspired by two general dental practitioners in Leicester who were also medically qualified.

> I suppose it was the glamour of this dental practice in Leicester that I had been taken to and their insistence to my mother that really dentistry is all right, but you'd be better off if you were medically qualified. There'd been a dribble of people through in Birmingham dental school who actually did a double degree. The great Humphrey Humphreys, was the man who had been everywhere and done

For a review of the historical relationship between dentistry and the medical profession see: 125 years of developments in dentistry, 1880-2005 Part 2: Law and the dental profession. Gelbier S. British Dental Journal 2005: 199, 470-473 and Dentistry - The dependence upon Medicine and Surgery for Professional Status. Stanley A. British Dental Journal, 1994 176(2) 448-450.
48 Memorandum on Post-Graduate Education. Addendum to the minutes of the Annual General Meeting of the British Association of Oral Surgeons 1st April 1966.

everything, was doubly qualified and was Dean of the school.[49]

So this was nothing to do with the present double qualification to do oral and maxillofacial surgery?

No, nothing to do with that.

Sir Paul had attempted and failed to get onto the combined dental/medical course at Birmingham so having qualified in dentistry and turned down the opportunity to work in practice with his mentor and inspiration Harold Round, he wanted to get a place in the medical school [1946].

Harold Round offered me a place in his practice, he said, 'I've been talking to Professor Bradlaw and he reckoned that the FDS made it unnecessity to go into medicine. Now, will you come?' This was very flattering to be asked by this mighty man to join his practice, but I said, 'I'm sorry, not going to do it; I'm going to do medicine, do it properly.'

So I went to the Sub-Dean, who was an absolute pig of a bully. He leaned back in his chair and said, 'No, we're not taking you back.'

I said, 'Excuse me, Sir; you've probably got my dental record in the office.' He said, 'Yes, I have.' I said, 'Well, would you look at it?' He pulled it out, looked at it and said, 'Right,' this was the middle of July. He said, 'If you can dissect arm and leg and submit yourself to a whole body anatomy exam, that is to say the full MB exam, which would take place in early September and if you pass, you can come into third-year medicine.'

He set me an impossible task, but I did it. The ridiculous thing is you do things in a hurry, you can't remember a bloody thing about them; just learnt all the mnemonics for the stuff round the ankle joint and all that sort of thing, and branches of the external carotid artery, all the mnemonics. So I did it, so I joined the medical course and I had a wonderful time there.

Gordon Fordyce decided on a career in oral surgery without going to medical school. He took the advice of the professor of anatomy, who

---

49 Humphrey Humphreys was medically and dentally qualified and became the first Professor of Dental Surgery in Birmingham in 1951. His father John Humphreys had been an instigator of the first BDS degree in the UK, in Birmingham. See: Anderson, R. J.. 'John Humphreys M.A., PhD., MDS., FSA., FLS., FGS.' Dental Historian 1990; 3-8.

taught him as an undergraduate [1948].

I became interested in anatomy. And the professor of anatomy was David Dow, and he was very kind to all of us dental students. When I came out of the army, I went to see him and said: 'Look Professor Dow, it looks as if I should do medicine.'

And he said, 'Well, hang on a minute.' He had been to a meeting in Edinburgh and heard that the College there, the Royal College in Edinburgh, was going to introduce a new examination for dentists whereby they would be awarded a Fellowship, FDS Edinburgh.[50] 'And that would be the future and the ladder for people like yourself, three years training in the army hospital experience, a little bit of max-fax experience, that would be the right way and much better for you because you're now getting on in your years, you're going to think about getting married, and to go back now and do medicine would not be really necessary if you could pass an FDS.' So I said, 'Right, Professor Dow, I listened to you a lot for many years and I will go along that path.' Which I did.

This was backed up by Paul Bramley.

The Faculty of Dental Surgery in the College of England had created the FDS with the principal desire of making it unnecessary from the point of view of knowledge and experience to get a medical qualification and that's why the English college was always very much oral surgery or pathology based because of that concept. Edinburgh was different. That was a general dental qualification, basically in classical restorative dentistry.

Gordon worked as registrar and subsequently senior registrar with Ben Fickling at Hill End and subsequently Mount Vernon Hospital. Ben Fickling was the dentist who worked with plastic surgeon Rainsford Mowlem on war injuries at Hill End. He was dually qualified and had an FRCS. Gordon asked him if he should do medicine [1949].

I had mentioned to Ben I wanted to do medicine, and this was after I'd been three years in the army and I'd been working with him for a

---

50 The diploma of Fellow in Dental Surgery of the Royal College of Surgeons. The Royal College of Surgeons of Edinburgh started the FDS in 1949, the year after the Royal College of England, this replaced the Higher Dental Diploma in Edinburgh which started in 1919. See: 125 years of developments in dentistry, 1880 - 2005. Part 5 Dental education, training and qualifications. S Gelbier. 2005 British Dental Journal.,199 685-688.

few years, and he said: 'no, no, you are a dentist. You must stay as a dentist'. Speaking, as Ben would have said about this, he would have said a dental qualification should have given you enough in the training to look after most of the straightforward medical complaints, and if you couldn't do that, you shouldn't be a dentist. That was Ben's point of view, and MacGregor and Paul Toller.[51]

So why was Fickling medically qualified?

Well, his father had told him to do it.

So what was the point? Gordon:

It had become traditionally an issue because the young dentists coming up were keen to get on the staff of a teaching hospital. That was important, a teaching hospital, because of this connection: they introduced a whole lot of people of their own age who would support their practice when they went and opened their rooms in Harley Street.[52]

Paul Bramley agreed.

Well, I think if you were working in London that was right. Yes, how dental hospitals were run before full-time academic teachers was the honorary consultant system. That meant you gave your services free, but you got the student contact for future referrals, to your private practice in Wimpole Street or Harley Street or thereabouts. That was the payoff, and it may well be that the medical qualification was part of that.

Mike Awty was a senior house officer at East Grinstead. He wanted to do a wider range of surgery than was being done by the department at the time. Sir Terence Ward was the chief [1954].

Well, I realised at Grinstead we would not stay doing the little that we did. I'd had my horizons lifted enough there and read a bit of the American books and things and I thought, no, this isn't on, I've got to have a better background so I can be confident doing more. People weren't confident because they hadn't got the background or the

---

51 Alex MacGregor and Paul Toller also worked as consultants at Hill End when Gordon Fordyce arrived as a registrar. MacGregor was dually qualified and was soon to leave to become Dean at the Birmingham dental school.
52 Fickling also worked at St George's Hospital as well as his dental practice in the West End of London.

training, so then I knew I had to do medicine. Terry Ward insisted. He said, 'It's no good, forget it if you're not going to do medicine,' so I went back.

I went back to the medical school, Guy's, which had some superb administrators, Jimmy Goodliffe and Mr Somebody Else and Miss Farmer, who ran the place as if they were father figures. I spoke to Goodliffe about getting back into medical school and he said, 'I'll see what we can do.' And then he said, 'Well yes, you can.'

Miss Farmer and I imagine Warner the Dean, were quite supportive I think because I'd looked after him well as his house surgeon. It was just arranged that I would come back and start.

Laurence Oldham had been declined a place for medicine when he had applied from school. Later he was working in Uganda with Sir Ian McAdam, a General Surgeon [1968].

Sir Ian McAdam said to me, 'Why don't you do medicine here. You can practise and do medicine at the same time?' Get an east African degree.

I had always wanted to do medicine. But it would have been difficult because we had two kids and it was becoming hairy in east Africa because Amin, that dreadful politician who was coming up through the ranks and eventually ruined the country. I could see this coming so I said no. So I came back home and realised that medicine was out.

Khursheed Moos had originally won a place to study medicine at Oxford but did not get a scholarship so could not afford to go. He went to Guy's as a dental student but hoped and expected he would be able to do a dual degree [1953].

Originally I had expected I would do dentistry and then go on to do medicine, as it had been implied at the interview. I accepted that that was going to happen. Everything went smoothly, and I had passed all the exams and the tests but then discovered that I would not be going to do medicine because they appeared not to want me even though I had been number one or number two in my year all the way through.

I found this rather difficult to accept. I felt perhaps they were prejudiced by my coming from a mixed racial background, my father having come from a different part of the world, India, and that may have been a factor. I could only think this was the case. I found it very strange because I was very much one of two students who tended to get top marks all the way through and more 'excellents' at restorative work than others, and two did go on to do medicine. I had had good marks in paedodontics and the prize in orthodontics when there, so I was quite surprised.

After dentistry at Guy's he became a senior house officer at Brighton [1958].

From Brighton I went to do medicine. I had hoped to do that in Guy's but that was not to be and so I applied to University College, London and I did my second MB there. That was the pre-clinical course. With a dental qualification, I was given some reduction in time, so instead of 18 months I could complete it in nine months.

Just before the examination I was called up to do my National Service, which rather surprised me because I thought I would have been exempted from that; but since it was coming to an end, there was a certain amount of pressure to get people in before it completely finished. I said that I was taking exams, but they did not seem to take much notice so I wrote to my MP and said I thought this was not a good thing and he agreed to help. So I was given time to complete that examination before going in and immediately after finishing second MB, before the clinical part, I started national service.

I lost my clinical place at University College Hospital because when I came out of the services they had already filled it so I applied to Westminster Hospital and they accepted me and I had a most stimulating time there. It was a much smaller medical school which pleased me, and I found I got on very well with everybody. There were none of the problems I had had at Guy's.

Russell Hopkins had initially failed part of his higher school certificate and after retaking 'A' levels he turned down a place at medical school because his confidence has been knocked. Now he was working at St Peter's Hospital Chertsey, where the chief was Norman Rowe [1959].

We went to meetings, and I could see from Germany and other places like that, that things were moving into a much wider field than we had been doing.

It was in the second year that I was at St. Peters, and I used to teach the house surgeons how to sew. And I remember there was a guy from St Thomas' (and they're even more arrogant than the Guy's people), and I was showing this particularly clumsy guy how to sew carefully and later he said, 'But you're only a bloody dentist, how can you do this?', and this used to rile me, that I was only a bloody dentist. And I thought, if I'm to make a career in the hospital side, and if I'm to go up in oral surgery, I'm going to have to do medicine. I wasn't married, and I thought, this is the time to do it.

I applied towards the end of my second year when I knew that I would have to leave my registrar job. I applied to Newcastle, and to the Royal Free. Several places said they couldn't take me because I'd already got a degree. The Royal Free was interested in me because I was a postgraduate and a male[53], and they were increasing the number of males, and they liked people with degrees, and who were sensible and who they thought would treat their female students reasonably well, and I applied to Newcastle because that was my old dental school. They accepted me, but they said you must do the MB, so it was going to be, with a year off second MB a four-year effort, and the Free was prepared to take me to do the conjoint. So I went to the Free. I did the first year in nine months and then 27 months clinical.

John Bradley did not become medically qualified.

There were a number of dentists at that time who felt, particularly if they were going into specialist practice, that medical training would be a considerable advantage. At one time, Guy's ran a combined dental and medical course. It was the only school to do that, I believe. This was quite difficult in a way because a lot of people said to me why didn't I go on it? I said well I really didn't know what I wanted to do when I started. I wanted to do dentistry, so I started and I had no idea about the wider aspects of all this, hadn't a clue. So it's the sort of thing you would do with hindsight, which is a wonderful tool of course.

However, taking medical degrees for hospital practice was regarded as not being essential at all. You could perfectly well practise, and a lot of my colleagues in Burnley, in the early days, said quite unnecessary, I was darn good at my job and I looked after my patients meticulously, and medical degrees were unnecessary, they thought.

John worked at St Thomas' as a house surgeon in oral surgery with John Hovell and at the Westminster as a senior house surgeon with Rupert Sutton Taylor. Both consultant dental surgeons had medical

---

53 The Royal Free had previously only taken female students.

qualifications and there were other well-known people such as Kelsey Fry, Ward and Norman Rowe. Did he know why, what was the advantage to them? [1959].

I think it was just a personal thing, largely. They felt that if you were going to take on a patient, you had to take on the whole of that patient, his complete care.

Did he think there was any element of snobbishness about this?

There was an element, yes, and one got this from the general dental practitioners, believe it or not. It was inverted snobbishness. They didn't like the hospital people, particularly if they had medicine because that was sort of almost a betrayal of the core profession of dentistry, which of course was a bit of nonsense, really.

I remember going with Norman Rowe to a British Dental Association section meeting down in Putney one time. We were treated rather like something that the wind had blown in. And I quietly complained to Norman about this, this most charming consummate man who, in his day, was probably the name in international oral surgery. He really was at this level. And he said, 'Never mind John, they will never understand.' I always remember him saying that and just smiling, and didn't bother to challenge it.

The British Association of Oral Surgeons (as the British Association of Oral and Maxillofacial Surgeons was then called) recommended that dual qualification should be mandatory for oral and maxillofacial surgeons in the early 1980s (it became mandatory in 1991). John Bradley was a member of council and sat on the Education and Training committee.

This was when I was already on the council, the British Association of Oral Surgeons as it was then, and they set up an education and training committee. The reason for that was the practice of oral surgery in hospitals had been radically changed, almost overnight, by an act of parliament, where it required every car driver to wear a seat belt. So almost overnight people being thrown through windscreens disappeared completely.

We were the first specialty in the whole of medicine and surgery to define a career pathway for a junior coming in as a houseman and finishing off as a consultant. There was a time scale, including medicine, and we did it. We planned it out for 12 years, which was pretty good going. It needed a lot of co-operation from medical schools, which was mixed. The best one was in fact Leicester school, they were very helpful.

A report with recommendations for training had been produced in 1973.[54] It is interesting to note that this report quoted that of patients receiving treatment in oral surgery departments 40% were having minor oral surgery and another 40% were having 'routine dentistry for patients with systemic disease'. At a council meeting in April 1976, John had put forward the possibility of formal medical training taking place during in service training. The present method of obtaining full medical training was wasteful of manpower and of finance; some of the brightest of the dentally qualified medical undergraduates were moving into other medical specialities.[55]

Mike Bromige was a member of council and Secretary of the British Association of Oral Surgeons when the discussions over making a medical degree mandatory were taking place.

The major issue at the time was that it was established that you needed dual qualifications. That was being discussed, and if you think of Paul Bradley who was a contemporary of mine he went on and did medicine and I didn't, and people said, 'Are you going to do medicine?' and I was advised in Birmingham not to because Birmingham tended to be a 'medicine not necessary place', although a lot of the consultants had medicine interestingly.

I think I was probably wrongly advised, although I got through without it and it didn't really interfere with my career. By the time I was secretary of the British Association of Oral Surgeons it had become established; but the main hurdle was getting a shortened medical training for dental graduates. And so a lot of our work was done in persuading Deans and getting the shortened medical course. That was one of the major issues.

John Williams had been a senior house officer in Plymouth for just over a year. He had been inspired by his chief, Paul Bramley [1962].

In that time it was quite obvious that this is what I wanted to do. Jill and I were married when I was a student and we had our first child

---

54 Report of a Sub-Committee for Training in Oral Surgery. British Association of Oral Surgeons. British Journal of Oral Surgery 1973 10, 360-371.
55 British Association of Oral Surgeons Council minutes 8th April 1976.

and were expecting a second one. I decided I wanted to go back and do medicine. So I went up to Guy's, and I had an interview the next day and was offered a place to come that autumn.

At that time there were plenty of people around practising with a single qualification, so what motivated John to apply for medicine?

Well, it was how the specialty was practised in Plymouth. I wasn't equipped to deal with the problems in quite the way I could see was necessary. If you were going to be part of that scene, you needed to have that broader experience; you needed to understand more about the body than I had at that time. And it was because working with somebody like Paul who could demonstrate that to you.

I did the second MB in nine months because they said you can spend as short or as long a time as you like doing it, but it meant then I had a period from the whole of the summer until about October before I could pick up a clinical programme. And the clinical programme had to be 36 months to get your degree. There was no shortening on that, at that point.

John passed his FDS when still a Medical Student.

I did my FDS in '66. Peter Leopard, Clive Rowe and I, we all did it together.

We'd got to the stage where we were doing electives. That's the first time I was exposed to Norman Rowe, because thanks to Paul Bramley I contacted him and asked whether we could go down there to Roehampton, Peter and I, in an honorary attachment position. So we became honorary supernumerary registrars during our medicine time. We'd done our obstetrics, and you then had a two-month period when you did whatever you chose to do, and from our point of view we chose to do this, and that was quite legitimate as far as the medical school were concerned because you were studying an aspect of medicine. And we took our final Fellowship at the end of that period. That was 1966, so we'd been doing clinical work then for the best part of 12 months before.

When we started the clinical period, the three of us had a lot of clinical experience. And we joined with three guys who had come down from Cambridge who had all got firsts, and we thought if we do that we're going to have that academic stimulus from them and we've got the clinical knowledge. That worked absolutely superbly. It was a really good balance, and we graduated in '67.

David Vaughan was a dental student in Cork and had been inspired by a plastic surgeon, JSP Wilson's lecture on about oncological surgery [1965].

I finished dentistry, and I did a couple of months' practice and got into med school. I finished my FDS whilst I was a clinical student, and when I finished medicine I spent four and a half years at the Regional Hospital in Cork doing general surgery, with the object really of becoming a head and neck surgeon. Dentistry was good to me in the sense that it paid for my medical fees because I worked as locums everywhere that I could.

John Langdon was a registrar in oral surgery at the London and Honey Lane hospitals when he decided he wanted to do a medical degree [1967-68].

By that time I knew that I wanted to do max fax. And I knew I was going to be a cancer surgeon. So the writing is on the wall. Interestingly, I talked to Gordon Seward about it, and he was not saying, 'Oh, well, if you're going to do that, you've got to do medicine.' In those days about half of the trainees were doing medicine and half weren't. And he wasn't necessarily committed to doing medicine. Now, whether he thought that was because I wasn't going to make the grade and it would have been a waste of time, or what, I don't know. But I knew myself that I wanted to do medicine.

I applied to a whole range of medical schools. I had about three interviews and was offered places at Charing Cross and the London. It was done through UCCA, the predecessor of UCAS in those days.[56]

Andy Brown qualified in dentistry at Guy's and wanted a place in medical school. Presumably for a career in oral surgery? [1969].

It wasn't so much that. What I took an interest in was getting a medical degree. The consultants in the dental school were termed 'consultant dental surgeons' and were all medically qualified, and they ran the teaching clinics and they ran the operating lists.

I first worked as a house surgeon for a chap called Jimmy Mansie, who was an amazing guy. He looked about 85 but was probably only about 55. He was one of the Guy's 'characters' and I said to him, in

---

56 UCCA. The Universities Central Council for Admissions.

the early months I was working for him, that I was thinking of doing medicine. 'Oh' he said (he had a rather strange mumbly way of talking) 'oh, that would be very good Andrew'. So I said, 'Thank you sir, I'm going to put an application in', which I did to do it at Guy's because they had a combined course.

He rang me up at home the day before my interview for medical school to remind me he was going on holiday the next day and he just wanted to check there were no problems with the patients, so I reassured him, and he said 'Oh, by the way, congratulations!' So I said, 'Sorry sir?' He said, 'Congratulations on getting into medical school.' And I said, 'No, I think you've got it wrong, Mr Mansie sir, it's actually tomorrow, my interview for medical school.' He replied, 'Yes, I know that, but I've just had lunch with the Dean!' That was how preferment was done in those days! It was a case of 'not what you know, but who you know'. So that's how I got into medical school.

The consultant dental surgeons at Guy's were mostly medically qualified, why?

I think it was a tradition that almost went back to the founding of the dental school, by a chap called Newland-Pedley. I'm not sure if he did medicine first and then dentistry, but quite a lot of those early pioneers did a medical degree as well as dentistry; and there was a long tradition of that at Guy's.[57] By the time I'm talking about in the late 1960s there were one or two consultant dental surgeons at Guy's who were not medically qualified, in particular Don Gibb. I can remember the other consultants being a bit concerned that a non-medically qualified consultant had been appointed!

Now, this was not a time when they used their medicine to extend their surgical training. For example, if Jimmy Mansie, who was the guy I worked for, had a patient with an ameloblastoma that needed a bit of jaw removing, he sent them to the general surgeons to do. He didn't do it, but you could go along and watch. There are other places like Manchester and others, that didn't have that tradition and that spun on into how oral surgery developed, which then became oral and maxillofacial surgery. In the 1960s and 1970s, there was the big debate

---

57 Frederick Newland-Pedley (1855-1944) qualified in dentistry in 1880 having studied at the Royal Dental Hospital, Leicester Square and medicine in 1881 having studied at Guy's.. See: Plarr's Lives of the Fellows. Royal College of Surgeons of England. On-line.

about whether you really needed medicine to work in our specialty.

Brian Avery was at Guy's Dental School [1965].

In my first year at dental school, a notice was put up on the notice board inviting people to apply for a combined medical and dental degree course. About eight or ten people applied for this course, and I got a place. They didn't take many, about one person every other year, and so I was very pleased. I don't know why I applied; I just felt that I wanted perhaps a bit more than dentistry once I'd got there. It was really due to start the very next year because the order of the combined course was that you did one year second BDS, and then a very tough year when you did second MB, and then you went back to clinical dentistry and then finally you went back to clinical medicine and the whole thing took about eight and a half years.

What was the reason for this course?

At that time more and more people were getting medical degrees on top of their dental degrees and the main purpose was to use the two degrees for maxillofacial surgery.

Brian went on to become a member of council, secretary and president of the British Association of Oral and Maxillofacial Surgeons.

As secretary of the Association, I went with the then president Peter Leopard to see the Chief Medical Officer, Professor Sir Kenneth Calman. We had two meetings with him and we tried very hard to persuade him to persuade the medical schools to take dentists universally for a three-year medical degree to try to shorten the training. Sir Kenneth was very helpful; he wrote to the council of the Deans of Medical Schools and persuaded them to provide three-year courses.

Shortly after the two meetings that Peter Leopard and I had with Sir Kenneth for a while every single medical school was taking dentists for three-year courses, one or two maybe for four. But that soon fell into disuse because the medical schools were changing their programmes and they felt that people couldn't get the whole programme completed in the three years. I think it led eventually to Guy's providing their three-year training course for dentists who want to do a medical degree and they've introduced now a three-year training course for doctors who want to do dental training courses, which as far as I know is still going on and that's provided many of our trainees for the profession.

Rob Hensher was at Dental School in Liverpool [1971].

My mentor, the late Lawrence Finch, who was a consultant there, said if you're going to do oral and maxillofacial surgery, the way the wind is blowing, we need to be doubly qualified, he was, and he said it's the way it is in Europe, and the United States will undoubtedly follow us.

I went to see Prof. Lawton, Sir Frank Lawton, and I explained about this and he said, well, if you want to, you can apply to do medicine here, Liverpool. He said because you had adequate A levels to get in if you'd applied to do medicine, and maybe if you do well in finals? Anyway, they ended up offering me a place and a house job at the dental school. I crossed the floor of the house, and in six months I was a medical student again. So, I did medicine there, always with the idea of doing oral and maxillofacial surgery.

While I was waiting to go to medical school, I had six months when I went to work in a couple of practices as a locum, sometimes in the evenings or at a weekend. They were often practitioners who were peripatetic teachers within the dental school, which I thought was a great thing because you could be taught by them one day a week, but then you'd work in their practice.

I did pretty well in the finals, well enough anyway to get a professorial house job. So, I worked for a chest physician and then the Professor of Haematology. Then I worked for Averil Mansfield and Raymond Helsby, vascular and general surgery. Then orthopaedics, then A &E. I reached the stage of being a very, very junior surgical registrar and then I went backwards. I went back to oral and maxillofacial surgery; I moved to London, and I got a job at Whipps Cross as a senior house officer in oral and maxillofacial with Denys Brock.

Adrian Sugar was a registrar on Teesside [1972-76].

The unit had two consultants and both of them were singly qualified. I think it's important to appreciate that at that time I had never worked for anybody with a double degree. And I don't think I'd ever even been to a national meeting, so I'm not even sure that I'd even met anybody with a double degree. So, that it's not surprising therefore that I wasn't particularly influenced in that direction.

By 1979 Mike Davidson had been dentally qualified for a couple of years, had a year and a half oral surgery experience as a house officer at the London and as senior house officer in Brighton.

I had passed my primary FDS, and I'd talked to many people both at the London and Richard Juniper in Brighton and the bottom line was if you're going to take this seriously, you're going to need a medical degree. You might try to wing it and get through, but many people whose advice I respected said, 'To be honest, you're going to need a medical degree.' And I could see that, especially having talked to people in the more advanced units. So towards the end of my time in Brighton, I applied for medical school.

I applied only to London schools because by this time I was married, and we decided that we didn't want to leave the Greater London area. I only had an interview at Charing Cross and the London, and I got a place at the London.

Chapter 9

Medical Training: Paying For It

'I also got a job in the resident band at the Top Rank suite'

At the time that most of my interview subjects were at university, students were entitled to 'maintenance grants' from the local education authority of the city or county council where their parents lived. The universities charged fees, but the councils paid these as well. These were grants which did not need to be repaid, rather than loans. A certain sum of money was set as the amount a student would need to live off, which was higher for London than the rest of the country. Parents normally had to contribute to this depending upon their income so that only students from less wealthy homes received the full grant. Grants were replaced by loans in the early 1980s.

However, councils were not obliged to fund second degrees, but some did; this was discretionary. Thus some dentally qualified medical students did get some support for their medical degree but most not. Most did locums and/or work in dental practices. Some dental practices, in London particularly, used to have a permanent position for dentists studying medicine, and these jobs were often passed along by word of mouth.

Paul Bramley started clinical medical studies in 1948.

I went into dental practice because it was 1948, that the Health Service started and it was easy to get patients.

I found, through a girlfriend, that her father had died about 12 years before; he used to run a dental practice in Hadley Road in Birmingham but nobody had taken it on. They didn't sell it, it just was there, it was vacant. I said, 'Well, look, I'm thinking of starting a practice, do you think your mother would be interested?' 'Oh, come and see her.'

So I went to see her. And there was this ancient Ritter unit, which 20 years before was the thing to have. An ancient chair, carpet on the floor, a mahogany thing with pullout drawers that all the instruments were in and a boiling water steriliser. And what's more, a very matronly person, dressed in a classic maid's gown was there. She had been his old chair side assistant, and she was looking after the family.

So I went into there. and I got one of my medical colleagues in the same year, who had done some dental assisting in the Royal Army Medical Corp, I said, 'Do you want to earn a bit, Ken?' He said, 'Yes.' I said, 'Well, come down on and assist me.' So there were two medical students attending about two evenings a week and weekends, who used to come over on a motorbike.

I had no problem. I moved about in a circle of people whom I had qualified with as a dentist, who were doctors, who were now teaching us as new medical students. A lot of the staff came over and we had a very distinguished clientele, which I treated on the Health Service. What the quality of the work was, I really don't know. I did the best I could.

So that put me in a position to enjoy a big social life because of all the contacts I'd had in two generations. Evening and weekend practice gave me enough to buy a really ancient 1946 Ford 8, which eventually I had to back up hills because the fourth gear wouldn't work the right way round. And I had a foreign holiday. And what's more, I found out much later in life that my years in that practice counted towards my entitlement of the years served in the National Health Service for my pension.

Mike Awty [1957-1961].

I was trying to think how I was going to finance it. I got a bit of help from the County, not much, because they said, 'Oh, it's your second degree, we can't.' They gave me a little bit. And then John Aust, one of the ex-Servicemen in our dental year, had a practice with spare surgeries up in north London and he said, 'Oh, you can come and work here.' So every spare minute I trekked off up to this practice, usually two nights a week and all day Saturday.

By then I was reasonably quick. Not dishonestly quick, but I'd had two years' experience of dentistry as a general practitioner, so I was fairly practised. He was quite generous, he didn't take much of the earnings. He was doing very well himself with other assistants. We'd been pals together as dental students. I made enough to live on, just about.

Khursheed Moos [1961-1964].

Just after I had started at Westminster my future wife was back in UK nursing at the Brompton Hospital and I was a student living in a Westminster Hospital student hostel. We married and with an army friend's help we had a small flat in Battersea. I used to travel by bike or scooter in those days. As I had to pay my way, I used to work at evenings in a dental practice in a rather downmarket area in New Cross. It was a big practice which took others doing similar things to me. Trevor Redpath[58] was one of my oral & maxillofacial surgery colleagues who also spent time there.

The person who managed the practice was a senior dental nurse who was in charge of everything. Her brother was the dentist, supposedly in charge, but he was rarely there; we saw little of him. There were certain peculiarities about the place because they also had a trained State Registered Nurse who looked after patients who were having minor gynaecological surgery, including abortions done. On one occasion a patient died there because of severe haemorrhaging when the nurse was away, I believe on holiday or ill, and there was a furore after that.

I was lucky that most of my patients were students and nursing staff from Westminster and other places, who knew me and for the dentistry I did there. I enjoyed doing dentistry, particularly doing endodontics and any surgery that came along, but I knew there were problems within the practice itself and just after I left the death occurred. Both Trevor Redpath and I had difficulty having our name plates removed from the practice; it was illegal to keep them up after we had stopped working there. I believe it apparently gave some credibility to the practice as we had dental fellowships. Almost all the work was National Health Service, and that was fine. It suited me and helped to pay my way through medicine.

Russell Hopkins

My medical school fees were paid by Sunderland County Borough, my old town. My living costs were paid for by working in a dental practice in Kingsbury for a chap, AJ Seymour, who employed people who wanted part-time work. They did all the work, and he did all the paperwork, and we were paid a percentage. I can't remember what the percentage was, but it was enough for me to run a motorcar, which I think was an MGB in those days, and to live reasonably well.

Initially, I lived in 140 Harley Street, on the fifth floor, so I used to call it upper Harley Street, and I shared a flat with a chap who was

---

58 He became an oral and maxillofacial surgery consultant in Southampton.

dentally qualified and had a practice in Harley Street. He was a medical student at UCH who became a pathologist and sadly later committed suicide. I then joined up with friends I'd made at St. Peter's at Chertsey, and around in the tennis club at Weybridge, in a house in Walton Street in south west Kensington owned by Cadogan Estates, five of us lived in this house, which was at the tail end of a lease, so we got it fairly cheaply. They were junior doctors and one was a businessman and I was a medical student. I used to go up from there to work in Kingsbury on Wednesday afternoons, Friday nights and alternate Saturdays, all day.

John Williams [1963-1967].

Jill and I were married when I was a dental student, and I decided from the very beginning that we would invest in a house. So we borrowed money from the bank which was as a 99% mortgage and all I did was to pay the interest on the monthly mortgage until we sold that house with a profit and invested in a house in Coulsdon. At that house I converted one bedroom into a dental surgery and Jill was my dental nurse. She's a physio. We ran this practice together. We did it in the evenings, got the children to bed early, and if need be on a Saturday morning.

John Langdon [1968].

Unbelievably, I got a second grant. I was interviewed at County Hall on the Embankment and was given a second grant that paid fees. I lived at home, so I was subsidised. And I did evening practise in Highgate in a practice owned by a guy called Neuberger. It was in Highpoint, the famous block of flats that had been designed by Lubetkin in the '30s. He had a duplex apartment with the practice on the ground floor and his living accommodation was upstairs.

Brian Avery [1971-1974].

Having got a place on the combined course, I already had a student grant. My home was in London and so I had a student grant from the Inner London Education Authority. A few weeks after I got a medical place, I was still in my first year of dentistry; I got a letter from the Inner London Education Authority. They said, 'We've had a letter from the Dean, Mr Fred Warner, and he said that they've taken you on a combined course and he asked us if we would give you a grant for the whole eight and a half years.' They said they were happy to do so. I tell my children this nowadays and they can't believe their ears.

I qualified in dentistry in December '70, did a house job and then in September '71. I started clinical medicine, and that was a very busy three years. I was doing the equivalent of two whole days a week earning my living. I did all day Saturday and two evenings, and I worked for a dental practitioner called Marks who had a big dental practice in Brixton. For most of my medical undergraduate career I was working in that practice, although I did some children's dental clinics for the local authorities.

I can remember one particular period when I'd been about two years into clinical medicine and I did primary FDS. By this time I was recently married so I was juggling a new home with a medical degree, with two days in dental practice and trying to do my primary FDS. And I can remember that I sat the primary FDS, which was a very difficult exam in those days, and I had to ask the hospital if I could adjust the internal examinations, psychiatry, ENT, eyes and fevers I was doing around the primary FDS while I did it. That was very stressful. I'm happy to say that I passed, but it was not something I'd like to repeat.

Rob Hensher [1974-1978].

I did a few locums, and I was very fortunate, and I got a series of scholarships on an exam basis which paid all my tuition fees. And, I suppose I saved up and did a bit of work to pay for things as I went, and that was subsistence. I also got a job in the resident band at the Top Rank Suite. A guy who was playing the piano had been an undergraduate at Liverpool, and he said they were looking for a bass player. Anyway, I got the job and that helped me sustain my life.

Mike Davidson [1979-1984].

I did enough studying to survive. I would turn up to the lectures and to dissection, but I did nothing extra because I was also working in dental practice to get some money coming in. So on Wednesdays and Saturdays I would work in practice and in the gaps in term time, I would either do locums or more dental practice to earn money.

So in the undergraduate time I was entirely focussed on trying to get some money in and do sufficient work to make sure I passed. I wasn't interested in a BSc, honours or anything. I kept my contacts with the oral surgery family via locums and for a couple of years I was an honorary lecturer in the oral surgery department teaching undergraduates. That was mainly extractions and a bit of oral surgery and oral medicine.

By the time I got onto clinical medicine I stayed up in London part of the week to save having to commute because we were living in Sussex. My wife Kath was working in dental practice in Sussex in Burgess Hill, because we'd bought a house. That was another reason for me working before we went off to medicine, because I knew getting a mortgage when I was an undergraduate and Kath being a self-employed dentist was going to be incredibly difficult, so we got our mortgage before I went to med school.

Burgess Hill was one of the cheaper parts of Sussex, and I was commuting every day up to the London, getting off the train at London Bridge and cycling across London to be there on time. So I shared a house up in London and I did it with three mates. There were four of us in the house, and it was smack next to the London, and I would go up on a Monday and dependent on what was happening during the week sometimes I would come back during the week, but most of the time I was up there Monday through till Friday.

And I had three great flatmates. I was almost back to being a true old-fashioned undergraduate. We would go to the pub and cook together and things like that. So, it was quite a strange life; I was married and owned a house, but I didn't live there for whole chunks of the time. And then, of course, you would get sent out on rotations, so you'd be going all over the place. By this time, I had a motorbike, so I would zoom around on my motorbike.

Ian Martin [1982-1986].

I didn't get a grant, so I had to go into dental practice in the evening. I started off in a practice in Crofton Park, which is south London, doing something like two or three evenings a week and Saturdays. Roder and Ziman's was one of these factory type practices. But I could earn enough then to live on, actually relatively comfortably by comparison with having been on a full maintenance grant when I did dentistry. Because of parental income, I had qualified for a full grant for my dental degree. I was better off when I was doing my three evenings a week and Saturdays at Roder and Ziman's. I did this for a couple of years and then moved to Rom's, which was in Brixton, another big National Health Service dental factory; again, I was doing two or three evenings a week and Saturdays. In fact, I think quite a lot of people who had gone on to do oral max-fax surgery worked there. A lot of us who did the dual degree worked to pay our way.

And then whenever I got the opportunity, I'd also go off and do locums in oral surgery. King's was very good, very liberal; they would let you go off and do stuff. Most of the locums I did during med school were on the London hospital circuit. I got my FDS in '84, a couple of years into medical school, and that was quite a big thing at the London because they had a rule that you weren't allowed to operate on your own without your FDS. There were quite a lot of registrars at the London at the time who didn't have their FDS; people who struggled to get their FDS weren't allowed to operate on their own. It was silly because they were far more experienced than I was.

Chapter 10
Medical and Surgical Experience

'This woman's dying and I haven't a clue what's going on'

Paul Bramley went to work in a mission hospital in Kenya after qualifying. He met his future wife Morag while he was at medical school. She was a student a couple of years ahead of him [1952].

She had been in correspondence with a Church of Scotland medical missionary in Kenya and he, through his two sons, tried to get Morag to go out there to help as a sort of locum with somebody else she would bring with her, medically qualified, and take over this hospital. He had to come home for a whole year because his wife was ill. And she said, 'Well, what about it?' And so I said, 'Yeah, we'll go.'

There was nobody going to be there except an American trained nurse and an administrator of the whole mission compound, a head teacher who was white, no other doctors at all. And we said, 'All right, we'll come.' She had to go out early to do a takeover because I wasn't going to be allowed to go. I had qualified in the College just before that Christmas.[59] So I went into the Dean and I said, 'Look, I want to go out to Africa on February the 16th.' He said, 'I advise you very strongly not to do that. You really must finish your MB ChB degree in June.' He said, 'When your name's in lights, we want to see MB ChB. Birmingham after your name.'

We got married, early February, and after a few weeks Morag left for Kenya and I got back into medicine and finished off. I then went out after with her and we had a massive time of surgical, medical, tropical medicine experience, all self-taught except for the handover period when we were given a few aphorisms to work on.

It did us an immense service because we learnt about independence; about making up your mind, are you going to operate or are you going to let him die? And what's going to happen if, etc? Dealing with emergencies, dealing with fear, drawing blood and so on, I got through at the price of being a butcher, and I realised it was a

---

59 Sir Paul had qualified with the 'conjoint' examination MRCS LRCP at the Royal Colleges. Medical and dental students could qualify with conjoint six months before they took their university degrees.

butchery, I've got photographs to show that. Morag did all the obstetrics and the gynaecology and some of the operating as well. There was a lot of medicine in the crudest possible form, but it worked. It's an amazing story.

We were there just about a year. That got us through the bloodletting and the fear. I even did a thyroidectomy on an acute thyroid, and she inevitably had a thyroid crisis after that. I looked up the emergency surgery under thyroidectomy and it said, 'Thyroid crisis: In any well-managed case of thyroidectomy, thyroid crisis does not occur.' That's all the help I got out of that book. But she survived.

We'd had no salary for a year, so when we came back we lived with my parents and I earned a living in the school dental service, which I enjoyed doing, I had never done it before, and I also worked part-time employment in maternity and child welfare clinics.

And then there were two jobs that came up at Roehampton and East Grinstead. Senior registrar and registrar jobs were as rare as hen's teeth.

Mike Awty qualified in medicine from Guy's [1961].

I did pre-reg medical job at St John's Lewisham and Lewisham Hospital, where I did general medicine, a bit of physical medicine and skins, and there were a few paediatric beds too. The children used to frighten me to death because I had very little support. The consultants weren't very much in evidence, and the registrar wasn't either. Well, he was working too hard anyway, had much too much to do, he'd come if I was desperate. So I learned rather quickly.

It was a time when the consultants felt themselves to be honoraries, really. They were quite helpful, good teachers on their teaching rounds, but it was difficult to get hold of them out of hours. The registrar was supposed to deal with that, but he was running around catching his tail, really. So that was really quite a very hard six months in Lewisham. There were a lot of very sick people there and it was very poor in '61.

Then I went to work at the Metropolitan Hospital in Kensington, the ENT Hospital, and I had five or six consultant ENT surgeons to work for. They all had their various interests, which I joined in. There was a very good registrar, who taught me quite a lot. The ENT surgeons, once they realised that I wasn't a callow youth anymore, would let me do quite a lot, and I was very happy doing sub mucous resections and all that sort of thing, and tonsils, always carefully because I had to deal with them if they bled, the consultants didn't come in. And at Christmas time I became an absolute ace at epistaxis with boozed up colonels from the depths of Kensington. They poured in around Christmas time with epistaxis.

Russell Hopkins qualified from the Royal Free [1964].

I did perhaps one of the best surgical jobs I could have done, at the Bolingbroke Hospital, where my consultants, four teaching hospital consultants, were JM Pullin from Thomas', Rex Lawrie from Guy's, Peter Phillips, a urologist from Charing Cross and George Pinker from Mary's, who was a gynaecologist. So I did general surgery, gynaecology, some ENT, and urology. I also did casualty.

Whilst I was on call, I had all those emergencies coming in and I learnt an enormous amount about a lot of the body. Because of my seniority, I actually did about 20 to 30 appendectomies in the time I was there, on my own, and I could do them in 20 minutes, I could do them almost faster than I could do a wisdom tooth. I did hernias, varicose veins. Every alternate Saturday I used to do a list of about eight to twelve abortions, incomplete abortions and dilate and curettage them. The other Saturday we'd do bougie clinics and pass bougies up the penises of first world war veterans who had got strictures from gonorrhoea, which was really the best clinic that I've ever done. And full of humour and goodwill, and I thought that was a wonderful job.

I did my house physician job at Croydon with a physician, Dr Baker, I learnt a lot of good general medicine there. There were two wards with 30 beds each. I was on call alternate weeks. It was a tremendous amount of work, a tremendous amount of pathology, but great education.

Khursheed Moos qualified from the Westminster and became the house surgeon to Professor Harold Ellis at the Westminster Hospital [1965].

I gave up my locum dental work because it was not possible to do that as we were totally committed to the hospital. In fact, I only left the hospital on two nights in the six months, which was the routine. That was when the Prof. was away overseas in the United States. Apart from that, I met a lot of interesting people. I was very lucky; I operated much of the time with Professor Ellis himself and he let me do all sorts of things because presumably I had some surgical skills already from dentistry, which was very advantageous. I was given much more to do than most other house surgeons would have been. This covered everything from burr-holes to thoraco-abdominals, GI tract to vascular.

Also Roy Calne was the senior lecturer there, and he was doing the first of the renal transplants and I used to have to go round the wards or intensive care unit looking for patients who were dying and everybody hated my guts because they thought this was the wrong thing to do; anything like that, taking organs out of patients immediately after death! That was quite tricky, but I coped and it worked out well.

After I finished that job, it was suggested I should apply for the professorial medical job with Professor Milne. In fact, I didn't apply for it because it was again a total commitment post which I thought would be very difficult for my wife. I had not been home for more than two nights in the six months and I did not want to get into a similar situation.

For my medical job I went to Warwick Hospital where I had done an elective studentship and I acted as house physician for Dr Stephen Whittaker, who was a brilliant teacher and very high in medical politics generally, and for Dr Vivian Weinstein who was a younger consultant interested in rheumatology & endocrinology.

Stephen Whittaker was a censor for the membership of the Royal College of Physicians examinations and I learned a huge amount from him such that I found it quite difficult deciding whether to do medicine or oral and maxillofacial surgery because I had enjoyed the challenge of trying to do things by making a diagnosis and working things out during that time. I also had quite some contact with the paediatric department there when on call and also the ENT department.

The ENT Surgeon knew I was interested in that type of surgery as well as in the general surgical side. I had a very good time there, and I enjoyed that very much and it was difficult leaving.

John Williams graduated from medical school in 1967.

I did the ENT House job at Guy's. Omar Shaheen was the first person who I did parotidectomies with, and we were doing quite a few. I don't think Omar had had a dentally qualified house surgeon before, but I think the others must have. With my background, I got a lot of extra experience. It was because of what I'd got, like the tracheostomy thing, beforehand with Paul. A lot of the routine work was stuff that I'd been on the fringe of. We'd been doing the closure of oro-antral fistulae, so I was familiar with the antrum and doing intranasal antrostomies and so on. Doing ENT I saw it from a different perspective, but it was the same work.

Then I did a general medicine job. It was linked with Guy's, it was part of New Cross Hospital and in the last part of it I did geriatrics as well. The acute part of it was very acute because it was during one of these bronchitis episodes in London with all the smog and we had repeated respiratory failures to deal with and I was having to bronchoscope people in their beds and suck them out, which most house physicians wouldn't dream of doing. I even did tracheostomies in their beds, which again surprised people a little bit. You could do it and treat the patients in a much more aggressive way, which was supported very much. I got a lot more out of my house physician job than I might otherwise have done.

Afterwards I went back to Plymouth. I knew the people that I would like to work with down there. I wanted to do casualty, orthopaedics and general surgery, and I saw this as an opportunity to do all three. I went back as a casualty officer; that was a busy job. There were only three of us, and we did a three-day rotational shift system with one day off in three weeks. That was fascinating, hard work, because you worked the whole night through. You very rarely got to bed when you were working. You went home for an hour, came back on at ten and worked till two, by which time you collapsed into bed. There was no A&E department between Exeter and Truro apart from Plymouth. So we were dealing with patients who had travelled a long way.

If you averaged it out, you put in a central venous pressure line every shift, that's how seriously the injured were. And of course they never came in singly, did they? You were on your own, but you'd get a carload of people who'd run into cattle on the moor. And so you'd get all these different injuries, the child who'd hit the dashboard, the father who'd hit the steering wheel, the mother who'd gone through the windscreen; you had all those to deal with at the same time, which was an interesting challenge.

What support did you have?

Nothing. Nobody to call on. We had a senior hospital medical officer, who came in and did A&E from ten in the morning until about four, but he was far more interested in his farm than A&E and we didn't see a huge amount of him. You didn't even have another casualty officer with you a lot of the time. You did during the day from ten in the morning till two in the afternoon. Two of you there in that period, but after that, you were on your own.

Then I went down to the orthopaedic hospital in Mount Gould and I was senior house officer there to Michael Salz, who was probably the senior of the orthopods and the person I had been impressed by when I was in Plymouth before. There was just me and he, I was therefore doing all the hips that came in and every bit of trauma I was perceived as being capable of doing. I always had him available on the phone, but he wasn't always sitting there on the side of the table. Most of it was road traffic accident stuff and a huge amount of it, motorcycles. We're talking about pre-seatbelts, pre-crash helmets and the face/leg syndrome was very common, tib and fib, and face, and I had a whole ward full of individuals at one time that I was responsible for that were face/leg syndrome.

Then I went into general surgery for six months. The one job I wanted to do in general surgery was with Michael Reilly, a tremendous surgeon. He'd been one of the first people involved in vascular surgery and we did a vascular case every week, so I got vascular surgery experience with him, which was very useful. He was a tremendous teacher, always taking you through things and he made me get on with lists on my own, taught me how to do cholecystectomies and said, 'Right, now I'm going to be next door but you get on with doing this list of cholecystectomies.' So I got a lot of good experience in surgery from him.

Paul Bramley had told me that at some stage in Plymouth John had taught the general surgeons how to do parotidectomies?

Yes, I did. Mike Reilly said, 'Okay, anything below the clavicles is mine, anything above the clavicles is yours.' So I had to do the thyroids, and I had to do the parotids, and so I was teaching Michael Riley how to do a parotidectomy, and I did quite a few parotidectomies with him. So that's when I was developing the expertise that I had learnt doing my ENT work with Omar Shaheen.

I finished general surgery and then I went back into the max-fax side there as Paul Bramley's registrar.

John Langdon qualified in medicine from the London Hospital. Had there been anybody in particular during the medical course who inspired him [1973].

There was a senior surgeon, A.M.A Moore, Dinty Moore, he was called, whose clinics I still to this day remember vividly. I can remember his aphorisms, his stories, his anecdotes, everything. He was a first class teacher.

The senior physician was like Dr Snoddy[60] in Doctor Finlay's Casebook. He had no empathy with his patients at all. I can remember doing an outpatient clinic with him one day. An old boy came in, coughing and spluttering. And he said, 'Go behind that screen and take all your clothes off.' There was just one of those mobile screens between him on the couch and us. He said, 'Of course he's going to die. He's got lung cancer.' In front of the patient; it was appalling. But of course you learn as much from your negative experiences as you do from the positive ones.[61]

Then there was the venereologist, Donald Dunlop, who was a first class teacher. The venereologists, as they were known in those days, were the most brilliant general physicians because they saw everything in their clinics. This was in the days where all our inpatients were screened for syphilis on admission, as part of the workup. So we saw a lot of very interesting disease then. While I was an undergraduate medical student, I was teaching dental anatomy in Turner Street. In those days at the London, the various side streets were still the tenement houses. But the hospital owned a lot of them and had converted them to offices and teaching rooms. And dental anatomy was in one of those houses in Turner Street. We would teach dental histology and dental anatomy, comparative anatomy there.

After graduation, I did both of my house jobs at Harold Wood Hospital. I chose not to do pre-reg jobs at the London because, having done a fair bit of hospital work as a registrar, I realised that doing a job at the London, was fine for your CV, but you got little hands-on. So I went to Harold Wood and did a surgical job with Mike Prinn and a medical job with Peter Cannon and had an absolute whale of a time.

---

60 A fictional character created by AJ Cronin.
61 This contradicts the opinion in his obituary, 'outstanding clinician with a real understanding of his patient's problems' and 'particular charm and manner'. See: British Medical Journal. 6 October 1984. Vol: 289 P: 929.

Mike Prinn was a youngish consultant general surgeon and a fair amount of head and neck would come into his clinics. He would always say, 'You'd better do this.' and just left me to it. I was doing parotids and submandibular glands as a pre-reg houseman.

Peter Cannon, who was the physician, was also a young consultant. We were just beginning endoscopy in those days. This would have been in '73, I suppose. And he and I learnt to do gastroscopies together, hand-in-hand. We were both equally experienced and skilled at it. We were doing all sorts of things, we did our own intra-venous pyelograms because the radiologist was an older guy who wasn't very fit was just happy to let us do them. The amount of experience I got as a pre-reg was incredible. In fact, I enjoyed it so much that although I went off to be senior registrar at the London, I took a month's leave to do a locum registrar in general medicine because I missed it.

The medical training gave the confidence to accept responsibility for the welfare of your patients, rather than always depending on a physician or an anaesthetist to tell you what to do or how to manage a case. And that so much of what we were seeing as oral surgeons was part of systemic disease. It was a time to mature and take a bigger view of surgery.

David Vaughan had decided that he wanted to be a head and neck cancer surgeon when he was a dental student. He qualified in medicine in Cork, where he had studied dentistry [1974].

I had realised that dentists cannot teach individuals to do soft tissue surgery, you've got to be taught by other people able to do soft tissue surgery. And that's the reason I went on and did general surgery. I felt I had to get a proper basic training in handling tissues before I could have any aspirations to be a surgeon.

When I started on my surgical rotation, I did nine months of neurosurgery. The neurosurgeon, Ted Buckley, was very kind to me; he let me do a lot because he realised I had this interest in the head and neck. But the guy who brought me on surgically was Prof. Brady; his background was vascular surgery. You started off, if you're any good, doing varicose veins. You were exposing these little perforators, clipping them, tying them, clipping them, you were doing it ad nauseam. Then you could move up to hernias, so you did direct and indirect hernias until the cows came home. These were standard procedures.

Then abdominal surgery, you started doing appendectomies. I remember as a surgical registrar I was seconded down to Kerry to the County Hospital there; the population swells to half a million during the Rose of Tralee Festival. In one weekend, this is no exaggeration, I did 37 appendectomies, and only two of them were Irish nationals. So you became very slick doing that volume of work.

And then he realised I had this huge interest in head and neck and he said, 'Okay, I've got this patient who needs dissection. Read it up and I'll go through it with you.' So for my first neck dissection, I was assisted by the Professor of General Surgery. And then they realised I was fairly safe, so by the time I finished in Cork, I'd done between 20 and 25 neck dissections. They were all radicals, by the way. So I had a fair experience of doing that type of surgery. I had done no sort of jaw or mid-face surgery, but I had the fundamentals.

David came to England to get more training in cancer surgery.

I had this long-term ambition to acquire training to enable me to participate in this type of surgery. As I became more aware, I realised that staying within the ambit of dentistry was a better option than either doing ENT or plastic surgery. I was a locum plastic registrar in my last six months in Cork, and a lot of it I didn't particularly enjoy. I wasn't moved by cosmetic surgery, that side of plastic surgery.

So I applied and got a job in the head and neck unit of the Royal Marsden. And I was very disappointed at the quality of the surgery that was being done there, apart from one individual, Nick Breach, who was at the time a senior registrar. By the time I went to the Marsden, I probably had done about 25 neck dissections in Cork, so I knew what I was talking about. Then I hunted around to see how I could get into oral and maxillofacial surgery, and I went to see Malcolm Harris.[62]

Andy Brown qualified from Guy's [1973].

I worked first for six months as a house surgeon in ENT surgery. Then I did a house physician's job at Greenwich District Hospital for six months. That was all you needed to do to register your medical degree in those days. There was no extra surgical training.

---

62 Professor of oral and maxillofacial surgery at the Eastman Dental Institute.

Brian Avery qualified from Guy's [1974].

So at the end of dentistry I'd got the BDS and the LDS, and similarly at the end of the medicine I'd got MB BS and then the LRCP MRCS from the College as well.

The first job was in ENT surgery, working with a chap called Omar Shaheen and a chap called Lawrence Salmon. They were a very good team, and I got to scrub up for a lot of head and neck oncology surgery. There were some amusing incidents there. I can remember at one time being on Lawrence Salmon's ENT clinic and he knew of course I was a qualified dentist, and a patient came in who was referred as an emergency. This patient had an injury to the columella of his nose. Lawrence Salmon saw him and it wasn't too serious an injury and he said to him, 'How did you get this injury? I understand you were at the dentist at the time?' And he said, 'Yes, I was at the dentist having a tooth out and the dentist slipped and caught me in the nose.' Mr Salmon said to him, 'Oh, and what did the dentist say to you when this had happened?' The patient said, 'The dentist told me I was a bloody fool because I moved.'

And then I did a job which was combined rheumatology, acute medicine and some geriatrics at New Cross Hospital which was just down the road, part of the Guy's group.

Whilst I was doing my second house job, which was mainly rheumatology, I was at New Cross and there were four senior house officers and we used to do a one in four rota and we covered for each other and for each other's wards at night. One night at about midnight I got a call from a senior nurse in the hospital saying would I go to a ward, because a patient had hanged himself.

So you can imagine I jumped out of bed and rushed over there. And when I got there, they took me to the patients' lavatories at the back of the ward and there was a patient hanging above the toilet. There was a bar above the toilet from which hung a chain and a handle so that patients with severe rheumatoid arthritis or whatever could pull themselves off the lavatory. The patient had stood on the lavatory, put a leather belt round his neck and round this bar and stepped off the toilet and hanged himself. By the time I go there, he'd been hanged for quite a long time. I can remember this bizarre and sad situation where I was standing on the toilet behind the patient trying to hold him up and get the noose off his neck while two policemen who had been called were holding his legs and they were looking greener and greener and looking very unhappy.

Eventually we got him down. Some months later there was a coroner's enquiry, and the coroner criticised the hospital for not getting this man down quickly enough. I should say that the police had asked me not to cut the belt so they could preserve it as evidence. That's one sort of incident that remains in your mind for the rest of your life.

What did Mike Davidson expect to get out of his medical training that would be of use to him in his future career?

You saw the patient far more holistically than if I'd purely done oral surgery without a medical degree, and I think you can communicate with colleagues better. Exposure to other disciplines made you realise there were potentially other ways of doing things. You form contacts and you understand how other disciplines work. Whether you need to do five years is subject to debate, but that was the rule. I did my final FDS in 1982 and qualified in medicine in 1984.

My house physician job was in Brighton and for my second three months I was the resident house physician at Hove General, which had general medicine, urology and general surgery. When you were on call, you were on call for the lot.

I learnt loads because the supervision was limited in Hove. It was the first time I had a death that I think I was contributory to. We weren't supposed to take patients from GPs, but it was in the winter and everything was snowed under, and I got told I had to take this patient from the GP, he insisted. So she came in and she was in a hell of a state. She was shocked, and I didn't know why, I couldn't get Venflon in, I couldn't get any support from anybody in the hospital and I phoned up a lad I knew from rugby days at Brighton who was a senior house officer in radiology but he also covered me when I was at Hove because that was part of his duties. I said, 'Look, this woman's dying, and I don't know what the hell's going on, I haven't got a clue here, she's in the wrong place.' Anyway, we got her transferred, but she died. She had septic shock from a urinary infection. So, it was a strange place. It was very isolated down there for the last three months.

I worked for a general surgeon whose main interest and love was thyroid surgery. We did loads of thyroids and para-thyroids. He was great but a bit of an academic snob, so he loved it that his senior house officer had a MRCP, I had a dental fellowship, and he kept having a pop at his senior registrar who had nothing additional.

He asked if I had any objections to private practice, 'I always ask my houseman are they happy to look after my private patients?' So I ended up doing that for him, and he would always give me a cheque. He said, 'I think you've seen five patients, here's a cheque.'

He was a really good boss, but in some ways, he was incredibly old-fashioned. AIDS was just coming in, and in Brighton we were AIDS-central. We had a guy come in with an appendix who was HIV positive, and the proverbial hit the fan. The question was, who was going to operate on him? And there wasn't exactly a queue forming! It was agreed that the senior registrar, and I scrubbed and rather gingerly took his appendix out. The consultant, who in many ways was a very generous, nice man, saw this as totally outside his remit, somebody who would develop a disease through deviant behaviour, as he saw it. He was very traditional, but that was the early days of HIV.

The on call was taxing. We were on a one-in-two; there were always two house surgeons on call, so the deal was that you would both keep going 'til getting on for midnight and then, if you could, you kept your mate in bed. We would take it in turns because we were nearly always on with the same person and would try to make sure that the other guy or lass got to sleep from twelve through 'til seven.

But the ward rounds were big, a lot of patients to look after, and all the prep was down to us, we had to do all the ECGs, take all the bloods and do all the cultures and gopher work, which now would be done by various other support staff.

But being a house physician or surgeon in those days was different. There was a lot more camaraderie. We had a mess which was very active, and you'd pop down the mess and there'd always be somebody there to say hello to, there'd be newspapers. For lunch, you had a separate little dining area, and you were served, the waitress would come and you would have a quick meal, and if you were on call at midnight, you could go to A&E and get a chitty and the canteen was open, a proper canteen, and a lot of people would meet at midnight and you could have some food, I think the chitty was worth the equivalent of a bacon butty and a cup of tea.

So, you would go up and do loads of business, you would bump into people such as the resident physician and you would say, Oh, have you seen that patient? Yeah, I've seen him, he's fine, you need to do this and this, and I've put him on the review round for tomorrow. We did loads of business like that. And you would see the anaesthetist, you knew everybody, and you could function well as long as you were a team player and you didn't let people down. If you let people down, word got around and your life would then become difficult.

I think it was a great era to be the resident. On the whole, the bosses looked after you; they knew you and were good people; they were interested in you. It was a very high standard. And some people I met were very bright, very gifted. It was a great time to be there; I enjoyed it. A good year.

Later he went to Chichester as a Senior House Officer [1986].

I started in A&E and that was, at times, hell from the volume of work, because at night there was only you. Chichester's fine in the winter, but in the summer the population doubles at least. At nights and at weekends you were just snowed under, and you were like a zombie by the end. The support often was minimal, so you had to make a lot of decisions. You quickly realised who was sick and who wasn't. So, if you're talking about forming me as a clinician, that six months was vital because you learn to think on your feet, you learn how to manage sick patients very quickly. That was, from that point of view, a valuable six months. Would I want to do it again? No.

And after six months he did orthopaedics.

Talk about the school of hard knocks, but it's often the patients that get the hard knocks. It's an era of clinical practice that has gone, and for the patients' safety, thank heavens it has.

I did fifty neck of femurs when I was a senior house officer in six months, and the oldest I operated on was ninety-nine. I would turn up on a Saturday and they'd say, 'There's four neck of femurs to do so far,' and you would just do them in the emergency theatre in and around general surgery, and you just plodded on 'til you'd finished. You would do fractured dislocations, manipulations, and I was trying to put plasters on. No-one had ever taught me how to put a plaster on, yet I was having to plaster fractured limbs, and they looked awful, I mean, the plaster technician would go loopy when he saw them, because they were untidy, but you weren't taught how to do it.

But what you did was learn surgical technique, but again often self-taught. The good thing though was when you went to theatres with the boss which wasn't that often, they were very good at teaching things, and so you learned, just maybe different instruments, how to harvest bone, different things that you wouldn't necessarily have learnt any other way in those days. So, it was again six months that at times was difficult, but I did gain something from it.

Ian Martin:

I qualified in Medicine in 1986 and did two house jobs at King's. I did a surgical job which was firm 1 which was Cotton and Berry. Cotton was the Dean by then, and he was a vascular surgeon. Berry's particular interest was thyroid surgery, so that was quite nice to get involved in nice clean surgery. Then I did three months of cardiothoracic. If you showed any interest, they would let you take all the veins out of the legs. I took a lot of veins out of legs, which was quite good, just general tissue handling and learning to handle vessels. Also, I looked after quite sick people on ICU.

And then I did firm C at King's which was renal and respiratory primarily, but also covered neurology out of hours. It was fairly high-powered medicine, and I really loved both the renal medicine and respiratory medicine, I found them fascinating. But you were dealing with a lot of pretty sick people, a lot of end stage respiratory disease, so quite a lot of death, it was quite philosophical. And then a bit of neurology.

At medical school you could do locums in your last year as a medical student. I had done a neurology job for a chap called Prof. Marsden, who was a very high powered professor of neurology. So I did those jobs, really enjoyed it and did loads of practical procedures, I was doing chest drains all the time. In renal medicine I was shoving central lines in all the time, I mean mainly subclavian central lines, catheterisation, suprapubics, all that sort of stuff. It was all heavy hands on.

These jobs in those days were all one-in-two, so they were heavy hours, you were resident in the hospital all the time. But they looked after you; you had nice accommodation, a lounge to yourself and a bedroom. There was onsite catering, and it was nice. At King's there were housemen in both the house jobs I did, and then a senior registrar, so there was a big hierarchical gap. And that was good because that meant as the houseman you had a lot of responsibility; you were seeing and often managing a lot of these sick patients in A&E on your own with occasionally the senior registrar coming along to support. You barely saw a consultant in medicine as they were very rarely there. On the renal side, I also got to assist for quite a lot of renal transplant stuff.

I'd decided that I didn't want to just do oral max-fax FRCS I wanted to be the equal of any other surgeon, proper surgery. There were people that hadn't got a general FRCS, but David Vaughan had a general FRCS, and I decided that to make sure that I couldn't be criticised as a surgeon, I wanted to have the general FRCS like everybody else. So to do that you needed to do a two-year rotation in surgery.

Somebody said to me, 'Oh, have a look at Plymouth because you get to do a lot more if you're outside London.' And I can remember at King's, things like appendices were like gold dust, everybody wanted to do an appendix because there weren't very many.

So I was persuaded to go off down to Devon for this interview, not really expecting that I would go there. But I got on the train and went down, and the first thing was it was the most idyllic train journey I can remember. You got on this train from Paddington and it went down along the South Devon coast. There were waves crashing over the railway line, and the coastline was absolutely beautiful.

I went to the interview at Derriford, which was the modern hospital. There were several hospitals in Plymouth. I was interviewed, and they were charming, and offered me this two-year rotation to do surgery, which was plastics, trauma and orthopaedics, vascular, and general surgery. So I thought, yeah, I'll do that. And I loved it.

My first six months were doing plastics. I got to do loads of flaps and stuff. I loved that. So you were given a lot to do; there was loads of work. Then I did the orthopaedics, and again a big hierarchical gap, so I was doing total hip replacements, dynamic hip screws, all sorts of really quite big orthopaedic surgery. I didn't particularly like orthopaedic surgery, it never really stimulated me, but it was quite nice to be doing quite a lot of hands on surgery.

And then I did the vascular/general job. I did quite a lot of anastomoses; I had lots of hands on doing vascular stuff. And then my last job was with a very nice chap who did everything from urology through to a bit of vascular. He said, 'Oh, well, you'll want to do parotids and thyroids.' So he put parotids and thyroids on for me to do.

I was allowed to do my own gall bladders and hemicolectomies. This was a senior house officer. If you think about it you can't imagine these days as a senior house officer being given a list to do and do a gall bladder and a hemicolectomy, can you? But, yeah, they were very supportive.

So that was the last surgical job I did, and then I applied to come back and do registrar level oral and max-fax surgery.

Chapter 11

Applying for Jobs and some Reminiscences of Professor Homer Killey

'There was quite a lot of booze and food laid on, and that was my interview'

There were times when getting a job was simple. If you were 'known' and had a 'safe pair of hands' you had an established entry card. Gordon Fordyce was a registrar at Hill End Hospital. This is how he became a senior registrar [1950].

There was an Irishman, whose name I have forgotten, who was the senior registrar, I was the registrar. I hadn't been there many months when the Irishman, a very nice chap, had to go back home. I had done a year as a registrar and Alex McGregor said to me one day, 'Oh, Paddy's having to go home, I'll look into having you promoted to senior registrar,' which commanded a salary of £1,000 a year. The registrarship was £775, so this was an improvement. So I was pleased with that.

It was not uncommon for the previous incumbent of a job to be tasked with finding his replacement. This was how John Williams got a senior house officer job at Plymouth with Paul Bramley [1962].

The reason I went to Plymouth was because of a chap who had done the house job at Guy's I was doing with Alan Thompson a year before me had gone down to Plymouth and worked with Paul. And Paul had commanded him to find another senior house officer; that was how people did in those days. And he came up and saw me and said would I be interested?

It was also not unknown for a registrar to make the assessment of a candidate for house surgeon or senior house officer job. It made sense as it was with the registrar that they would have the most professional interaction. Mike Awty was a house surgeon at Guy's Dental Hospital, from where he had qualified, when an opportunity arose at East Grinstead [1953].

A chap who had been a house surgeon at Guy's before me and had gone to East Grinstead, came and said to me that the man who was following him had been called up for National Service. He'd rung up

Terence Ward and said, 'I've got a good chap here, could he fill the place in because I know him?' And the message came back, 'Yes, send him down on Sunday.'

So I duly caught the train the following Sunday and went down and presented myself. I met Willy Gray, who was a registrar, and I was ushered in to see the great man. I had about two minutes' talk and he said, 'Go round with Gray.'

So I was taken round, then sat down with a bottle of sherry, just Willy and I, and he talked about what I wanted to do and what I'd done; he was sizing me up, really. And then I went to see Sir Terence, and I thanked him for the hospitality. I said cheerio, got on the train and went back and I thought oh well, cross our fingers. On Monday morning, John Gresham came up to me, 'I've just heard from Terry, you've got the job.'

Soon afterwards, I went down to start.

Paul Bramley applied for the senior registrar post at St Thomas' with consultant John Hovell. He turned it down [1952].

They gave me a very condescending interview, which I did not like. There was a problem. It was a joint job between St Thomas' and Westminster. Hovell was at St Thomas' and Rupert Sutton Taylor at the Westminster. I said it's very important for me to decide how this is going to be apportioned and where was I going to get my training from. 'Oh, you can't ask that question, we haven't decided yet,' that sort of thing. So I thought, well, get stuffed.

So I cleared off and three weeks later Hovell was coming down the steps at some College of Surgeons meeting and I was going up with Norman Rowe. And Hovell came down the steps and said, 'we'd like you to come to St Thomas'. I said, 'I'm very sorry, Sir, but I'm booked.' And I thought well that's one for you, but you should not be surly to your candidates and then try to offer them the job at the last minute, at least after the last minute.

Paul Bramley had taken a registrar job with Norman Rowe at Rooksdown House Basingstoke. He was subsequently appointed as a consultant in Plymouth from this registrar job without having been a senior registrar!

John Williams had worked as a senior house officer for Paul Bramley before he went to medical school. Later, when medically qualified, John returned to Plymouth as registrar to work with Paul again. But Paul had just been appointed as a professor in Sheffield. In Plymouth the other consultants wanted John to replace Paul Bramley, even though he was only in his first year as a registrar. John [1970]:

I was back as a registrar with Paul. His decision to go to Sheffield had been made and his job replacement was up, and the day before the applications closed Paul came in to me and said, 'You've got to put an application in.' And I said, 'Really?' He said, 'Yes. You've got to put an application in because if we don't put an application in we can't keep the other buggers out,' those were his words. So I had to shove in an application on the last day, and that resulted in my getting short-listed for the job and stopping an appointment being made.[63]

I'd only just started the registrar job with him. But when it came to the interview, Rupert Sutton Taylor was the College assessor, and he said, 'You can't have John Williams, he's not trained enough, he hasn't done his proper training. It's not fair on him, it's not fair on you.' And they said, 'Well, if we can't have him, then we don't want anybody else.' And he said, 'Well, you can't have him.' Quite right, I mean I wasn't trained. I'd done a lot, but I wasn't trained; it stopped any appointment at that stage.

They hadn't got a single applicant who would match up to Paul, no doubly qualified person, nobody with experience. There were a lot of people who didn't do medicine at that time, but Paul had set the standard and he knew they needed to have somebody who had got his background and more, to take Plymouth further forward. Now inevitably next time round I wasn't short-listed, quite right.

Rupert Sutton Taylor grabbed me at the end of the interview and said, 'Laddie, I've been told to tell you to apply for a job at the Westminster Hospital.' 'Yes, Sir.' And of course that was with Norman Rowe and Rupert Sutton Taylor who was retiring. Rupert Sutton Taylor's replacement was in line for his job, and that was the senior registrar John Bowerman. That opened up a senior registrar position to which Monty Reitzig was appointed and that opened up a registrar appointment, which was the one I went for and was appointed to. Paul Bramley was very keen that I worked with Norman Rowe.

Some got jobs by just turning up and asking. After medical school Andy

---

63 I suspect that there was an application made by someone that Paul Bramley did not want to inherit his legacy.

Brown was a pre-registration medical houseman at Guy's, [1975].

So, halfway through my medical house job when I realised I was going to be out of a job in three months' time, I made an appointment to see Pat O'Driscoll, a consultant at Guy's. He said, 'I would talk to Professor Killey at the Eastman Dental Hospital and get his advice.' So I made an appointment to see the great Professor Killey, whose name I knew as the co-author with Norman Rowe of the major textbook in facial trauma - Rowe and Killey.[64] He was also author of some Dental Practitioner Handbooks, as they were called in those days - on minor oral surgery and other things. So I went to see him. You could have a whole tape of reminiscences and anecdotes about Homer Killey. Anybody who worked for him has got their Killey stories! And I suddenly realised, at the end of just having a talk, that I was being offered a job as registrar at the Eastman Dental Hospital. I hadn't bothered to cast around and consider anything else! I stepped straight out of my pre-registration year and started life as a registrar at the Eastman.

A digression. John Langdon had been a senior house officer in oral surgery at the Eastman in 1966, he remembered Professor Killey.

Paddy, as we all called him, was a great character. He was always around, sort of in the background, he was a constant presence. And we would go to theatre with him and assist him, and also with Norman Rowe, who had sessions there.

Paddy Killey very rarely operated. He would let his senior registrar and registrar do all the surgery and he would just be sitting on a radiator and reading the Times newspaper. And the senior registrar when I was there was Malcolm Harris, and the registrar was Peter Banks, so it was a fairly lively period. And I can remember Paddy sitting on the radiator with the Times in front of him, apparently taking no notice of the proceedings going on. But clearly, he was listening to every word that was said by the operating team. He would sort of give a commentary if one of them said, 'Oh, the wisdom tooth is loose.' 'Oh, we're all loose, old boy.' He would make odd comments like that.

Occasionally, if something went wrong, he'd scrub. And he was a brilliant surgeon. People never realised it because he so rarely

---

64 Paddy Killey had left Rooksdown House to become Professor of oral surgery at the Eastman.

operated. But he was one of these people where instruments came naturally to his hands. And his handling of tissue was just elegant.

The other thing I remember about Paddy Killey, he was a chronic depressive. He would sit in his office in the dark for hours. And if you had to see him or ask him a question or something, you'd knock on the door and he'd call you in. And he had a party trick. He'd be sitting at his desk and there'd always be to hand a copy of the British Dental Journal, which in those days was rolled up in a paper sheaf to go through the post. And, as you walked into the office, he would just pick up this copy of the British Dental Journal, sling it over his shoulder and it would land, fair and square, in the waste bin. And, clearly, he practised this for hours on his own.

Andy Brown [1975-76].

When I was at the Eastman as a registrar with the famous Paddy Killey, I don't think I saw him operate in all the time I was there! He used to sit in the corner of the operating theatre and let you do the interminable wisdom tooth lists yourself. He was a bit of a surgical nihilist. Whenever we tried to persuade him to do something more adventurous, he would always say it wouldn't work. For example, when we had a patient who needed a mandibular set back or something like that, he'd find some excuse such as they always relapsed, or that there was no point in operating because it was interfering with the gene pool and all sorts of crazy things like that.

He was a remarkable man, however. I say I never saw him operate, but I did see him do a very small amount of minor oral surgery. People who worked with him in his younger days, before he settled into his later years as a professor, said he was certainly a remarkably slick dento-alveolar surgeon. And I'm sure when he worked in facial trauma with Norman Rowe, back in the days of Rooksdown House after the Second War, he built his reputation as a surgeon, writer and teacher. So I don't think I saw the best years of Killey, but he was great fun to talk to.[65]

Paul Bramley had been a registrar at Rooksdown house, Basingstoke with Rowe and Killey [1952-54].

Killey lived in Rooksdown House, he was a single man. And 'Where

---

65 See: Obituary Professor Homer Charles Killey. British Journal of Oral Surgery, 14 1976 185-186.

are the X-rays of X, Y and Z? We'd hunt high and low for them. 'They must be under Killey's bed.' He was hoarding all the records for the book,[66] all the records and X-rays of past patients we wanted, and we inevitably found them under Killey's bed. Anyway, he did no operating, I didn't get on with him at all, I think he had a very negative view of life; he was rather cynical.

Andy Brown continued:

I worked at the Eastman for about a year and a bit as a registrar but realised that if I was going to train in the wider aspects of oral surgery I needed to get out of the Eastman. It was a great institution to pass exams like the FDS, which I took while I was there. But if you wanted to see the wider world, you had to get out of the postgraduate dental school. It was still very dentally orientated rather than surgically orientated.

So I went to talk to Killey about applications for senior registrar jobs but he tried to put me off because he wanted me to be a senior registrar at the Eastman and pulled a few strings to make sure that I could take the FDS early so I could be appointed. It was all strange and difficult because I didn't want to upset him. He persuaded me to start as a senior registrar at the Eastman on the understanding, which I made clear to him, that I would probably apply to go elsewhere.

And within six months or so, two jobs came up at two of the premier units close to London. One was at Queen Mary's Roehampton and one was at the Queen Victoria Hospital, East Grinstead, which were two of the old wartime units that had built a reputation as centres of excellence in oral surgery. And then I was in a difficult situation because I thought, do I really want one of these jobs or both jobs or either of these jobs? I'd sort of got it into my mind that I'd rather go to East Grinstead than Roehampton. Norman Rowe had just retired from Roehampton, and he was basically the star in the specialty universe at the time.

I had visited East Grinstead because when I was a senior dental student we used to have day trips arranged by Guy's. They rented a coach and you could sign up on a sheet on the dental school notice board to go down for a day to East Grinstead where we had some lectures and some operating demonstrated. I remember being very

---

66 Fractures of the Facial Skeleton.

impressed by the whole setup.

In addition, somebody who later became a very good friend of mine, Peter Banks, had recently been appointed to East Grinstead and was writing quite a lot and developed a reputation as a new thinker in the specialty. He is a 'character' but he was also one of the junior stars coming into the universe. He was down there with Michael Awty, who was the more established but who had already developed quite a reputation as a teacher and organiser and promoter of the specialty. I decided I would only apply for East Grinstead.

The Roehampton interview was about two days before the East Grinstead interview. To my horror, I was told that Peter Banks had let it be known to the then senior registrar that he wasn't going to have another registrar from the Eastman and Guy's! He was apparently fed up with having Guy's and Eastman people who had rather 'trodden a path' to East Grinstead and he felt they needed fresh blood in the unit, and so he was looking elsewhere. I suddenly realised that I would not get this job at East Grinstead and that I'd probably burnt my boats!

To my joy, the guy who had virtually been promised the job at East Grinstead was appointed to Roehampton, which left the way open for me at least to have a fighting chance at East Grinstead. I ended up as everybody's second choice. Peter Banks said to me when I first met him on my first day there and introduced myself as the new senior registrar 'Oh, you know we didn't really want you, don't you?' And that was my welcome! Fortunately, I ended up at the end of my career with him as one of my greatest friends.

That was in the days before all the current political correctness whereby you have to tick all sorts of boxes and allow people to see their references, etc. Most of the things in those days were done by telephone calls between units. You know how it went, 'I've got a good chap here' - and it almost invariably was a chap not a girl because the specialty was dominated by men - 'I've got a good chap here, he'd be good for your registrar job, are you interested?' or 'I see you've got a senior registrar job coming up, I can recommend John Smith' or whatever. So there was a lot of the old boy network and many people complained about it, but on the whole these were experienced consultants selecting out what they hoped were the pick of the crop to be allowed to go onto the next stage, and that's how training took place.

It was a pyramidal, hierarchical system, and some people dropped out on the way and went off into general practice or other specialties, or languished for years as a senior house officer or some such. It was how medicine worked in those days. When you were actually fortunate enough to get a senior registrar job, that was when you more or less relaxed and said, 'That's it, I'm home! If I just serve the time and keep my nose clean, I shall probably get a consultant job at the end of all this.' The only problem then was the manpower planning and making sure that there were enough jobs for enough people, so there were little hiccups, but you did get a job.

Brian Avery also went straight to the Eastman after his medical house jobs [1975].

It was a sort of slightly bizarre situation in fact the Eastman was quite a bizarre set up. I approached Professor Killey and said, 'Is there a job and can I come as a registrar?' He said, 'Okay, we'll interview,' and he took me on. They liked to take people who'd gone through this process of medicine and dentistry at Guy's and house jobs and then move on to registrar posts with them. And that's how I got appointed.

After a year at the Eastman, it was time for Brian to move on. It was quite common for decisions on appointments to be made before an interview. On this occasion it was a complete waste of time, but not for Brian [1977].

I'd decided I wasn't getting anywhere, and I applied for a job at Roehampton, which was with Norman Rowe and John Bowerman. I went for an interview at Westminster Hospital, and there were three candidates. As my surname was Avery I was interviewed first as we were taken alphabetically.

They interviewed me and then and there, before I left the interview and before they'd interviewed the next two candidates, it was arranged when I would start the job which was going to be the 1st of January 1977. I went back into the interview waiting room and I had to keep mum while they interviewed the other two.

That's how things were done in those days. So the other two just didn't have a chance of getting the job. I'm pleased to say that both those chaps are very nice and they eventually ended up as consultant oral and maxillofacial surgeons and had successful careers.

He later went to Canniesburn Hospital Glasgow [1978].

My wife spotted in the British Medical Journal a job advertised at a place called Canniesburn in Scotland. Now I'd never heard of this hospital. My wife's a Scot and we were going to go up to Scotland to visit some of her aunts and uncles. I thought what I'll do is I'll pop in and have a look at this place. I'd never heard of it, and I rang up and I arranged to go there.

I arrived at this hospital and as I walked around the wards my eyes popped out of my head, I couldn't believe what I was seeing. I was walking down rows and rows of patients who had had orthognathic surgery, cranio-facial surgery, and trauma cases.

Right there and then, I said, I'm going to apply for this hospital. Happily I got a lot of support and applied for the post and I was interviewed in Glasgow with Peter Ward Booth and several other people. When we got there, they announced they had two senior registrar posts available, and they appointed me and Peter and they gave me the option when I could start. I took the first job starting in September 1978 and Peter started a couple of months later in November.

A bad reference was sometimes an advantage. Tony Markus applied for senior house officer job at Barts [1973].

I went to Barts for an interview. I was interviewed by TT, as we call him, Theo Schofield, Frank Coffin and Derek Winstock. TT was wonderful. Frankie, who had a terrible stutter, asked me a question and said, 'Are you p-p-p-punctual?' I said rather foolishly, 'Yes, I think so, sir.' And he said, 'Ei ei ei either y y you are or you are not.' I said, 'I am.' I've never forgotten it.

I got the job. And years later, after I'd got my senior registrar job, I went to have tea with Theo Schofield in his room, 1A Upper Wimpole Street, and he said, 'Dear boy,' he said, 'you had the worst reference I had ever seen when you came for that job.' He said, 'It was so bad I thought I've got to give you this post.' It came from the Dean of the dental school in Newcastle who didn't know me from Adam, a chap called Maurice Hallett, and I don't know why. But anyway, it did me no harm.

Maybe somebody wrote on his record that he had fitted dentures to a patient at the try-in stage? (see chapter 3) Tony:

Yes, maybe.

Or as he had admitted to me just five minutes before that he did little work as an undergraduate?

Yeah, absolutely.

I mentioned that he went poaching when he was a student. Maybe they put that in?

They didn't know about the poaching. But yeah, Maurice Hallett had given me this awful reference, and Theo Schofield thought this is perfect. So rather like the Jesuits say, 'Give me a boy at the age of seven and we'll you give you a man at the age of 17,' I think he felt that give me this chap and I'll make a man of him.

Later Tony was a registrar at Guy's and applied for a senior registrar job at University College Hospital [1977].

Robin Bret Day made me dictate my own reference, terribly embarrassing, but a very good exercise. I gave myself a wonderful one, but he made me dictate it in front of him and he would stop me and correct me; it's quite difficult but we have a degree of reserve. One doesn't generally go around bragging about oneself.

It was the first senior registrar job I applied for. I started at UCH in May '77, working for Ray O'Neil and David James.

John Langdon was a senior registrar at the London Hospital when he had to take several weeks off work to have back surgery [1976].

And during that time rumours had started spreading around of me being gay and having affairs with various members of staff around the place. That I was gay wasn't untrue; but all these rumours of liaisons and affairs were totally and utterly untrue. Anyway, I got back to work and there with all these rumours blowing around, which made life totally intolerable. I reached the stage when I said, 'I can't take this anymore. I'm resigning.' Gordon Seward sent for me and tried to persuade me to withdraw my resignation. Which I did, and I lasted another ten days, and then left with no job to go to, but I was just relieved to be out of the atmosphere. It was totally toxic, it was impossible.

Anyway, I was at home with no job and no income. And out of the blue I got a phone call from Malcolm Harris, who at that time was senior lecturer and consultant at King's. He didn't go into any background or anything, he just said, 'I gather you're looking for a job.' And I said, 'Yes, I am.' And he said, 'We've got a senior registrar coming up here at King's. The interview's in two days' time. Are you interested?' And I said, 'Yes, of course I am. But the closing date was two weeks ago.' And he just said, 'Are you interested?' And I said, 'Yes.' And he said, 'Be here at...' Whatever time it was in two days' time. So I turned up and the interview panel was him, Ian Gainsford, who I'd known for donkey's years because he was at the London originally and was by then Dean at King's, and Geoff Forman. They interviewed me, along with other people, and on the spot offered me the job. So they salvaged me. And they never asked any questions at all about what had gone on at the London. They never even made a reference to the London.

When Malcolm rang me up and said, 'Be here in two days' time.' I said, 'What shall I do about references?' And he said, 'Go and see Gordon Seward.' And I said, I can't ask him for a...' 'Go and see Gordon Seward.' I went there, and he handed me a reference. He didn't say much, and he'd already written it, just handed me the envelope. So Malcolm had obviously been onto him.

Mike Davidson finished his medical and surgical pre-registration house jobs in Brighton [1985].

I forgot who, but somebody said, 'Oh, why don't you go to Chichester because this guy Williams down there, who I had heard of, tees up six months orthopaedic, six months A&E, and then you become his registrar?' I thought, that sounds pretty neat, Chichester's not far from Burgess Hill, we wouldn't have to move far, I could go and sniff it out.

Anyway, I went down and we're talking very informal interview. I wandered in to John Williams, and he said, 'Well, we can't offer you a registrar job yet, but I can tee you up with a house job in A&E and orthopaedics, but you must go and meet them.' So, I did, I went off, and I met the orthopaedic head who was a guy called Elliot, and he said, 'what have you done?' And I told him what I'd done, who I'd worked for, and he said, 'That's fine, that's good, yeah, well, we'd like to offer you a job.' No adverts, just literally he was filling in slots on his rota. Then I went to A&E, and I met a guy, Reg Weeks who was a single-handed A&E consultant. 'Yeah, if John Williams says you're alright, you're in,' and so I was in. And I'd got those two jobs, and I thought, great.

Anyway, I pulled up on the first day, there was the induction and everything, and I was in the mess and this guy comes up to me, he says,

'Hey, is your name Mike Davidson?' I said, 'Yes,' he said, 'Are you thinking of being max-fax surgeon?' I said, 'Yeah.' He says, 'My name's Dave McPherson.' And John Williams had two of us there, but there was only one registrar job in a year's time. So, John Williams had got two of us there doing orthopaedics and A&E, and we literally swapped at six months, so that's the first time I'd met Dave McPherson.

So, there I was, I'd moved house to near Chichester, I now had two children, and I was in a job that after a year might all go belly-up and they might decide they want Dave and not me as the registrar, so that was a bit of a surprise to the system.

Well, as we were moving to the end of our year, both David McPherson and I realised that we both want to stay in Chichester. And both John Williams and John Townend[67] realise that now. So, the job was advertised and we both were duly short-listed, along with one other. And the College examiner was from Guildford. I'd done some background checking on him, and I found out there was a registrar job coming up in Guildford. And I said to Dave, 'I bet you, he will offer one of us to apply for his job, whoever doesn't get down here.' Anyway, we were interviewed and, for whatever reason, I was offered the post which I accepted. And sure enough, Dave McPherson, more or less without an interview, was offered the Guildford registrar job. So, he went to Guildford, and I stayed in Chichester.[68]

The appointments process could be quite informal. Ian Martin had finished his surgical training and was looking for an oral and maxillofacial surgery registrar post. He applied for a locum senior registrar job in Newcastle [1989].

I found myself unemployed. There was a locum advertised for a senior registrar post in Newcastle. And not thinking I'd get anywhere, I applied.

What I didn't know was that two of the consultants had retired from Newcastle at more or less the same time, and they'd advertised for locum consultant posts for these two and had got nobody. So they'd downgraded it and see if there was anybody around for a locum senior registrar job. So, not thinking I'd get it, I applied, and I was the only

---

67 Oral and Maxillofacial consultant at Chichester.
68 David McPherson subsequently became a consultant at Chichester.

person.

I was very flattered that they paid for me to fly up from Plymouth to Newcastle and I turned up to Arthur Hind's leaving do, where there was quite a lot of booze and food laid on, and that was my interview, and I was given the job.

Chapter 12

Higher Training

'Oh my God, that's the end, the dentists are doing rhinoplasties! It's the end of the world.'

Gordon Fordyce was appointed as a senior registrar at Hill End hospital after less than a year as being registrar. Rainsford Mowlem, the plastic surgeon, was in charge of the unit [1949-52].

Alexander MacGregor, Ben Fickling and Paul Toller were the dental consultants. We had no defined programme. We just did the work, and we were busy. Rainsford Mowlem would come Wednesday morning and do a ward round, and in the afternoon he was in the theatre. And then Friday he would come to do theatre and if anybody wanted him, they could go take him to the ward.

Hill End was linked to Barts; that's where our nursing staff came from. There was an orthopaedic unit, a neurosurgical unit and a general medical ward. That was good because we worked closely with the neurosurgeons on several things. Orthopaedics helped as well because they looked after broken legs and arms and things. We had two wards each, two in neurosurgery, plastics upstairs and downstairs, with wings on either side. But I think part of the hospital was still a mental hospital. I don't know how much of it was.

This was four or five years after WWII but there were still some war injuries around. Mowlem and Ben Fickling had looked after a number and they would still come back, their prosthetics needed doing again and flaps had to be fiddled with, nothing very serious. The more serious items, which were around because Mowlem was there, were facial reconstructions, such as syphilitic patients who'd lost their maxilla completely. I remember one, I'm not too sure I didn't publish it, which we had to restore prosthetically and Mowlem grafted areas so we could make a complete removable acrylic maxilla with teeth. And during the war of course, in London many hundreds of people had their faces damaged or burnt, and a lot of them were still having fiddling little operations to make life easier for them.

The other big group that Mowlem attracted were facial distortions, birth injury type things, ankylosis of the jaw, and all that sort of thing. This was teamwork because so many of them required prosthetic work done. And we learned from them how to do grafting so that we could recreate a dental sulcus properly with skin grafts and extend the prosthesis by filling up areas you couldn't do otherwise. This was the buccal inlay.

Mike Awty at East Grinstead was advised by Sir Terence Ward to go to the Eastman Dental Hospital as a registrar [1962].

Going to the Eastman was the best way to get the sort of registrar job I needed to get my fellowship because Killey and Bradlaw [69] would have given me enough teaching to get through. I went to see Killey. He said, 'I haven't got enough money to pay you so I've arranged for you to go into perio for a few months,'[70] and it wound up as being three or four months, just to pay me. And after four months I moved to oral surgery, and I did clinics with Killey and general oral medicine with Bradlaw. I saw all the patients, wrote them up, made a tentative diagnosis and passed them into his clinic. He would teach on them, and if he disagreed with your diagnosis, you'd have a full and frank discussion about it, which he won, always.

It was good because you saw all sorts of things, no trauma but mainly general basic oral surgery and oral medicine, just right for a Fellowship. And then I moved on from there to be a senior registrar at East Grinstead.

Laurence Oldham graduated in 1954 and after a house surgeon job in Birmingham and two years National Service in the RAF became a lecturer at Manchester. He was not impressed [1960-65].

When I was there, we had all our inpatients on ward S2 at the Manchester Royal Infirmary. The biggest thing we did was mandibular fractures, they used to be admitted and wired. We did no malignancy, we did cysts, fractures, wisdom teeth, that was the total repertoire, which was very limited.

Russell Hopkins [1959-60].

Whilst I was at Nottingham I applied for a registrar job in St. Peters, Chertsey, in the South West Metropolitan Region, at which my

---

69 Robert Bradlaw had been a professor of dental surgery at Newcastle but in 1960 moved to become the professor of oral medicine and pathology at the Eastman and Director of Studies. He became the first Dean of the Faculty of Dental Surgery of the Royal College of Surgeons of England.
70 Periodontology department.

boss was Norman Rowe.[71]

St Peters was essentially run by George's and Thomas's doctors. It was the A&E centre. It had been an American casualty hospital so it was a series of concrete huts. The doctors' mess was one hut, the nurses' accommodation was relatively adjacent, two or three huts. The wards and A&E were huts; it was spread over a long, wide distance. My job covered St Peter's, Chertsey, the Holy Cross Hospital in Haslemere, where we had beds for elective surgery, St Richard's Hospital in Chichester, Aldershot General and Woking General.

So, I had an itinerant job, and I bought myself a Triumph TR3A, which was a wonderful two litre Triumph sports car and I did two or three thousand miles a month up and down, and I earned enough money on my petrol expenses to pay for buying the car, and to pay for the petrol. I ran my car on the job, hood down, I had seatbelts put in, not like the modern seat belts; I had shoulder and waist straps.

That was a wonderful job. In Roehampton the plastic surgeons caused a lot of trouble to Norman, and they were very jealous of anything that Norman tried to do. So he did all of his more advanced stuff down in the Holy Cross at Haslemere.

After his medical training, Russell got an unusual job [1964].

I went to sea as a ship's surgeon on the Union Castle. One chap I met, who was very influential in my life was Bill Heald, who became vice president of the College and is perhaps recognised as one of the premiere colorectal surgeon in the world, who's changed the treatment of cancer of the colon,[72] but he was the RSO[73] and he had already been to sea, and I used to do relief trips once a year wearing his uniform. That was a tremendous experience, not only a wonderful way of life, but much more work than I expected and much more complicated because you had 1600 or more people on board the ship, 400 in first class. Passengers would fall, have heart attacks, break a wrist or leg, or fall over the side of the boat.

The crew were mainly homosexuals, and they would beat each other

---

71 The plastic and dental surgeons at Rooksdown House had moved to Roehampton Hospital as their main base in 1959.

72 Professor Bill Heald first described Total Mesorectal Excision for rectal cancer in 1982. See Wikipedia 'Total Mesorectal Excision'.

73 Resident Surgical Officer (usually a general surgery registrar).

at frequent intervals. So I was constantly working with medicine but living a life of Riley, because I had my own dinner table and my own steward, I loved it. I did that for six years on and off until I got married. I used to save up my holidays and then do one trip down to Cape Town, up to Durban and back again, which takes five and half weeks.

I was away for five and half weeks after I'd finished my house job, and after that I'd been appointed the senior registrar in the Royal Victoria Infirmary in Newcastle. I applied for Newcastle because the consultant in charge had this reputation as a go ahead professor who did great clinical surgery, and had written lots of papers and I believed I was going to work for a person who was going to set the world on fire.[74]

When I was interviewed, he gave me a bollocking afterwards because I was not absolutely sold on the idea and therefore treated it somewhat lightly. He said, you treated it as if it was a joke, and you were laughing and everybody else was laughing, and he said it almost cost you the job. If I hadn't got the job, I wouldn't have been broken-hearted because then I would have looked for a job around London, where I lived. However, I got Newcastle and bought my first house for just over three thousand pounds.

I was there for two and a bit years. I left Newcastle because I was not getting any training. I discovered that this chap who was describing all these cases, was actually doing them with the plastic surgeons, he wasn't doing them himself at all. Whenever he did a case with a plastic surgeon, which was not very frequent, he would hold the retractor and I would look over the top, I wouldn't get to see anything. I remember plastic surgeons did a condylectomy, and I couldn't see what they were doing.

I was very angry that I was doing all the trauma that came in, but I was using all my skills I'd learnt as a registrar and as a senior house officer; he never came in. He didn't do much of the stuff. I remember we did a submandibular gland on the list, and he started doing it. He cut the facial artery and he couldn't clip it and he threw the clip down and walked out of the theatre and said, 'You finish it.' So that was the training I got from there and so I thought, well I'm wasting my time, I've either got to look for another senior registrar job but Cardiff came

---

74 Professor Geoffrey Howe.

124

up. [75]

John Bradley, after a year as senior house officer at the Westminster, went to Salisbury as registrar from 1961 to 62 and then returned to Roehampton as senior registrar [1962].

I was still pretty young for the senior registrar job, but Taylor [76] *wanted me. So I went for the job and I was exceedingly lucky because by then most of the senior registrars had got a medical qualification and I hadn't. If I hadn't been appointed, I would have understood why. But anyway, bless him, I was appointed.*

It was an incredible experience working under Norman Rowe at Roehampton, the other consultant there was Ian Heslop. Taylor was also on the staff at Roehampton; he was the senior consultant. Westminster was the major hospital and Roehampton was subsidiary. It had got this very famous plastic surgical unit, founded by Gillies, and the senior man there was Patrick Clarkson. He was a big, very dominant man. So I was coming into another totally different experience.

Roehampton hospital was an old Ministry of Pensions, war pensions, hospital and it was part of the military then. The department was a 1914/18 Nissen hut. The hospital had a big orthopaedic unit. There was a big limb fitting and construction factory there. We had quite a large ward; we had our own high dependency ward; it was two beds. So that was a major referral centre for severe trauma for around south west London and going out into Surrey. We used to get patients in from Guildford and Redhill and even up from the south coast from time to time. I learnt an enormous amount. I saw just about every variant of facial injury at that place.

Correction of facial deformity was developing and Rowe's innovative developing skills and mind came into full flow. When we started with all this, they were only just about beginning to do sagittal split osteotomies, which I think is a superb operation for correcting relatively minor deformities on faces.

Taylor usually operated on either a morning or an afternoon, usually mornings. Ian Heslop used a half day operating list as Rowe did. But if we had a big case, then we would operate all day if we

---

75 The consultant job in Cardiff that he was appointed to.
76 Rupert Sutton Taylor.

needed to. The boss man was always there. Dento-alveolar surgery would tend to go on a registrar's list. The consultants were very conscientious; they were very much hands on and they always made themselves available.

On a typical list, Norman Rowe would deal with quite a lot of benign pathology in the jaws. They would be referred from way outside south west London. Or he would get patients from all of the south of England coming in with fairly rare pathology of one sort or another. We had the dento-alveolar work and he would do some of it, depending on what he felt like. But if he had rather pressing things to do, if he felt he could delegate it, then he did so, which was fair enough.

We didn't tend to do much cancer. Mostly cancer was dealt with by doing a biopsy and then went out to the radiotherapists and the oncologists. When it failed, and they had breakthrough tumours, it went to the specialist general surgeons. There was surgeon called Stanley Lee at Westminster, a very nice man. Westminster was a very big cancer centre. The guiding light there was Sir Stanford Cade, who was a Russian, and a very dynamic man. I assisted him on several occasions, dealing with tumours of the upper jaw.

We did a moderate amount of special care dentistry in the hospitals because there was nowhere else for them to go. Simple straightforward restorative dentistry, usually using amalgams.

Khursheed Moos became a senior registrar in Cardiff, not long before Russell Hopkins became consultant. The job involved rotation to Chepstow [1967].

There was not much surgical experience; very little maxillofacial surgery was being done at Cardiff and the work in the dental school was essentially dental extractions, third molars surgery with some minor pathology; and the trauma was limited.

Trauma had to be treated, but the senior lecturer there who had come from East Grinstead had difficulties taking on board major surgery. I'd had quite a bit of experience before going there, but largely unsupervised, and I was happier carrying out surgery with junior staff assistance, and I was usually left to do that. I really learned little there until latterly.

I was becoming increasingly unhappy because I was not really learning anything or gaining much surgical experience because of the restrictions on what one could do there. Part of this was because of pressure from plastic surgery in Chepstow who controlled most of the major trauma in the south Wales area and all the orthognathic surgery and much of the hard and soft tissue surgery.

I was concerned that I did not really want to go to Chepstow where it would not be an easy scene as I am not a very aggressive person when it comes to having a fight with plastic surgeons. I thought about a move from the area, hopefully to get a job somewhere else before I needed to do my two-year rotation to Chepstow.

However, very fortunately for me, Russell Hopkins was appointed as a new consultant. He came with a background from the Roehampton maxillofacial unit and he and I immediately got on well together.

Mike Bromige qualified from dental school in 1958 and became a house officer at Selly Oak and later a registrar.

I was three and a half or four years registrar at the General Hospital with two housemen most of the time. There were two occasions when they didn't or couldn't appoint and life got a bit difficult then, particularly with this large number of casual attendances coming in at night or in the evening. When there weren't housemen they used to employ a local practitioner to come in and do sessions, seven till ten or something like that. But the trouble was that at 10 o'clock there used to be the rest of the queue and I used to get rung up by the sister and say, 'What are you going to do about this queue?' so I had to go in and clear it, and that used to happen not infrequently. But it was all good experience because with things coming in off the street you're never quite sure what to expect.

The consultant at the General Hospital was Tavener, he'd taken medicine part time. He was employed through the war at the General Hospital which received a lot of war casualties, and somebody said, 'You really ought to get medicine to do this,' and so he signed up for a part-time medical course and got his degree after the war. He was a very able man, but he was often absent and I was on my own.

Professor McGregor,[77] the Principal of the dental school had operating rights, and so did Dr Mitchell the Superintendent. Dr Mitchell didn't enjoy operating, so he'd attend, but I would do it. Prof. McGregor came in twice, that's all I can recollect, in the three or four-

---

77 Alex McGregor who had been a consultant at Hill End.

year period.

The only orthognathic surgery I saw was Professor McGregor doing this one bilateral osteotomy of the mandible. And otherwise it was pure dento-alveolar work, cysts, impacted teeth, extractions, clearances and trauma. There was a fair amount of trauma. I did quite a bit of soft tissue work in A&E. I used to go down and suture things up. But otherwise in the department of oral surgery it was pretty humdrum. But a lot of basic experience.

Cancer work was mainly done by either one of the general surgeons or an ENT surgeon who was appointed whilst I was registrar. I used to work with him and we did a few maxillectomies, as I remember, and a glossectomy. But it was the first time he'd done them as well, so we were actually propping each other up. The rest of it I'm sure went to the plastic surgeons and the ENT surgeons at the Queen Elizabeth Hospital. They were based at the plastic and jaw surgery unit out in Wordsley, Stourbridge,[78] but had sessions and beds and operating time at the Queen Elizabeth Hospital.

Mike became a senior registrar in Birmingham [1963].

It was a split job based with RO Walker and Pusey at the Queen Elizabeth Hospital, who also went to the Birmingham Accident Hospital, as it was then. We were the only outside specialists who went into Birmingham Accident Hospital, otherwise they were self-sufficient. There was a lot of trauma there. I was also senior registrar at the plastic and jaw unit at Stourbridge under Maurice Jones and Colin Brady. They were two separate units, and I worked between them. I did outpatients and operating lists at Wordsley at the plastic unit and similarly at the Queen Elizabeth Hospital, and then did the trauma work at the Birmingham Accident Hospital. A lot of travelling around. I often used to go to Stourbridge and the Queen Elizabeth Hospital and do a ward round or operate at the Accident Hospital in one day.

All trauma that came into the Queen Elizabeth Hospital via the Accident Hospital was dealt with by our unit, including soft tissue. The Accident Hospital had three teams, each containing two consultant surgeons, two anaesthetists and all the junior staff, and they were on for 24 hours at a time, so they dealt with a lot of things. But for

---

78 Wordsley Hospital, see Appendix 2.

anything to do with the face, we were called in; we had a very good relationship with them. I spent three months with Peter London, the senior surgeon at the Accident Hospital, doing anything but oral surgery and he was very good to me and I did a lot of bone work and suturing and wound work with him. I lived in for that three months.

There was a great rivalry between Stourbridge and the Queen Elizabeth. RO Walker was a difficult, intensely jealous man and life was quite difficult as a senior registrar. The one before me had been dismissed for some demeanour and I think it was carrying a procedure that had been developed at one hospital into the other. It's all a bit murky, but certainly I went in with a cloud over the unit because Bruce Jackson had been dismissed. The senior registrar before that was Joe Moore, who had run it like an army unit, allegedly where the housemen and the registrar weren't allowed to speak to the consultant other than through Joe Moore, the senior registrar. So I followed fairly odd predecessors, and you just had to be very careful what you said and what you did. Quite unlike today.

At Wordsley the plastic surgeons did the cancer, and we did the prosthetics for maxillectomies. There were four maxillofacial technicians at Wordsley, and they were doing the prostheses for noses, eyes and maxillectomy obturators, for a very wide area. We're talking about the West Midlands unit, but it covered an area going right over the border into Wales. We would have people coming from Hereford and Wrexham and places like that for cleft lip and palate surgery, for instance, and also for malignancy.

John Langdon was a senior registrar at the London [1974-76].

Gordon Seward was an immaculate operator. I mean, he wouldn't spill a corpuscle. All his operations were conducted in complete silence. These interminable operating sessions would go on for hour upon hour without a break, with very little being said apart from asking for an instrument. He did all the surgery; I have a great deal of respect for him, but he didn't teach. He was very shy.

I suppose it was the attitude of that period. If the consultants, except Terence English, were in theatre, they did the surgery. If they didn't want to do the operation, they weren't in the theatre. So you didn't really get any formal training. Nobody ever took you through anything. Gordon Seward was more or less the first max-fax surgeon, oral surgeon, to do parotid surgery, facial nerve dissections; I must have assisted him in dozens of them. But he never once let me operate. The biggest operation I ever did as a registrar was in my last week, when Terence English let me take out a submandibular salivary gland and do the whole operation.

But when you were senior registrar at the Royal London, did you manage to get on and do cancer surgery?

No.

Despite not having any supervised surgical training, John was expected to pitch in to treat private patients.

Patrick James became infected by Hepatitis B and was off work for about six weeks. Out of the blue, he went off sick. He rang me up, no preamble, 'You're running my practice while I'm out of circulation.' And I said, 'What do you mean, I'm running your practice?' 'Well, there are a certain number of patients and operations I can't cancel. I've cancelled most of it, but you'll have to do the rest.'

For six weeks he was off sick, in my lunch hour I had to race up to Cavendish Square, where his rooms were, and see patients, and get back to the London to do whatever I was doing in the afternoon. So I was driving from Whitechapel to Cavendish Square and back. In the evenings I had to do the odd operation for him. And he had the temerity to say, 'There's no need to tell them you're not me.' So I was there fraudulently seeing patients and operating under his name. When he came back, he just handed me an envelope, and it had a cheque for seventy quid in it. It didn't even cover the cost of the car parking in Cavendish Square. Never a word of thanks or anything.[79]

Andy Brown applied and was appointed as a senior registrar at East Grinstead, having been there as an undergraduate from Guy's [1976].

I think what is fascinating is to realise that I had worked at the Eastman Dental Hospital and had basically only carried out intraoral surgery. I had really no experience beyond being, somewhat by force of necessity because of my training, a fairly adroit dento-alveolar surgeon. But I had done nothing major, and nothing extraoral. I hadn't even scrubbed in on a single osteotomy by the time I started my senior registrar training, let alone done one. It's as if my training was back to front, as it was for many oral surgeons. Essentially, I did all my

79 Another of my interviewees has subsequently told me that he too was compelled to see his private patients in Cavendish Square.

basic surgical training at the end of my career, not at the start of it! So I came through the door at East Grinstead very green.

Mike Awty and Peter Banks had done a lot and if they could see that you had a bit of ability and interest, and had, as Mike Awty would say, 'sharp elbows' and could elbow your way to the table, then they would let you operate freely under their supervision. So at last I got supervised training. But people of my generation were training when the specialty was expanding in scope and depth; so all of us, including the consultants, were pushing the boundaries and entering areas that we hadn't been into before. So self-teaching, or being self-taught, or reading an operation up and then having a go, was quite common.

I believe today that the best surgeons are going to be self-taught in the sense they always want to read up an operation before they do it, if it's a new one. Even if they are going to be shown it by somebody else, one hopes that they've learnt up the basic anatomy and indications before they get to the table.

I saw my first sagittal split osteotomy done on the mandible at East Grinstead. They were also doing submandibular gland surgery; although they weren't doing parotid surgery or head and neck cancer surgery, that came later. But they were doing quite a lot of extraoral surgery, temporomandibular joint approaches, ankylosis and the like. The other thing that I think we were getting into was pre-prosthetic surgery, which was a whole area which has now almost gone completely with dental implants.

Mike Awty and Peter Banks were the only two consultants there. They were major influences on me and have remained so throughout my career.

David Vaughan was a registrar at the Eastman Dental Hospital [1979].

I only spent five months in the Eastman. I got a job at East Grinstead as a senior registrar, between East Grinstead and King's. And I was in a hurry at this stage, because I wasn't getting any younger, I would have been about 35. So I went down and had a very funny, interesting interview with Mike Awty. He was very suspicious of me.

'You've got an FRCS and you've done all the surgery, why do you want to be an oral and maxillofacial surgeon?' And I said, 'I'm reasonably happy with my understanding of the surgery of head and

neck cancer, but I have no experience in trauma, dento-alveolar surgery or for that matter deformity surgery, and I understand that this is a very good unit for that type of thing.' So I got appointed. And I spent my time with orthognathic surgery because I hadn't a clue about it, genuinely I hadn't.

I must give Andy Brown lots of credit for pulling me through it, because I wasn't that interested in it; I thought it was cosmetic surgery to be honest with you. He was the substantive senior registrar; he didn't move anywhere, whereas of the other two senior registrars, one rotated to Guy's and the other one to King's. I found it a very humiliating place to work, in the sense that all the cancers we picked up, we doffed our cap and brought them over to the plastic surgeons and gave them to them. But it was a very pleasant place to work otherwise.

Brian Avery also became a registrar in oral surgery at the Eastman after his medical jobs [1975-76].

I worked there for a year and a month and I have to say that that was a pretty bizarre set up. I learnt how to do a lot of dento-alveolar surgery, but really nothing else went on there. I remember doing one sagittal split osteotomy with one boss at St Mary's Hospital, but otherwise it was basically dento-alveolar surgery and wiring fractures if we got them and we didn't get many. My bosses then were Professor Homer Killey, Mr Lester Kay and then there were some other chaps, John Canniff, John James and John Eyre. It was very bizarre. Homer Killey was very nice, you couldn't help but like him, but he had some very strange habits and I think he was rather a lonely man. After I'd been there a year, he died whilst I was his registrar. Lester Kay was also there, and I think he was already suffering from a degree or pre-senile dementia. Again, a very nice man, very interesting, lots of anecdotes, but I didn't learn anything there.

Brian moved on to become a registrar at the Westminster Hospital [1976].

It was a rotation between Roehampton and Westminster and I have to tell you it was very famous, Roehampton. I started off at Westminster and I was doing okay, there wasn't a lot of oral and maxillofacial surgery there but there were a couple of head and neck surgeons. There was a general surgeon called Westbury and a plastic surgeon known affectionately as 'Tiger' Wilson, and they were doing a lot of head and neck surgery. I used to go to the lists, and I got on very well with them and they let me do more and more. And although I was not doing the neck dissections, I was doing a lot of other things, such as a lot of the resections. They were very good, and I was getting on so well that in fact my boss asked me to stand back and not get involved so much because the senior registrar there, who I shan't name, was getting rather jealous because the two chaps were inviting me to do the operating and he was getting left out; he'd fallen out with them.

Well, I was disillusioned at this point and I have to tell you I was looking at adverts for careers in ENT surgery. I was not happy; I wasn't getting the training. I went to Roehampton, and it got a lot better, and John Langdon was doing a lot of things and making it much more interesting. Norman Rowe was doing quite a lot of orthognathic surgery, John Bowerman was doing things and I was becoming a lot happier then and so that was quite a good experience. I was there for just over a year, and during this time I was applying for jobs as a senior registrar in the south east and London.

But he became a senior registrar at Canniesburn [1978-83].

The chiefs in Canniesburn were Khursheed Moos and Amir El-Attar. But there was also a very famous team of plastic surgeons. I think Canniesburn with no doubt at all was the most famous plastic surgery unit in the UK. It had Ian Jackson doing the cranio-facial surgery, Ian McGregor doing the head and neck oncology, and two or three others doing lots of interesting surgery. It was just unbelievable what was going on there, and that was a busy job.

I got little if any training in oncology but so much training in dento-alveolar surgery, trauma – we were dealing with 800 fractures a year – orthognathic surgery, and some salivary gland surgery but very little oncology. There was quite a lot of hostility between the max-fax surgeons and the plastic surgeons, particularly over oncology. The plastic surgeons regarded the head and neck oncology as their fiefdom to the point where you couldn't really do it.

Adrian Sugar qualified from Leeds, did a house job and a short while in dental practice and then took a registrar job on Teesside [1972-76].

The unit had two consultants, Brian Summersgill and Richard Pratt, and both of them were singly qualified. I was a registrar there for about four years.

There I became very proficient at dento-alveolar surgery and facial trauma. I learned a lot about facial skin suturing from one of the plastic surgeons Charles Viva and about clinical neurosurgery from Patrick Clark. Mr Clark was outstanding and went on to become President of the Society of British Neurological Surgeons. Those were the days before CT scans and diagnosis was mostly clinical. I spent plenty time on his ward. I also learned about head and neck oncology attending the regular multi-disciplinary team meetings at the radiotherapy hospital and sometimes operating with the ENT surgeons where I performed my first tracheostomy.

In Teesside (Middlesbrough General Hospital) I was more or less 1 in 1 on-call, just getting alternate weekends off, unless we were short staffed when I was on-call all the time. I never received a penny of on-call payment. The rules were written in such a way that you had to do so many days on-call before you qualified for payment. Nobody did more hours than me but I never qualified for any payment. I worked hard and enjoyed the work and became chair of the junior medical staff. It was around that time that we along with most juniors in the country took national action and at last won on-call payments.

I finished my registrar job in Teesside, and then I took another six months looking after a single-handed dental practice. I quite enjoyed it.

Adrian then got a registrar job in oral surgery in Leeds [1976].

Although this was basically an oral surgery job, I had to do a rotation into paediatric dentistry. And the Professor of paediatric dentistry, who was a guy called Jackson, was very understanding, and he set up a rotation for me so I also did paediatric medicine with the professor of paediatric surgery and paediatric oncology, including work on the paediatric wards. That was fantastic; it enthused me immensely.

There were two registrars in oral surgery but my fellow registrar disappeared and so I worked all the hours that God gave and it was a very busy two years. The trauma was very much to the fore, so it was in that job that I and two senior registrars developed a close working relationship with the neurosurgeons. It was probably one of the first units in the country that was actually very aggressively treating primary cranio-facial trauma; that was '76 to '78. So we'd have patients who'd be brought in within half an hour of a major injury. I was also starting to do some orthognathic surgery, not really anything on cancer, and very little on clefts, and so it was a radical change in the sense that every day we were doing things new to me and that I was enjoying, and that we were doing quite well. The consultant oral surgeons were supportive, but not really involved.

While I was there, two senior registrar jobs came up in Leeds, one academic and one hospital. I was asked to apply for both of them. But although I had learned a great deal, I also knew from that what maxillofacial surgery was about, and I knew I was poorly prepared for it. I knew that there wasn't much else that I was going to learn there. I had to go somewhere where I could learn the other things.

Adrian left Leeds and was appointed as a senior registrar in south Wales [1978].

I don't know how many applied. I know that there were only two of us shortlisted. At the time we were the generation of the bulge when we had many more senior registrars than there were consultants jobs coming up. It was quite difficult to get jobs at senior registrar and consultant levels, and you were competing mostly with the same people.

That job was a senior registrar rotation between Russell Hopkins in Cardiff and John Gibson in Chepstow. I started on the Chepstow end. I did a day a week on a Thursday in the dental school with Brian Cooke and Murray Walker doing oral medicine and oral pathology.

In Chepstow, I spent one year assigned as first assistant to one of the plastic surgeons, Michael Green, one day a week in 1.5 theatres. We did major cancer resections and reconstructions most weeks including tracheostomies, local and neck resections, forehead flaps, delto-pectoral flaps[80] and pectoralis majors.[81] This was in 1979/80 before microvascular flaps were being used. We also did primary cleft surgery and general plastics including skin cancer. I did a lot of surgery and learned a lot.

After one year, Adrian rotated to Cardiff and Russell Hopkins [1980].

In Cardiff with Russell, we did a wide range of almost everything, especially trauma hard, soft and cranio-facial with the neurosurgeons. We did orthognathic, pre-prosthetic, salivary and temporomandibular joint surgery. There was a wide range of cancer

---

80 Fasciocutaneous flap from the upper chest based on perforating mammary arteries.
81 Pedicled reconstruction flap consisting of pectoralis major muscle and overlying skin, formerly a commonly used technique for reconstruction following oral cancer resection but replaced by free tissue transfer.

resections and flaps but no neck dissections. I attended a weekly multi-disciplinary team meeting and enjoyed the surgery for head and neck cancer and looking after the patients on our ward. But cancer was never going to be a major interest for me.

When I started there was about three or four weeks when I was obviously on some kind of probation. It was then made perfectly clear to me by Russell, that I could fly, and I had a great time and we got a lot of work done. In the latter year or two, I was doing most of the surgery, but there were still things that he would do for example, Le Fort II and Le Fort III osteotomies that I helped him with, but which he did.

He was very good at doing parotids. It was a hard job for me to get trained to do parotids, but I got there in the end. I had to be devious, though. I tried to get him to teach me and that had gone nowhere, so I did a deal with one of our regular anaesthetists in Cardiff. We used to start the list nominally at eight-thirty, but Russell would rarely come in before nine-thirty. I organised the lists, and I put a parotid on first, and we started at eight o'clock, so I was operating by eight-thirty, so I was halfway through if not three-quarters of the way through by the time he came in at nine-thirty. because once I'd done one, and I'd identified the trunk of the facial nerve, and I was dissecting the branches he didn't even scrub. He said, 'You'd better finish it then,' and he went and sat down and drank coffee and I joined him shortly afterwards and we finished the list.

Tony Markus was appointed as registrar at Guy's [1975].

Shortly after I started they opened the Guy's Tower, so we were transferred to the 23rd floor of the tower where I had a beautiful office that I shared with a couple of other registrars. We had en-suite facilities and I could look out over the railway lines as they exited from London Bridge Station and watch the trains coming in and out, and going away into the distance. I worked for Pat O'Driscoll and for Dick Haskell and also for Rod Cawson, with his terrific intellectual breadth, not just about oral medicine and pathology, but anything else, a terrific man. I worked for a chap called Tom Lehner who was the professor of immunology. He did part time, and I had an attachment there for a short period.

The other surgeons there were Don Gibb and Robin Bret Day, and there was a lovely chap called Cyril Hagger who ran the dental emergency unit and also taught me how to take out teeth properly under general anaesthetic.

At this time the method of payment for being on call changed to UMTs, Units of Medical Time. They introduced the A units and the B units. And Guy's said that to be paid A units you had to be actually in the hospital, and B was if you were just somewhere outside. And it was a huge difference, I think an A unit was one-third and a B unit was one-tenth of basic pay. Anyway, we, the poisons unit and the psychiatrists, took them, with the backing of the British Medical Association, to a tribunal which was heard somewhere near Elephant and Castle, so I presume it was somewhere at one of the Department of Health buildings. And we won and so we were given A units, although I lived in Richmond.

With Cawson in oral medicine we tried to cure recurrent oral ulceration, I can't remember what the drug was, but that wasn't so important because you learnt some of the mechanisms, as we understood them in those days, behind the diseases that presented to us later as consultants in district general hospitals. Rod Cawson would be referred these refractive cases of lichen planus or any number of vesicular bullous lesions. He would look at them and he would say, 'Well, my dear, I know what you've got but I'm afraid we can't cure it.' And that was a fantastic lesson, we can manage it of course, but we couldn't cure. And we're no different now, 35 years on.

Tony started as a senior registrar at University College Hospital in May 1977.

I was working for Ray O'Neil and David James. The job also involved Great Ormond Street. David James and Ray O'Neil didn't get on at all, and David had to prove himself. He was not aggressive in an unpleasant way, but he was aggressive inasmuch as he wanted to establish a jolly good surgical practice and prove himself, which he did. If you had a patient with a fractured malar when you were on call and you rang O'Neil up because you wanted to lift it, he'd tell you to do it through an infra-orbital approach and vice versa. Without seeing the patient.

I was at UCH for 18 months before I rotated to Mount Vernon. There was a good atmosphere at Mount Vernon; but rarely was there a consultant there. Occasionally Dickie Dawson[82] would appear, I

---

82 Senior consultant plastic surgeon.

remember the first time I got a surgical emphysema when I'd just lifted a fractured malar, just at the point when he was being inflated, and the air had got in and tracked around the orbit and I'd literally just turned around to put my instruments down and I turned back and this thing was happening. And I just then glanced to my right and there was Dickie, this was ten o'clock at night, smoking a fag, standing outside in the corridor outside the theatre, but we had glass windows there so he could see what was going on, and he just laughed. And so he opened the doors, and he told me what it was. And I knew what surgical emphysema was post-elevation of a malar ever after. He had that habit of turning up just at the right moment.

They were changing the rotations a little bit and there were too many senior registrars around to get jobs. There weren't enough consultant jobs. So they changed things around, and so I had this opportunity to work at St George's and the Royal Dental hospitals. The Royal Dental was in Leicester Square and St George's at Tooting. Our inpatients, plastics and maxillofacial at the time were at St James's in Balham, up the road. I used to go up and do outpatients one morning a week at the Royal with Derek Henderson and David Poswillo was around at both hospitals.

John Towers was hugely confrontational with the whole world, very belligerent, never out of trouble with the gas man or the electricity board, many problems. But he had a terrific mind but and was sometimes very difficult to pin down. He'd ring you up in the middle of the night and say, 'E lad, that osteotomy we're doing in the morning, I think we ought to do it this way.' So a plan we'd already agreed was changed in the middle of the night, and we did it that way. We always had our once or twice weekly tutorials in the pub on the Wandsworth common after we'd finished operating.

Then there was Derek Henderson, and that was just wonderful because I learnt how to do down fractures quickly and effectively and his whole approach combined with what I was beginning to learn from Delaire[83] was really becoming consolidated. It made my life easier in assessing these patients and what they needed. David Poswillo fired me up. He wrote nice papers with lots of very interesting stuff and was a great support. So it was just terrific to go there after UCH and Mount Vernon, that was essentially the end of my training, and it was the real

---

83 Jean Delaire, French Surgeon, see chapter 20

icing on the cake.

Mike Davidson became a registrar at Chichester after his medical jobs [1986-88].

As a registrar you were first on, on a one-in-two on call rota for Worthing and Southlands, which is the best part of twenty miles along the A27 along the coast. Yet you were second on for Chichester when you were on call, and of course you were living in your home because you were non-resident. I don't know how many miles I did while I was a registrar because you literally traversed the county. At one point, three of the staff had had accidents.

Chichester was a very close, friendly unit. For all its stresses, for all its hassle, I loved the doctors' mess at Chichester. There was a really good tradition that at weekends everyone on call would eat together; the physicians, the orthopods, and the general surgeons. Traditionally, the house surgeon and the house physician on call would prepare the meal, but while they did that their pagers were carried by their registrars. And the quality of people they got was high. It was a popular place to be, so a lot of the trainees were good people and I learnt a lot from chatting to them.

John Townend had a clinic somewhere in central Sussex. He had arranged it so that his clinic was literally next door to the dermatologist. The dermatologist loved it because she could say, 'Will you biopsy this? And my job was to hang around doing this biopsy clinic, all skin and little excisions and flaps.

John Townend was very generous because he would talk about what I'd done that day over a cup of tea at the end. But the downside was, suddenly, you'd get these cases 'Just take a piece out of this,' and of course it wasn't just head and neck, it was off legs and all sorts of things. Again, no formal training, but hey ho, that was a great learning experience. You'd always have about three or four cases booked, but you'd always get one or two added. At the time, very few people in oral and maxillofacial surgery were getting access to skin tumours, and I got shed loads down there.

But then Mike went to Leeds as senior registrar [1988-91].

I started there in April '88. I sat the Edinburgh FRCS in the summer of '89; I was appointed in Leeds despite not having the fellowship, because a lot of people didn't but the important thing was I was eligible and ready to roll.

I'm tempted to say it was three years where I marked time in many aspects of my life. To call them totally wasted I think is harsh because I did learn something even if it was, I mustn't do this. What I did do in Leeds was a lot of dento-alveolar surgery, a lot of supervising dental undergraduates. I did quite a bit of oral medicine.

The dental school was one of the most incestuous organisations I think I've ever functioned within. There were only some people there who I think were worth their salaries.

I saw a moderate amount of trauma. The only salivary gland work I did was a parotid. The boss had deliberately arranged to be on holiday, so I was doing it unsupervised, but I'd done quite a few in Chichester.

But there was no skin, temporo-mandibular joint not really, salivary gland not really, trauma yes, but very much self-taught, loads of dento-alveolar, and some orthognathic, but it was pretty good the orthognathic, the clinics and the orthodontics were good, and although there wasn't a vast number, they were well done. Oncology, I could observe the plastic surgeons, but literally observe, I barely got to scrub. So, I would have a great chance to watch the plastic surgeon spend all day doing a free flap and join in the applause at the end.

One of the NHS consultants was doing free flaps and did them very nicely. But I never did any, I never did a neck dissection in its entirety, so my career from a professional point of view was static. I wasn't going forward, in fact, in some ways my career was totally on-hold and some skills like skin were slipping backwards because I wasn't doing it.

I did a lot of teaching and I quite enjoyed that, undergraduates, and also preparing people for dental fellowship. I got to appear on television because Jimmy's[84] was being filmed and that was the first week I arrived. The consultant said, 'Oh, have you seen this thing Jimmy's? They want to do a case of ours and we're going to do a temporomandibular joint ankylosis.' I said, 'Okay.' It was on a child, and he said, 'Have you ever taken rib because I don't want to have to

---

84 'Jimmy's' was a television documentary series broadcast on independent television between 1987 and 1996.

have another department coming and taking it because we're on television?' So, I said, 'Yeah, I've taken rib,' he said, 'Right, you're taking rib then.' So, my first major case at Jimmy's was appearing on television taking a rib whilst it was filmed.

The professor signed me up for my accreditation, and we had to have the formal interview. He had a list of procedures, 'Have you done this during your training?' And we went through the list and by the time we got to about the end thing, I said, 'Yes, I have. Well, to be honest prof., shouldn't you know if I've done this?' And his attitude was, 'What are you whingeing about? I'm going to sign you up, anyway.' It was just a farce, really. Again, socially he was a nice enough chap, but to be honest, his contribution to the field, to my training and to the education of undergraduates in oral surgery was pretty minimal.

In many ways, Yorkshire was disappointing and in hindsight, I wish I'd never gone. Although socially it was fine and academically, I learnt a few things; I made some good friends, but professionally taking the first senior registrar job that came that I stood a chance of getting was a mistake. I had learnt far more in my eighteen months at Chichester than I did in my entire three years in Leeds. I learned that I didn't want to be anywhere near a teaching hospital and certainly not a dental school ever, professionally.

After his time in general surgery as a senior house officer in Plymouth, Ian Martin applied for oral and maxillofacial registrar jobs and was appointed on the Merseyside rotation [1989].

The Liverpool job came up, with Vaughan and Pospisil, and, obviously, I'd worked with David, and I knew he was doing cutting edge stuff. I didn't know much about Pospisil at the time. It was actually a rotation, Walton, Broadgreen, and Chester with John Cawood.

Initially, we lived in the nurses' home at Alder Hey; we were put up in a single bedroom at the top of the nurse's home. The beginning of our married life really was pretty dire. And opposite it was a Chinese restaurant which we spent a lot of time in. It was a nice Chinese restaurant, actually. A lot of the film crew from Brookside, which was the precursor of Hollyoaks, and all those sorts of things, used to turn up into this restaurant. So we were among celebrities as far as we were concerned, in this little restaurant.[85]

But the thing that struck me about Alder Hey, when I first moved there, was there was an off licence, and unlike any off licence I'd ever seen before in my life, it was like a bank. All the bottles were encased in reinforced Perspex stuff; there was a bank teller's thing, and you had to say, 'Oh, I'd like that bottle please,' and he'd get it. And then when you'd given him the money, hand it out through the thing. So they, obviously, had so many robberies in this off licence that they had to protect all their bottles.

I spent my first four months with John Cooper and Harry Alty at Broadgreen. Both real gentlemen. Harry Alty was very old-fashioned. John Cooper was a really nice meticulous, singly qualified surgeon, did lots of orthognathic stuff. He also got into arthroscopy, and we kind of learnt arthroscopy together because I think he was new at it, and I had done a tiny bit in Newcastle with John Hawkesford.

I did four months at Broadgreen, four months at Walton, and four months at Chester. And then I did a second term at Broadgreen and Walton, but I never went the third time to Chester, so I did about twenty months as a registrar.

I got lots of practical experience. At Broadgreen you would get to do half of all the osteotomies with John Cooper. Harry Alty didn't do that much really, he was still doing things like a closed condylotomy, I can still remember him with the Gigli saw and as he took the Gigli saw out there was this almighty spurt of blood which hit the light. He'd gone through the maxillary artery or something. And Harry was as cool as a cucumber. He just put his finger on it and he stood there humming to himself for about fifteen minutes with his finger on it, and it stopped.

There was a lot of trauma at Broadgreen. I got more than my fair share to do. It was busy. I'd had lots of surgical experience as a senior house officer doing plastics and quite a lot of general and vascular surgery. So I was a reasonably competent, generally trained surgeon by the time I went there, and I think that made a difference.

Ian went to East Grinstead as a senior registrar [1991].

I started in East Grinstead in '91 and my first attachment on the

---

85 Brookside was a soap opera shown on channel 4 from 1982 to 2003 and Hollyoaks is a soap opera shown on channel 4 from 1995. Both filmed in Liverpool.

firms was to Mike Awty's firm, but Mike Awty had retired a couple of months before and so they had a locum there. And he was a sort of Walter Mitty character, really. Apparently, according to him, been the head of the service in Dubai or somewhere. He was singly qualified, and was one of the worst surgeons I've ever seen in my life. He was awful; he was dangerous; he had no judgement whatsoever.

Peter Korczak was on the other side of the rotation with me. Peter was a delightful chap, and we got on very well together. We spent most of our time trying to rescue these poor patients from what this locum was trying to do. He wanted to open every clicky temporo-mandibular joint and stuff like that, and so Pete and I would go round the wards before he arrived and have a word with them and discharge them. He was terrible, and I spent quite a lot of time dealing with his cock ups.

There was a patient who came back after he had taken her wisdom tooth out. It was a distoangular wisdom tooth in this middle-aged woman. It was low down, and he had taken three quarters of the mandible away to get this out and surprise, surprise, she came back in with a fractured mandible. Oh god, it was awful; I mean, I had to put something like a ten hole plate on. He was just awful. Oh dear.

Mike Awty:

When I learned that this person was looking after my team I was shocked, really. I want to record that I strongly disapproved. How he got the job I don't know.

Ian:

Peter Banks was the senior consultant at East Grinstead, I had a great time with Peter. I mean he was a difficult character, a terrible temper, but a temper that lasted for thirty seconds and then everything was fine and he'd move on. A very generous character, very hospitable, very bright, terrible hands. By his own admission a very clumsy surgeon, which he found intensely frustrating. But he was a really interesting boss to work for.

He was very self-conscious and actually, in some ways, I think probably a bit shy, and this was a reaction to being watched by plastic surgeons doing stuff that he felt a bit uncomfortable about. That being said, of course, he'd made his name really with two things, the post-condylar grafting, where he was shoving bits of lyophilised cartilage behind the condyle to treat class two deformities, which was an interesting concept. And he did it in a very odd way, using bits of wire and K-wires, and washers, to stop it cheese wiring though the graft.

The other thing he did was quite a lot of secondary cleft work. He had a series of about 100 Le Forts Is done on clefts, which were quite bad. And the reason they were bad was the primary clefts were done largely by an old school plastic surgeon and had produced massive scarring. So they all had fairly severe maxillary deficiency and needed a lot of pulling forward. So he had a big series of secondary cleft stuff, and we looked at the stability of his clefts over time. One of the interesting things was it didn't matter how long you put them into fixation for, it made no difference in terms of stability. But Peter was actually quite reluctant to let you do some stuff, he wasn't happy to have cancer cases done on his lists, he didn't like that because he didn't feel very comfortable with it himself. I think he always felt slightly out of control if senior registrars were doing stuff that he didn't feel comfortable to get them out of.

My main contribution as a senior registrar at East Grinstead was to persuade him to come on the Bull rhinoplasty course with me.[86] And he was uneasy about it because, of course, that was mainstream plastic surgery territory. But I said to him, 'Look, if you're doing maxillary osteotomies on people with facial disproportion and they need their nose doing, we should do it.' And he kind of accepted that.

We went on the Bull course together, and I can still now remember the first rhinoplasty that we did. It was a bit of a disaster; it was the wrong case to do. The woman had a big droopy nose, and it wasn't a great result. But we went on to do quite a lot of noses after that, particularly secondary cleft noses, and he was quite good at that because it was fiddly stuff that he was quite interested in.

But in East Grinstead in the theatres you had the operating list on a big board, and everything was glass, and you could see through it, so the plastic surgeons would wander round and see what the dentists were up to. And so we had to think of creative names for these rhinoplasties like reposition of superior maxilla, and stuff, we weren't allowed to call it rhinoplasty on the operating list because he didn't want the plastic surgeons looking too closely at what he was up to. But John Bennett, who he was great friends with, was one of the senior

---

86 Professor Tony Bull was an ENT surgeon who ran a rhinoplasty course at the Institute of Laryngology and Otology.

plastic surgeons there. I can still remember one day he wandered in and Banksy and I were doing a rhinoplasty, and it was just a bog standard rhinoplasty and John Bennett wandered into theatre and he looked over his shoulder and he said, 'Oh my god, that's the end, the dentists are doing rhinoplasties. It's the end of the world.' And walked out again. Oh dear.

So he was fun. A very generous host, we'd often go round to his house for dinner and parties, and all sorts of things. Yeah, a great time, a great character.

Andy Brown has been a chairman of the Specialist Advisory Committee in Oral and Maxillofacial Surgery. I asked him to give me his observations on the changes and developments in training that took place during his career.

The changes in training that have occurred can't be separated from how the specialty has expanded its scope and latterly, in the mid '90s, how the specialty flew the dental nest as its primary link and became recognised under the European guidelines as a medically based specialty, with maxillofacial surgery being the medically based specialty and oral surgery remaining as the dental specialty.

I think the European Directives were a big change because we then had to make sure that our training was transportable; that we had parity of training with other European countries so that there was the ability for mobility of labour, which was all part of the wish list of the European Union. So the biggest changes in training came from the mid '90s onwards.

When I was in so-called training, it was very much a classical apprenticeship system of learning. You followed your boss around, or if you were a junior registrar, you followed your senior registrar. You were drip fed things and picked them up on the run as you went, supplementing that by your own personal reading and by attendance at meetings.

The Faculty of Dental Surgery had set up a Speciality Advisory Committee in four dental specialties. I got a certificate of completion of training, which sort of just arrived! I was quite surprised when I suddenly had a letter from the Faculty saying I was going to be awarded my training certificate. I got that towards the end of my training under the dental regulations, but I hadn't had to keep any log books or anything like that.

The training was overseen by the Joint Committee in Higher Training in Dentistry and the method used was to inspect a hospital and to accredit a training unit as being 'fit for purpose'; thereby assuming that everybody who came through that unit would be properly trained! So it was slightly the other way round from assessing the trainee and saying whether they were meeting the targets and being trained properly. Instead, you looked at the unit that trained them and gave your accreditation approval to them.

And so every five years we were inspected and I can remember when I was at Guy's as the senior registrar having to pull out all the facts and figures because the Specialist Advisory Committee was coming round and we all had to try to cook the books and make sure that we were doing enough work to justify continuing the training!

In those days the registrar posts were split between registrar and senior registrar and entrance into senior registrar training, which was tantamount to saying you were going to get a consultant job unless you did something seriously wrong, was by getting the Fellowship of Dental Surgery under your belt and completing a successful time as a registrar with reasonable references.

The only problem then was the manpower planning and making sure that there were enough jobs for enough people, so there were little hiccups, but you did get a job. Actually, once you were a senior registrar, you didn't have to keep a logbook. Many people kept a record of things, but we didn't <u>have</u> to do that. We didn't have annual assessment meetings where we were assessed and looked at and where we had to present the papers we had presented, or the log books that we had, so nobody found any hiccups then. That came in the late '90s and into the 2000s.

I was in the thick of it all at that time as I was chairman of the Speciality Advisory Committee for two years and we had to write down our curriculum in much more detail than we had before. Instead of saying 'Well, what we do is surgery of the mouth and jaws' we had to break it down into a much more detailed, descriptive level of different operations and then classify those operations into areas of difficulty from the routine through to the most difficult; and perhaps select some out to be part of super-specialty training or post-specialty training and things like that. The whole codification took an enormous amount of work, which I remain to be convinced was really worthwhile, although the reasons behind it may have been good.

146

The juggernaut rolled on and it was possible to keep a log book so that, almost by creative accounting, you could tick all the right boxes. We were setting the bar a lot of the time at the lowest common denominator. I still think it was of limited use to go through all this exercise.

The biggest change in training in my specialty has been the move from being dentists with a little of surgical training through to being properly trained surgeons with dental knowledge and accepted and classified as a surgical specialty.

Chapter 13
Kaduna and Elsewhere Overseas

'The Russians are wanting to take over!'

Between the 1960s and 1980s, when some oral and maxillofacial surgeons were expanding their remit, enthusiastic trainees were hungry for new clinical experience. In some areas, particularly cancer, they were competing with other specialties and sometimes with each other for surgical experience. Many went for attachments to hospitals overseas. Like several others, I visited the cancer hospital at Maharagama in Sri Lanka.

The most established arrangement was to Kaduna in northern Nigeria, where for many years the East Grinstead senior registrars went, each for six-month attachments. The maxillofacial unit there had been set up principally to deal with war injuries sustained in the Nigerian civil war, but it continued to function after the ceasefire in 1970.[87] Mike Awty told me how it came about and how he set it up [1968].

One of Sir T's[88] oral house surgeons, an Iranian called Robin Shamiaia, went to work for the Colonial Medical Service in Nigeria. He had been to America and been befriended by a plastic surgeon who taught him quite a lot of soft tissue work, thinking that this lad was going to go back and work in Africa. He was a very good operator and very hardworking, but when the Nigerian Civil war came along, he was just snowed under.

He wrote to Terry to ask him if they could send some help. So Terry approached the government, and they said, 'Well, we'll think about it; go and have a look.' So he went out for two or three days and came back and reported that this would be a good thing to support. And then about a fortnight before Christmas he said to me, 'You better go'.

So I went out and set it up, and an Air Force team came and joined me, and they were very good. It was lucky that the Nigerian Chief

---

87 The war started in 1967 and ceased in 1970 and sought to separate the Igbo people from the Nigerian state into a state of Biafra. Nigeria had ceased to be a colony of Britain in 1963.

88 Sir Terence Ward

Dental Officer had been at Newcastle with Bradlaw[89], so we had immediate rapport and joked about the senior people in British dentistry. The Chief Medical Officer had been sacked as a house physician at Croydon for some reason or other. He quite liked England, despite all that. I was a bit apprehensive when I went because I thought as an ex-colonial power, what will they think? '68 that would have been.

I'd been a consultant for about three years. I reported to Terry that I'd got the premises organised and all the rest of it, so then he sent the Air Force team out. And that was a dentist who was all right, and two nursing sisters, who had been in Aden during the troubles. They were excellent; they worked their butts off and taught me a great deal of soft tissue treatment management. There was an anaesthetist who was an Air Force wing commander (admin), who realised that as he came near retirement he would need to augment his pension, so he re-mustered to anaesthesia and he came out with his golf clubs and did the anaesthetics. There were two technicians, who were a god-send. We set up 70 beds and a good number on the floors.

We collected the patients off a train. That came up at night, because that mad Swedish Count[90] was bombing the railway in the day, if he could, so a hospital train came up at night and tipped all the patients out on the station. I would take the truck down with an excellent vascular surgeon from Canada, who'd been trained in England, and we would sort through what we reckoned we could deal with.

My stuff was often quite major injuries. But of course, if they had survived that long, got back from the front and got loaded onto a train to get up to Kaduna, they weren't in immediate danger because they'd have been dead by now. I was immediately impressed that the more intelligent they were, the more inventive they'd been in managing their survival. A chap who had lost the bottom half of his face had fabricated a feeding cup out of a Golden Syrup tin and taught himself how to drink and feed, and so I admired them enormously. Anyway, we got them all into the theatre.

We had a German hospital which had been built with German aid, and of course it was air-conditioned so that none of the windows would

---

89 Sir Robert Bradlaw. He was then a professor of oral medicine and Dean of the Newcastle dental school and was very influential.
90 Carl Gustaf von Rosen - see his Wikipedia page.

open. The only problem was, the air conditioning didn't work and so it was really quite difficult conditions to work in. We could only have the operating theatre in the afternoon, the general surgeons had it in the morning. There was an excellent Indian general surgeon who had been trained in England. He helped me a bit when I got stuck on things; I was seeing things that I had never seen before, of course.

We gradually developed a work pattern with outpatients' reviews in the morning and operating in the afternoon, all the afternoon. Two X-rays were as much as we could use on anybody, and only if it was absolutely important that we had an X-ray. There was no blood and no fluids. The blood bank had bottles of water, I used to drink one for therapy and two for fluid replacement, after I had operated for five hours or so.

It was very helpful that I'd done my military service to run a military unit, which is virtually what I did. I had to get on side with a staff sergeant or a warrant officer to maintain discipline. The patients with maxillofacial injuries were otherwise fit men, and they were paid on Fridays just like the army in England, so they all went off to the pub or brought beer in; so we had some difficulties on Friday nights. Sometimes I had to run for it if they were all boozed up. I had a bodyguard of two big Tivs[91] at times. Tivs are built like tanks, they're huge men and they had riot sticks and they used to protect me if things got out of hand.

We were so stuck for equipment that we could really barely do two procedures for a chap. Our aim was to give them sufficient function so they could go back in society and survive. Really, it was as bad as that. I had to go down to Lagos and scour the medical warehouses for equipment. There wasn't anything. Dressings and sutures and things were at a premium; we'd use gloves several times. I had a truck down in Lagos that the Boy Scouts gave to the Nigerian Army, which I trundled round in, getting stuff from the warehouses. I put a chap in the back with a gun so it didn't get nicked. It was a learning curve, all right.

I went for a month or six weeks, I think it was supposed to be, and then the government said, 'Oh, you can't come home because the Russians want to take over the medical services.' I would deal with the Nigerian government's permanent civil servant and our ambassador,

---

91 An ethnic group from the north-east of Nigeria.

that was the sort of level we worked at. I sat in the ambassador's place on the seafront and we talked about my going back and he said, 'Oh, now, Michael, we'd better go into the secure room because that trawler out there is listening to our conversation.' A Russian trawler parked in the harbour. So we had to go secure and discuss when I could go back and when Peter Banks, the current senior registrar, would come out and follow me for six months. So that's how it worked. The Russians were trying to take over.

The Canadian surgeon was tremendous; we shared the hotel, such as it was, where we lived. On the first day we came back, I was absolutely exhausted having worked in these conditions, and he said, 'Michael, I did five Syme's amputations today and I haven't done one since I was a registrar in Edinburgh. And I didn't know whether I was going to sleep first or the patient; the ether was everywhere.'

When I came back home I was debriefed by the Overseas Development Organisation and I said, 'Look, the best aid that we can do is to second a chap there to keep it going, otherwise we'll lose face in Nigeria.' So they bought this, with Terry's support, and so we arranged for the Overseas Administration to second people there, and it went on for something like 16 years.

I would send the senior registrars, once they'd been in post for a year, so they were established. I didn't want them to go before because it was easy to get bad habits there with no supervision. So they went and on the whole enjoyed it all and learnt a lot. That gave us great feelings that you could do things way outside your field. I picked through a neck happily after a little while there, for big benign tumours and things. It wasn't worth doing anything about cancer because you couldn't follow it up or do anything. We got the big osseous lesions, you could really improve things and get them out. I used to do that sort of thing when there was a lull in the war.

Robin Shamiaia, the chap who had initiated the whole thing, was still there. He ran the dental centre, and he had some assistance, and they were very busy all the time with dental sepsis. The Army chaps were better, they were much fitter; they were the fittest members of the community really, and of course they paid to join the Army because it was a good regular job. I helped with the dental sepsis when I had time. We worked pretty hard.[92]

John Williams was a senior registrar at Roehampton [1971].

I was the first non-East Grinstead person to go out to Kaduna; there was nobody else to go. The last person who went was Richard Juniper, and Terence Ward had phoned Norman Rowe up and said, 'I want a boy to go to Kaduna, I haven't got one. Have you got one who will go? Tell me by tomorrow morning.' And so Norman phoned me up about ten o'clock at night and said, 'John, I've been phoned by Terry Ward, they want somebody to go to Kaduna to take over the max-fax there. And the promise is that you've an anaesthetist who will also be seconded out who will be a senior registrar from here; it's a six months secondment.'

I turned to Jill and said, 'What do we do about this?' We've got three children, the youngest was one, this was a single unaccompanied appointment and if I went I wasn't going single unaccompanied, we'd have had to pay for it ourselves. And we said, we couldn't do it, I mean it was just impossible. And about half an hour later, we said, 'Wait a minute, aren't we looking at this from the wrong end? Isn't this the biggest opportunity we've ever had in our lives? Yes, right, we'll go for it.' So a fortnight later after I'd spent a fortnight gathering all the instruments and everything I could together and shoving them into boxes labelled, 'X-ray plates, do not expose to light,' and all sorts of things like that to avoid the customs taking half of it, we met up again at the airport. Three children, Jill, I and a load of equipment and off we went to Kaduna.

I went in the last part of my time as a senior registrar and that taught me a heck of a lot about organisation, dealing with management and so on. So that was a very useful six month interlude, and it prepared me very well for having to do what I had to do to start with in Chichester.[93]

When we arrived Richard Juniper hadn't actually left; there were a few days of handover before he went. There was six months of absolutely fascinating work. You were dealing with the things that were gunshot injuries, similar to what we'd been dealing with at the

---

92 For more on the treatment of the war injuries see: Treatment of maxillofacial casualties in the Nigerian civil war. Awty MD, Banks P. Oral Surgery Oral Medicine Oral Pathology. 1971;31(1):4-18.

93 Where he was soon to be appointed as a consultant.

Westminster as cancer cases. And so you were looking at not a cancer case but a trauma case with the same reconstruction problems, but there was only you to do it all.

Most of the injuries I was getting at that stage, at the end of the war, were delayed; late ones coming out of the jungle, wounds crawling with maggots. Actually, it was the sort of broad experience that required you to draw on everything you'd done before in order to give the patients the best chance of success.

It was a fantastic stepping stone to a consultant job. Dealing with the administration, organising the unit, organising staff. I had six trained nurses to look after a 48-bedded ward and theatres, 24 hours a day. I had 40 Nigerian Army conscripts to select from to make into potential nurses, so intelligent, capable people. There were others who were just about fit to clean the latrines. So you had that to organise. And the whole thing was just amazingly good in terms of experience because it was all practical.

Getting your staff paid at the right time on payday was an interesting exercise because all the pay was done at the military hospital on the other side of the town, a couple of miles away. One day I went for lunch and when I came back there were no staff as they'd all disappeared because it was payday. And if they weren't there, they didn't get paid, and you couldn't go later and get it, they had to be there waiting for it.

The only way I could keep running was to go down and exert a greater authority over the officers at the table; you had to adopt a very senior officer position. There wasn't anybody else to do it. I'd say, 'You will pay those men now, immediately,' and they would have to be paid there and then in order that they could get back to work. I insisted on it and fortunately, with using a bit of authority, it worked.

That was a tremendous experience.

An illustration of the level of benign disease that the Kaduna visitors encountered is seen in John's 1973 paper on Fibrous Dysplasia.[94] Trevor Redpath wrote a paper on his experience of mandibular reconstruction at

---

94 Fibrous Dysplastic Lesions of the Jaws in Nigerians. Williams J. Ll. And Faccini J. M. British Journal of Oral Surgery 1973, 11, 118-125.

Kaduna.[95]

Brian Avery [1979].

That was a wonderful time. I was a senior registrar in Canniesburn and as you know the people who went to Kaduna tended to be the senior registrars based on the Queen Victoria, East Grinstead rotation. I got to hear that they had a gap. They didn't have enough people to send one senior registrar every six months, so I asked my bosses if they'd mind if I took six months out and went off to Nigeria. They agreed, so I approached the East Grinstead people and they were only too pleased to have someone.

I went out in December 1979 with my wife. It was a British Government appointment, Technical Aid, and it didn't cost the hospital anything. The Government paid your salary and your superannuation while you were there and they also paid you a very good living allowance, so it was financially very good as well.

We flew out to Nigeria on a British Caledonian flight and arrived in Kano, which is just up the road from Kaduna. It's where all the riots are going on now and where a lot of Christians are being murdered and Kaduna's the same at the moment. We arrived in Kaduna and there was a big hospital there called the Ahmadu Bello Hospital named after a famous Nigerian leader. It was a big hospital with a big max-fax unit. This hospital had been built in 1967 or thereabouts in response to the Biafran war. It was designed to treat injured Nigerians injured in the Biafran war.

When I started operating, I realised that the filtration system in the operating theatres didn't work any longer. The theatre was a design whereby air was sucked in through a central filtration unit on the roof in the middle of the two theatres, then it was pumped out under pressure into the operating theatre. All the doors and windows had gaps under them or round them so that this pressurised air containing all the bugs was pushed out. Unfortunately, not long after the hospital had opened, this central filtration pump had broken down and when I went in 1979, a good many years later, it had not worked for years. Consequently, the gaps under the door provided an intro for dust to come in because there was no pressurised air forcing the air out.

---

95 Mandibular Reconstruction in Nigeria. Redpath T. H. British Journal of Oral Surgery 1971, 9, 85-90.

They had to completely redecorate and clean the theatres whilst I was there. While that was happening, over a period of weeks, because nothing happened quickly in Nigeria, I ended up operating on the ward. That was a very interesting experience because we were always running out of everything, including anaesthetic gases. Doing major surgery on a ward was quite difficult.

This sort of thing happened all the time in Nigeria; they just didn't maintain their machinery. Unfortunately, the leaders of the country had been trained in western countries, in Germany, UK, America, Russia, some of them, and they all came back bursting with the latest technology and ideas. When they became leaders of their hospitals and ministries they would never accept what they thought was second best, they always had to have the latest technological advances. But of course if something broke down and didn't get repaired, then they became just the opposite. They weren't the leading technology they were the worst possible technology you could have. The wards had no anaesthetic gases, ran out of drugs, ran out of everything, but yet they always ran two large cars per ward driven by ward assistants who used to go out and moonlight as taxi drivers with them. To us, they seemed to have their priorities wrong.

However it was great fun, and while I was in Nigeria, I became the medical officer for the rugby club and for the polo club. The Nigerians were fiendish polo players, they really used to go haring around the fields, which were really rock hard sandy ground. They'd go haring around on these ponies, playing with two teams of four in front of a large crowd. Unfortunately, if someone fell off a horse and got a head injury, there wasn't much you could do, and they often rode bare headed. There was no neurosurgical service the nearest one was 1,000 miles away in Lagos. And because they were Muslims and Lagos was Christian, even if they got them down there, they would never get treated, anyway.

So I used to sit there drinking Pimm's and at the end of a chukka saying, 'That was a damn good chukka, don't you think?' That was really my only contribution towards the medical care, it was just being there. Fortunately, I didn't have any serious injuries whilst I was the medical officer.

Mainly I was dealing with tumours, but most of them benign or intermediate tumours like ameloblastomas. The catchment area for this maxillofacial unit in Kaduna extended hundreds of miles. It extended north into Chad and Niger and into the northern part of Nigeria, and patients would come hundreds of miles to seek treatment. Now if they got a malignant lesion, a mouth cancer or a lymphoma, by the time they arrived at the unit they were usually absolutely beyond treatment. So you saw people with myxomas, ameloblastomas, giant cell granulomas, very neglected, but the patients lived.

I can remember a girl of about 20 who arrived. She had an ameloblastoma of her mandible, which extended down to the fourth rib. I asked her how long she had had it and the answer came back 12 years. And it had just grown and grown, untreated.

When I say untreated, all these patients tended to have scars externally on the skin. These were where witch doctors had tried to let out the evil juices by draining it. Of course it had never worked. You'd end up resecting nearly all the mandible. In fact, on two or three occasions I resected the whole of a patient's mandible from condyle to condyle, one massive tumour. No reconstruction, you didn't dare put a tracheostomy in because the nursing staff wouldn't know what to do with a tracheostomy. Sometimes they'd done a tracheostomy and the patients had been fed through a tracheostomy tube. Having said that, you cut out this lady's mandible from condyle to condyle, and the next day she'd be up staggering down the ward and coping very well.

Power cuts occurred nearly every day, and of course they occurred in the dark. I used to do the afternoon stint, which went from 2 to 8 o'clock. It got dark at about 5.00 or 6.00 pm, so the last two or three hours of the operating list were done after dark and the power would go. It happened at every operating list, suddenly everything would go black; the whole of the town was totally black and you couldn't see anything. I'd say to someone, 'Get a torch,' because you'd be in the middle of a major operation. There'd be a lot of cluttering and banging and you'd hear people tutting and then someone would say, 'Can't find it,' or, 'No batteries.' And this happened every day. Then you'd say, 'Go and get the man to put on the emergency generator.' and they'd say, 'He's gone home.' I'd say, 'Go and get him.' Then they'd get him and about half an hour later come back and then they'd say, 'Generator has no petrol.'

I used to go to theatres with an empty petrol can, and I would give one of the orderlies the petrol can and some Nigerian Naira, some money. There was a petrol station just outside the gates of the hospital and I'd send them. They'd come back with petrol, but probably siphoned half of it off for their car. Anyway, they'd put it in and then start up the generator and we'd get light, just enough light for the operating light but no more and you couldn't have the air conditioning on so you'd get very hot. This happened not occasionally, but every day without exception. Having said that, the people there were lovely, they were friendly, and they laughed a lot and they laughed at your jokes and they were very happy people. But it was not a place to run high technology operating theatres.

We got abscesses, but it was mainly odontogenic tumours that we saw. We saw trauma, often the trauma came to us very late. I can remember one little girl who had been hit by a lorry and she had a split right down the middle of her face. It was fortunately not the bones, but she had a soft tissue split from the forehead right down the side of her nose through her upper lip. It was several days old, and it was infected and I spent several hours debriding and sewing that up and she healed up. I think it was about a week before she got to us.

I remember doing a clinic, and there were patients that arrived the night before from hundreds of miles away, and they slept on a mat outside. They all had major problems; we helped most of them, but there were quite a few we couldn't help; bad burns are really difficult to deal with.

On one occasion a chap came and complained of pain in the side of his face. I examined him and arranged an X-ray of his jaw, and to my amazement I couldn't find anything wrong. It was the only patient I could ever recall seeing where there wasn't an obvious large lump or where the pathology wasn't immediately apparent. After a while I realised this patient had temporomandibular joint dysfunction problems and I'd never seen it on the clinics before and I didn't see it again afterwards either. A good example of how you can be caught out.

Remember, I wasn't being trained in oncology, but basically it gave me confidence to do things such as split someone's face open and take out their whole mandible. Resecting a squamous cell carcinoma years later in the UK was not a problem if you can take out the whole mandible from condyle to condyle. So it gave me a degree of confidence in dealing with major problems and also improvising.

Andy Brown [1977].

All the senior registrars at East Grinstead were offered the opportunity - and it was an opportunity you were encouraged not to *refuse, to go to work in Nigeria for six months. That was a great experience because it was 'in at the deep end.' I mean, I hadn't had a proper surgical training in the way that our modern trainees have. So that's really where I was having to open the book and treat cases I'd never seen before, such as massive ameloblastomas and malunited infected fractures.*

That six months was great fun! It was a bit frustrating working in an African situation where things didn't always work. It was also a great test of ingenuity because if you didn't do it there was nobody else around who could do it. You might accuse me of practising on patients, but really that's what you did, and that's what you had to do.

We had 60 to 70 beds to look after, most of the occupants having significant facial pathology. It was largely benign pathology, but it was significant pathology; large fibro-osseous lesions and ameloblastomas, for example. I came back from Nigeria much more confident, having learnt how to dissect tissues better, how to control haemorrhage, how to do all the things that most surgeons learn in their early years of surgical training. These were the sort of things that the plastic surgeons at East Grinstead at that time would have learnt in their early years of surgical training.

So I got my surgical training in a rather rough-and-ready way in Nigeria and came back more confident.

David Vaughan [1980].

I spent ten months at Kaduna; I had a ball there. There was a 100-bedded unit and I suppose I gave full rein to my surgical desires. Curiously, I did cleft, lip and palate, I used to do three or four a week, and when I came back I never did one again. I did a lot of parotid surgery; I did a lot of reconstructive surgery using delto-pectoral flap and forehead flaps, that sort of thing. It was a seminal time for me.

I had big difficulties in settling back to the UK. When you saw the state of the people there and what they were trying to live with, and you saw how cosseted and comfortable people were here, you just began to wonder whether it was worthwhile working here and listening to the people with temporo-mandibular joint pain dysfunction syndromes and stuff like that. So I had a bit of difficulty in readjusting when I came back. But it was a big milestone in my development, there's no question about that.

Having been the one to set up the Kaduna project Mike Awty reflected on his time there.

Nigeria was a game changer really, because I'd got confidence to go right outside our normal boundaries. Dealing with large fibro-osseous lesions in Nigeria, with health tissue around them, gave a very nice dissection field which gave me the courage to deal with it and repair it again.

Having got the experience of dealing with these massive lesions that went well down into the neck, when I came home I went on to do down fractures, Le Fort II osteotomies and debilitating developmental problems with confidence. That confidence came after that I'd been to Nigeria. I didn't feel so constrained as before I went out there. I was frightened to death to begin with but I got more confident.

Nigeria did it for me and I hope that it did it for the senior registrars who went there for 16 years. As time went on there were less gunshot wounds as the war had ended so they treated more pathology. The registrars also gained useful experience from having to run the show.

At Canniesburn Hospital the cancer was all done by the plastic surgeons, so Khursheed Moos arranged overseas cancer experience for his trainees.

Some of our trainees had already had training in cancer surgery elsewhere before coming to us. But we couldn't provide that at Canniesburn so we sought concentrated experience overseas to good units which colleagues and I had inspected ourselves.

A surgeon who was appointed to Monklands District General Hospital in Lanarkshire, Sri Pathmanathan had done quite of lot of surgery for malignancy in Sri Lanka before coming here. He was keen to help us with the training of our senior registrars in that field. I went with him to Sri Lanka and to several other major state cancer units in India where much head and neck surgery was being competently done. We looked at several units, about four to five, and the one in Sri Lanka with Tony Gabriel as the surgeon there was selected. He was an eminent cancer surgeon for head and neck and was keen to take our students, and so several of them went there for six months training.[96]

The only problem was we then had to fill the post at Canniesburn with unpaid locums, so we got senior trainees from the USA. We could

---

96 I was one of them. See: Obituary Anthony Gabriel. British Journal of Oral and Maxillofacial Surgery. 2008 46; P 89.

give them experience in mid-face surgery, cranio-facial trauma and major trauma since we were doing a full range of facial bone surgery in which they had little experience. They came from several major units in the USA, notably North Carolina, Ann Arbor and Dallas, Texas. We timed their arrival with the departure of our senior registrars who were going overseas and we used to find little bits of extra funding from various sources, notably courses when they needed help to travel overseas.

It was a great opportunity to do this, and I was really pleased we managed it. Some went to India; I think Joe McManners went to Ahmedabad, Leo Stassen to the Tata Institute in Mumbai, Peter Ward Booth to Sri Lanka and Brian Avery to Nigeria, and there were others. I can't remember where they all went but there was a steady flow during the 80s and 90s for them to go out. Later some went to the States for shorter periods.

Lawrence Oldham went on a Rotary fellowship to Philadelphia early in his career [1957].

My father was Rotarian, and he said, 'Why don't you apply for a fellowship?' which I did. I sent for all the dental school prospectuses I could get hold of and I looked through and I concluded that the surgical course in Philadelphia was the leading one at the time.

I went on the preparatory year which was designed for those going on as a resident in the States, well I didn't do the residency but I did the preparatory year. We dissected the human body, yet again, and we would work on dogs. We had to break a dog's jaw and have to wire it with an external Risdon incision,[97] and then we could see the dog the next day to see if we'd caused a haematoma. But I was very unhappy with that because I'm a dog person. At home we always had a dog, and I enjoyed looking after and taking it for walks and the personality of a dog was always very attractive to me. So it was very hard to inject a dog and then to cut it open and wire its broken jaw, unpleasant really, I didn't like that but that was how they used to train people in the States.

American postgraduate education is extremely good; they worked

---

97 Submandibular incision described by Risdon who used it for access for temporo-mandibular joint ankylosis surgery. See: Risdon F. Ankylosis of the Temporomandibular Joint. J Am Dent Assoc. 1934; 21: 1933-7.

very hard for the whole course and the reason for that was their futures depended on it. They paid a lot for postgraduate education; they had to finance it themselves and it was a very serious business, nobody played about. It was your life's dedication that counted at that stage and I'd never met this before; English people by and large are fairly laid back.

Later Laurence became a lecturer in oral surgery at Manchester, where there was a very limited surgical repertoire, so he went to Uganda [1965].

I stayed in Manchester till '65 which was five years. At the end of five years I got so bored and nothing was new. I said, 'I'll do a masters,' but the supervision was nil and I made no progress at all and I thought, this is ridiculous, I'm just marking time, wasting.

I went to the British Dental Journal where there was an advertisement which said, 'Ten years surgery experience in two, East Africa, dental surgeon wanted. I thought, that's just what I need, and learn some proper surgery.

It was totally carte blanche and of course the pathology in East Africa is absolutely horrendous and it wasn't long before I realised I was totally out of my depth. So the first thing I did was to get under the general surgical division and the professor was Sir Ian McAdam who I got on with very well; in fact I got on with all the surgeons very well. On the first Saturday morning I was there, I said, 'I'll join the surgical ward round,' and this had never been done before for a dentist to go on a surgical ward round and I showed great interest in all the conditions like Kaposi sarcoma, or the Burkitt tumour.

There were three surgical firms, and I got very close to all three, coupled with the fact that my equivalents were people from the UK; most of them were UK graduates in urology, ENT, plastics and so on. We all formed a very good sub-consultant level working department.

The medical staff committees were the best I've ever been to with McAdam in the chair. He ran the meeting in a way that you got the best out of everybody there was no hierarchy, everybody's contribution was welcome, you were all highly thought of, regardless, and I thrived in this environment enormously.

So I was able to do a whole gamut of stuff. First let's take infections. We had the most horrendous abscesses of the face, Ludwig's, enormous cysts, enormous ameloblastomas and malignancies of all sorts; it was a tremendous opportunity.

The advertisement had said ten years of surgery in two, and that was true. I was there for two years. For the first six months I was just useless; I observed but couldn't do anything. The second six months I was realising what was needed and the second year I actually contributed. I realised how deficient I was in the early stages, having come from a dental background and here was a challenge.

The prof. said to me, 'Is there anything you want?' I said, 'Well I've never been taught to do tracheostomies' so I got one-to-one teaching from a very good professor surgeon. I did the tracheostomy on an ankylosis patient of mine and from then on I could do my own tracheostomies and did them here in Taunton subsequently.

I also had to teach, and I used to go up to Old Mulago Hospital once a week and teach African assistants. They weren't qualified, but they were taking teeth out in clinics and I would have to run my own chair and teach them. Of course this was quite a challenge because extractions on African patients can be very different; they have very dense bone, big teeth, molars particularly could give a lot of problems and I gradually got better at that.

John Cawood went to the USA for a year when he was a senior registrar [1979].

First, I went to Miami, then I visited Seattle where Philip Worthington was an attending surgeon. Prior to that he had been a consultant in north Wales, and by sheer luck there was a vacancy in their programme. So I was fortunate enough to become a resident in Seattle for just about nine months.

Seattle made a huge impression on me and changed my outlook. Their three year training programme was highly structured academically as well as clinically. There was a prolific number of orthognathic cases, up to eight a week over two operating lists.

That was a huge milestone in my career. In those days Seattle was a leading unit in North America, and I worked mainly with Roger West who was a prolific surgeon particularly in orthognathic surgery. So I got a very sound grounding on the principles and practice of orthognathic surgery, and much insight into the orthodontic aspects of it.

Their philosophy was to obtain optimal function and form and involved close cooperation and teamwork with the orthodontists. Treatment took about eighteen months, 12 months pre-surgical orthodontics to level and coordinate the dental arches and 6 months post-surgical orthodontics to finalise the occlusion.

When I first met Roger West in his office, which was bare, I expressed surprise at the lack of a computer or other technical aids. He replied, 'eyeballs are the best computer'. Planning involved deciding the correct position of the maxillary incisor from which the antero-posterior, vertical and transverse relationship of the jaws followed. So I really learnt a lot from Roger and from Bill McNeil, who was the orthodontist, about planning and the surgery.

I got exposed to a lot of visiting lecturers, including Norman Rowe. Seattle attracted a lot of international interest, mainly because of Jim Hooley who was the chair; he had a very high profile, particularly in training and programme learning. Another exceptional individual who made a big impression on me was Michael Cohen, who was a syndromologist. He had edited the new edition of Gorlin's Head and Neck Syndromes, he was a phenomenon.

I really felt the difference between being part of a training programme as compared with just being a service clinician and picking up training as you go along in somewhat apprentice-like fashion and attending courses.

There was no concern about a medical degree, they were not involved in cancer and were highly regarded by the other surgical specialties

The residents in Seattle went to Arnhem in the Netherlands for six months. So I followed on from Seattle to Arnhem for three months, and that was another major milestone in my career.

In Arnhem there were three consultants, Paul Stoelinga and Henk Tideman, maxillofacial surgeons, and Hans de Koomen who was a prosthodontist. They were at a municipal hospital, not a university hospital, but they did a large amount of pre-prosthetic surgery and had an international reputation for it. They were working hand-in-glove with each other. So I learnt a lot about pre-prosthetic surgery.

I visited several units in Germany which were close to Arnhem and that afforded the opportunity to experience oral and maxillofacial surgery as practised in Germany. It seemed to have advantages over the UK. Firstly it had a long history and was therefore well established, it practised the full scope of oral and maxillofacial surgery including plastic surgery, the units were university based and were strong clinically and academically and the possession of a medical and dental degree was obligatory.

On my return to Liverpool, I realised how far behind the UK was clinically, academically, and politically and at that time we remained underdogs surgically.

Mike Davidson spent three months in the USA [1990].

I got sent to the States for three months and from a professional point of view, that was one of the most focussed, useful three months of my senior professional life. I got sent to Cleveland, Ohio, on an exchange with their chief resident. It's something that Mike Corrigan[98] had teed up, and it was excellent.

At Leeds I shared on call with Charles Lansley, the other senior registrar on a one-in-two rota, and he was the first one to do the exchange. The American guy who came across had only been married for a week when he arrived. And sure enough, after three days, he said, 'I can't do this,' and went home. Charles stayed in the States because that had been agreed, and so I was on a one-in-one for three months as senior registrar, and that was pretty tough.

But then the next year I went away for three months to Cleveland, at Case Western, which is the big university in Cleveland, in that part of Ohio. It's a private run medical school, and I was an associate professor/chief resident, and I was licensed to practise in Case Western. That was fascinating because I did a bit of teaching; I got exposed to a lot of temporomandibular joint and orthognathic work and did virtually no dento-alveolar. I learnt a lot about orthognathic surgery and temporo-mandibular joint work and different ways of doing things.

Trauma-wise they shared; oral and maxillofacial surgery took all mandibles and then on a one-in-three basis they shared the middle third facial fractures with either ENT or plastics. The reason for that was that both ENT and plastics had to do some middle third treatment as part of their board exams.

---

98 Consultant oral and maxillofacial surgeon at Leeds.

When I went across to the States, Kath was working and the children were in school. So I went by myself, so I was back being a bachelor working every hour God sent, but also going to the gym, being asked out for meals and being able to go, and exploring the midwest. It was a very formative three months, and I got a lot out of that. I made some good friends out there, which I still have. Prof. Jerry Goldberg took me under his wing a bit, and he introduced me to baseball amongst other things. I went with his dad a couple of times to the baseball matches to watch the Cleveland Indians.

Jerry said he'd got a research project he'd like to do. Would I come back and do it? It was looking at whether one could use hydroxyapatite things on canines to encourage bone transformation in clefts. We had these Beagle dogs, and I surgically created a cleft, and then put hydroxyapatite on the canines, and then at various stages these dogs were sacrificed to see what was happening to the bone. That was all teed up, and I went across for two weeks after I'd been appointed as a consultant, but before I took up the post. I took a couple of weeks leave from Leeds and went across and did it with Gerry. I presented it at a European meeting. I really enjoyed my time, because I like the States.

Chapter 14
Becoming a Consultant

'Out of about 20 applicants six were shortlisted'

In the early days of the National Health Service it was quite usual for consultant appointments to be part time. John Bradley was a house surgeon at St Thomas' where he worked for John Hovell and then the Westminster Hospital with Rupert Sutton Taylor [1958-59].

They were National Health Service consultants, but they did quite substantial private practice; they were both probably half time. Hovell was doing oral maxillofacial surgery, and also orthodontics.

They had their rooms in the Wimpole Street, Harley Street, Hallam Street area. In his private practice Rupert Taylor did nothing else but take out teeth, roots and buried teeth but others, Ben Fickling, for example, he did restorative dentistry in his own private practice. Most of them were very successful in private practice.

I did a job down in Salisbury after Westminster and the two consultants down there, Eric Dalling and Colin Wishart, were both full time National Health Service consultants. They had no private practice at all. This is what you found out into the regions, a majority of consultant dental surgeons, as they were known in those days, were full time in the hospital. Norman Rowe had no private practice.

Mike Bromige was appointed as a house officer at Selly Oak [1960].

This was also a time when all the dental staff in a hospital were paid less than their equivalent medical grades, significantly less, consultants as well. Then within a year or two the salaries were aligned with the medics, and this was immediately evident because every dental consultant went out and bought themselves a new car.

Most of the consultants were actually part time and also ran a practice in Birmingham somewhere. Those that had been appointed pre-war had been honorary appointments, and then they became official salaried appointments after the war. And then other ones were taken in as jobs were created. They were called consultant dental surgeons, and when fellowship became available, they took it.[99]

Consultant appointments were almost always made by a formal procedure involving an advertisement in the British Dental or Medical Journal and an interview by an appointment advisory committee.

There was a representative of the Faculty of Dental Surgery of the Royal College of Surgeons on the committee; he was there to ensure the candidates had received the proper training. There was normally a university representative and someone representing the Regional Health Authority. These would be consultants from outside the principal hospital where the successful candidate would work.

It was also usual for the candidates to be invited for 'trial by sherry' where they were invited for 'drinks' the evening before the interview. They would meet any consultants from the hospital who wanted to speak to them. They then fed back their opinions to the consultant representing the base unit. This was still taking place up to the 1990s since when it became extinct.

The job contracts were held with the Regional Health Authorities rather than individual hospitals, and they normally involved working at more than one if not several hospitals.

Sir Paul Bramley and Gordon Fordyce had explained to me how the honorary consultant system worked before the National Health Service started. Consultants attended the hospital one or two days a week for free and earned their living in their practices outside. Early in the National Health Service it was expected that the consultants would work in a similar pattern and only attend the hospital for a day or two. When Paul Bramley was appointed as a consultant in Plymouth he was only paid a salary for two days a week. He had to find other work to earn a living [1954].

---

99 The first Fellowships in Dental Surgery were granted by examination at the Royal College of Surgeons of England in 1948 soon after the Faculty of Dentistry was formed in 1947 and Edinburgh in 1949. See: Gelbier S. 125 years of developments in dentistry, 1880–2005. Part 5: Dental education, training and qualifications. British Dental Journal, 199, 10 685 - 689. Nov 26 2005. The first candidates to pass were: Norman Rowe, Homer Killey and Tom Battersby, seven candidates took the exam. See Russell Hopkins interview and The Faculty of Dental Surgery of the Royal College of Surgeons of England: An overview of the first 70 years of achievements. Stephens C. Dental Historian 2017; 62(1) 24 - 32.

I was paid for four sessions a week. I put up a brass plate in The Crescent, hoping to start proper specialist referrals. What I did get was dental treatment for the families of colleagues for free. It wasn't a good thing. They said, 'Well, you're a dentist, we know you,' I was doing ordinary dentistry, and I was doing everything that came, but most of it was courtesy work. I would see the private wisdom teeth; that's all I got. I only ever got one private fracture case, that was a publican trying to salve his conscience when he'd beaten up his wife.

Sir Paul also got a job working in the local authority schools' dental service. But he was doing much more than two days a week in the hospital.

Oh, far more, I practically lived in the place.

He needed to persuade the Regional Hospital Board to increase his contract to full time.

Well, they didn't. They thought that would do, that was enough; and I made sure it wasn't enough by giving it the right publicity. I did an immense amount of local lecturing, taking my trade round and saying, 'If you've got cases like this, here's the service,' throughout the South West.

I had a conversation with a man called Carter, who was the chief administrator of the South West Health Authority in Bristol. I set out the figures and turnover and what I was doing, and the work was there and had to be done and it was important work, etc. I needed them to have a look at my contract. He sent back a reply which was totally negative. I showed it to our senior ENT surgeon. He put his arm round my shoulder and said, 'Paul, you realise that anybody who has got a diploma in public medicine after their name is a two-faced twisting bastard.'

It was an encounter outside the children's clinic where he was eating his sandwiches at lunchtime that got results.

On one of my days at the children's clinic, it was in a place called Beaumont House, which was a Local Authority clinic, I saw this young medical officer, Henry Yellowlees. He had Plymouth under his control as well as doing another job centrally in Bristol. He was sitting outside on the concrete steps in the sunshine. And he said, 'How are you getting on, Paul?' I said, 'I'm not. Look, I got this letter you really must get something done about it.' And we had a good chat. And he said, 'I'll see what I can do.'[100]

Following the intervention of Henry Yellowlees, he got a proper maximum part-time contract.[101] On appointment as a consultant in Plymouth, Paul Bramley felt he had been inadequately trained to do the full remit of surgery he wanted to.

I was not trained to do any of the head and neck cancer cutting, nor were any other people at that time, or indeed anything major. I mean you couldn't even cut skin; you could not do because your boss wasn't allowed to do it. He was making his way in this ladder of training, so he spawned trainees, like myself, who were not equipped to do surgery of the skin, full stop.

So what did we do about it? Well, I had the experience of surgery in general.[102] So as soon as I was appointed I regularly took off a fortnight a year to go somewhere else where I could learn a head and neck technique. It might have been to Obwegeser,[103] it might have been to Rupert Sutton Taylor, he worked opposite the side of the river to John Hovell at the Westminster. I even went to John Hovell because he was doing things which nobody else was doing and possibly shouldn't have been doing.[104]

I also went up to Manchester to see the plastic surgeon, Champion, who was doing some jaw joint stuff. The experiences were sometimes very daunting, but usually I thought, 'Look, I could do better than that, you're not so hot as I thought you were.' I learned in a negative sort of way, self-confidence in doing various procedures which I brought into my own practice. At meetings I met others and found out that somebody else such as Roy Whitlock[105] was good on the gunshot wounds because of the troubles in Ireland; we were all trying to learn

---

100 Henry Yellowlees became Chief Medical Officer of The United Kingdom in 1973 and was later knighted.

101 Most 'full time' consultants had a maximum part time contract which was to do the same work as a full time but get 9/11th of full time pay. This entitled them to do private practice. Full time work was considered to be 11 'sessions' each of which was half a day. Saturday morning work was considered normal. However some sessions were usually awarded in lieu of being on-call.

102 He had practised surgery as a volunteer in Africa soon after his medical qualification.

103 In Zurich.

104 John Hovell operated at St Thomas' Hospital.

105 Consultant in Belfast.

from each other. We couldn't learn from one person because there was not one person really trained to do it all. All sorts of people were learning off other people and it was actually a marvellous development.

Gordon Hardman was up in North Wales He really wasn't trained; he'd been through East Grinstead. Terry Ward and company did no real cutting; they made a song and dance about it. He came out untrained, but he had the opportunity, as I had the opportunity, of going into a district general hospital where anything like an oral surgeon was never heard of. They didn't know what sort of animal you were, and you made your way. Gordon went and did quite a lot of major work. I don't know how well he did it, but he did it and he did it with confidence. A lot of people learnt from Gordon, who went to him; Americans particularly went over there because he was bold, he was straightforward, and he just got on with it.

There were a few people like that who were learning, while others at the same time were sitting in posts and doing nothing except wisdom teeth; well, pretty well nothing except wisdom teeth and mandibular fractures. That era in the development of oral surgery was not really understood later on where the system had got gelled. Later fully trained consultants did the stuff and churned out, like any surgical consultant, their own trainees who had had the practice.

By 1954 Gordon Fordyce had been a senior registrar at Hill End and Mount Vernon hospitals for four years.[106] He had risen the ranks quickly, because he didn't do a medical degree. The 'Department of Plastic Surgery and Jaw injuries' was headed by Rainsford Mowlem, the plastic surgeon. The senior dental surgeon (which is what they were called then) was Alexander MacGregor who went on to be the Dean of the Birmingham Dental School. The other consultants were Ben Fickling and Paul Toller; they were all part time as they worked in other hospitals and ran dental practices. The day-to-day work was done by the registrar and senior registrar. Gordon told me how he became a consultant. You couldn't make it up! [1954].

Finally my four years came up, and Alex was still there, and he had a sympathy for people that Ben didn't have. Ben didn't have a sympathetic side, he was so straight. Alex MacGregor used to come on a Friday afternoon, late, and do a quick ward round. Then we were off

---

106 The Hill End unit moved to Mount Vernon in 1953.

to the pub with Alex and played darts and talked about his garden. He was quite an authority on a number of plants and things. Nice fellow, good chap. And he had been to Cambridge as a student when he did his medicine. He was an educated fellow.

And he said to me one day, 'Look, you can't go on being a senior registrar after four years, people won't like it. What I'm sorry to tell you,' he said, 'we have to advertise your job. We don't want another senior registrar to replace you, we would rather if we could appoint you as a senior hospital dental officer.' So I said, 'Well, what does that mean? ' He said, 'Well, you get a little bit of a rise but not an awful lot, but it's better than having to go looking for a job somewhere else, because you're still very young.' But he said, 'Give it a try'. I was about thirty.

I looked at the Journal[107] and there was a job advertised in Scotland, Glasgow or somewhere, to be a consultant. So I thought, why not? So I went up there and by this time I had published two or three bits. Glasgow was very kind and after the interview I was called in. They said, 'Well look, we like what we hear about you, we liked your publications and things, but you're a little bit young to be made a consultant. There would terrible trouble if we did this, but do come back when you're over thirty two.

Then there was another one, Salisbury, and I applied for that and the same thing happened. So I told Alex about it and he said, 'No, no, we're going to advertise it, we'll advertise your job as a senior hospital dental officer and you can carry on doing what you have been doing. That's the way we would like it, let's see if you are appointed.'

I don't know what went on behind the scenes, but I had to go for an interview. And the senior registrar from East Grinstead was up, and he was doubly qualified. Nice enough chap, Gordon Hardman, quite a tough character, then went to work as a consultant in North Wales. He's a well-known fellow. But he didn't get the job. He was a little put out, I think, but not broken-hearted.

I think Alex MacGregor had made sure that the advisors on the committee were sensible people. So I then went back as an senior hospital dental officer until I was of a proper age and then applied for consultant jobs. And the first one I got was at the Royal Free, because

---

107 British Dental Journal.

the Royal Free dentist was singly qualified, so they weren't too fussed that I wasn't doubly qualified.

I applied for the Royal Free and was appointed; it was for two sessions a week. Then I went back to the North West Thames Regional Health Authority and said, 'Look here, I'm a consultant now, can we review my position at Mount Vernon, is there an opportunity to be converted into a consultant there?' So someone said, 'Well, how many sessions is it going to be?' I said, 'Well I've got two at the Royal Free.' And the north-west board treasurer said, 'As long as it's not going to cost us anything, we could offer you six sessions,' and that was done.

Then I was full time. They made sessions at St Alban's and somewhere else so it made it up to full-time consultant. It was working on a part-time basis in each one so I could do a little bit of private practice if I wanted. That was the idea.

Mike Awty was a senior registrar at East Grinstead and became a consultant there, but the move was not straightforward. There was a job coming up in Cardiff [1965].

Sir Terence Ward was trying to get a third consultant at East Grinstead, but it wasn't working out. And so he said, 'You better go somewhere else first.'

We drove down to Cardiff to meet Brian Cooke Dean of the Dental School, who I knew, of course, from Guy's.[108] And the new school was up and they were still fitting it out. I went to talk to Brian, and I put in a declaration of intent. Brian was very enthusiastic and very welcoming. Then you could look out of his window at the new medical school and he said, 'Well, you better go and have a look.' I said, 'Oh, good, I'll take Janet, she's very interested in new architecture.' And he said, 'Oh, no, no, I can't allow that.' And I said, 'Well, what do you mean, Brian, can't allow that? She's very interested in architecture, been around, she's not going to be frightened of the heights or anything.' 'Oh,' he said, 'the men might whistle and that's terribly degrading, it's not right for a woman.'

Mike did get appointed to East Grinstead.

Poor old Ryba, East Grinstead consultant, had a minor stroke, so I was told to put in an application and Ray O'Neil put in an application.

---

108 Brian Cooke had been a reader in oral medicine and pathology at Guy's before being appointed as Dean in Cardiff.

I didn't interview very well, I was a bit strung up for some reason or other. I was appointed, I think it was the devil they knew rather than the devil they didn't.

Russell Hopkins was the successful candidate for the Cardiff job. He had been wasting his time as a senior registrar in Newcastle with Professor Howe [1968].

So I applied for Cardiff; in fact, I applied for three jobs in a week and I was shortlisted at Nottingham and Stoke-on-Trent. I didn't get either of those, and I was shortlisted at Cardiff.

But at that stage he'd been a senior registrar for less than three years. What about College of Surgeons training accreditation?

It didn't exist then. I simply said I'd done medicine. I'd been a senior registrar for this time etc., I was the only doubly qualified chap on the Cardiff shortlist, all the rest were singly qualified. Gordon Hardman, who was a colleague up in North Wales, he was doubly qualified, and was a very strong character. He insisted that this medicine had to contribute to the time I'd spent as a senior registrar and had to be recognised, and so they appointed me. And by the grace of God! Because Cooke didn't want me, Cooke was the Dean. He wanted somebody from Guy's. I started on May 1st, 1968. I was 36.

Mike Bromige considered the job in Cardiff [1968].

I looked at Cardiff, I found the visit quite extraordinary, and being taken under the wing of Professor Cooke. They seemed to be very strange characters. I was warned off it actually by a couple of colleagues down there, friends, who said, 'You don't want this.'

Russell [1968]:

I arrived in Cardiff, a bachelor, to set up and I was appointed as a Consultant in Oral Surgery. That was my title. I had no work programme and no job description; it was simply advertised as a consultant in oral surgery. There'd been a guy there for a year, from Guy's, who'd resigned, and they hadn't been able to fill it, so I'd gone to a job against my previous professor's advice. Professor Howe said I would not get on with the Dean. He said, 'Don't go there', but it was a new hospital, to be the University Hospital. It was a huge hole in the ground with the foundations in and the metal scaffolding going up. I thought to work in a new teaching hospital has got to be a good thing to do. And I think I was right.

The dental school was actually open. That was built first, before the major teaching hospital, and the first lot of dental graduates graduated two months after I got there.

I had an office in the dental teaching hospital, and the oral surgery beds were in the Cardiff Royal Infirmary. There was a senior lecturer who did the teaching and did very little surgery. I had junior house surgeons, who were ostensibly there to look after the bleeding tooth sockets.

Professor Cooke, the dean of the school, regarded consultants, he said, as donkeys and they weren't academically brilliant and therefore they weren't suitable for teaching students. Because of that, when I got there, students weren't allocated to me, I thought this was bizarre. But they came to my clinics, and they saw the sort of work I was doing, which they'd never seen before. Then they came to my operating lists, down at the Infirmary, and watched us doing the stuff. And then they'd come to my clinics, and the numbers came so large that I had to limit them.

The vacant consultant job in Nottingham that Russell didn't get arose because Tom Battersby, who inspired him, had died. Mike Bromige was successful. He had been a senior registrar in Birmingham from 1964 [1968].

There was a glut of jobs in 1968. There was Stoke-on-Trent/Stafford, Bath, Cardiff, Nottingham, and I applied for all four and visited all four. I didn't continue with Stoke and Stafford because there was a very strong contender, Peter Leopard, at that time.

I was actually shortlisted for all jobs, but the Nottingham one was first and I went to Nottingham and got it. Russell Hopkins got the Cardiff job; he had been interviewed with me in Nottingham the month before.

I was appointed in Nottingham, and part of my job was to create a department in Mansfield. It was part time, it wasn't maximum part time, and I queried this and they said, 'That's all that's available.' And it was even stranger than that because the General Hospital was open in Nottingham and my colleague had beds there. The outpatients were in a building down the road detached from the main General Hospital, which had the A&E. But my beds were to be at City Hospital on the plastic ward there. I got on very well with the senior plastic surgeon, Wynn Williams. He was very kind to me and looked after me very well, so there no problems there at all.

I did Mansfield on a two session basis starting up from scratch. They'd had a practitioner going in now and then. When I got there they made some beds available to me and there was an operating list and an outpatient clinic. There were no instruments, so I went and knocked on the door of the hospital secretary who was a splendid man. He said, 'Oh we can't be having that, Mr Bromige,' he said, and he reached for the phone and dialled the Sheffield Regional Hospital Board and said, 'I've got a consultant here with no instruments, what are you going to do about it?' And he looked over and he said, 'How much do you want?' and I said, 'About £5,000 will do.' 'He says £5,000. Yes, thank you very much.' He put the phone down and he said, 'Go and order them,' and that was how it was done. Very efficiently. It was the Sheffield Region at that time and I was employed by the Region, not by the hospital, and all travelling expenses and holiday allowances went through the Region. That changed after a year or two and then I was employed by Nottingham area.

Peter Selwyn was my colleague. He arrived there as a locum for Battersby, because Battersby was ill periodically, he had enormous problems with osteoarthritis in the neck, so he went there as a locum. Then he stayed there and set up a practice and then he went into the hospital as an senior hospital dental officer and was upgraded to consultant the year before I arrived.

Battersby had established a very good clinical practice. I had a lot of things referred to me the moment I arrived that I had only seen and not dealt with in my career. Such as an adenoma at the junction of hard and soft palates that I recall, which I did with a rotational flap based on the palatine arteries. I repaired the soft palate which I was very proud of. And salivary glands, I'd done a few salivary glands. Colin Brady and I had done them behind locked doors in the theatre in Wordsley because a very powerful plastic surgeon called Oliver Mansfield would've hit the roof if he'd known.

Poor Laurence Oldham was a lecturer in Manchester and was desperate to leave [1968].

I came down to Taunton for an interview, having been primed, and I sat in the ante-room at Musgrove Park Hospital. Eventually I went in for an interview and I think because I'd had this East African experience and was therefore attuned to working on my own at quite advanced stuff they said, 'Right, we'll give him the job.'

There were seven or eight people on the interview committee; there were representatives from the university, the hospital and from the College. It was a very big interview. The medical officer of health for Somerset's first question was, 'Tell me Oldham, you're wanting to leave the university to come down here; won't you miss the academic environment and what do you really want out of life?' So I thought for a minute and said, 'Well, to be quite honest in the university, there's a lot of repetitive teaching and I've tired of it. I'd rather get on and do it, do the surgery rather than teach it, and I'm looking for that opportunity.' And somehow that seemed to fire them up and they appointed me.

John Williams got a consultant job in Chichester [1973].

Chichester had been serviced by Norman Rowe and Jim Evans, the plastic surgeon, when they were at Basingstoke, and they used to come down on their trusty motorbike, not frequently but they used to come down and do it. When Rooksdown House Basingstoke moved back to Roehampton, they hadn't got enough space at Roehampton to take the whole of the max-fax side. They knew that there was a desperate need here in Chichester.

One surgeon at Chichester had worked at the London, and so he was very well aware of what the scope of max-fax was because he'd been exposed to Gordon Seward and he'd seen Gordon doing parotidectomies. So the basis was that Chichester was a knowledgeable place that really knew what they were talking about.

When I was asked at interview how I'd organise it. I insisted on a link with the Westminster because of the Westminster background and my interest in oncology. I wanted a link with an oncology centre and I knew that Portsmouth did not have a good reputation for this.

I was appointed in August '73, but I spent six months pretty well getting instruments, organising the instrument trays, getting theatre trained, getting the outpatients setup organised, getting the equipment on board. When I started there was myself, a senior house officer and a technician, no secretary, no nursing, no instruments, nothing. Later I built up a team here with a senior registrar and a registrar.

There was no intensive care unit and so one of the first things that I needed to do was to establish with the cardiologists that I could utilise one of their beds occasionally; they were the only people who had any sort of intensive care facility. I may have used it more than I needed to because it was a policy to make sure that they realised the need for intensive care in Chichester.

I possibly used general anaesthetic more than was necessary from the clinical point of view, but there was a very serious reason behind it, and it worked. It also put our specialty in the front of the physicians so they could see what we were doing. The surgeons saw what I was doing in terms of borrowing beds from the physicians for intensive care, so it was all part of a strategy.

I was trying to make use of what I had to do teaching and getting the senior house officers involved in intensive care and in trauma so that A&E knew that max-fax people were frontline. You called them in the beginning; you didn't wait to have them seen by a general surgeon first. Before I had any of these people, they called me and I used to spend almost every night in casualty in my first seven years here. That was the only way to get over the importance of the specialty and to make sure that we got the trauma I wanted. And that's how we built it.

The first colleague I got was a registrar, about five or six years after I started. The senior registrar, which was the next thing, came almost at the same time as a second consultant and that was seven years after I started. That was a redistribution of a senior registrar in the region, but because of my regional involvement I was in a position, when I was asked about it, to say yes, because I was known and I was there. If I hadn't been, they'd have gone somewhere else. But that was when I got the first extra consultant, John Townend. David McPherson's appointment, which was the next one, was a long way down the line. That was the first real expansion of consultants because until then we were on call one in two and that meant we were one in one on holidays. So for 12 weeks in the year, when you've got two consultants away, whoever was on was on for 12 weeks. Basically, a quarter of the year you were one in one.

It was extremely busy, and there wasn't any time off. You had to do trauma at night, you couldn't fit it into the day, the day was full. I got the registrar to look after Chichester and the senior registrar to look after Worthing, so they had a bit more independence. There they could get on with things without me breathing down their necks all the time. It was good training for them.

John Cawood was a senior registrar in Liverpool and it was difficult to get a consultant job [1979].

In 1979 we got into a pickle because there was no apparent control of the number of senior registrars being appointed. That came to a head when there was an embargo on consultant expansion which affected our specialty.

I was involved together with my colleague Adrian Flower. I was on the Central Manpower Committee,[109] and Harry Alty was involved with the CCHDS.[110] There was a backlog of senior registrars because there were no new posts. Being a relatively young specialty, there weren't the possibilities of many vacancies arising through retirement.

We phoned round all the units in the country to identify how many senior registrars and consultants there were, mainly National Health Service but also honorary, and the age bands of the consultants. Then we did some number crunching, and we realised there was a big problem in manpower imbalance in the specialty. So we wrote a paper on that. Harry Alty wrote to Health Trends,[111] and I wrote to the British Dental Journal.[112] And we had quite a big meeting of the British Association of Oral Surgeons and I presented a paper about the manpower and there was a bit of a rumpus as we realised we had total imbalance.

I presented at the Joint Committee for Higher Training and the then Chief Dental Officer was present, and we put the figures to him. He was duly sympathetic. Ultimately, we got an embargo on any new senior registrar posts and at least a partial solution achieved. Because of this hold up in our training, virtually all senior registrars became time expired, so our contracts were extended on the proviso you applied for every post that came up. So there were quite often fifteen or sixteen senior registrars appearing for interviews. We all got to

---

109 The Central Manpower Committee was formed in 1972 by agreement between the professions and the Department of Health to monitor hospital medical and dental manpower. See: The Work of the Central Manpower Committee for England and Wales: some personal observations. David Brown. British Medical Journal. May 8th 1976.
110 The Central Committee for Hospital Dental Services is a 'craft' committee of the British Dental Association concerned with working conditions for hospital dental staff.
111 Manpower imbalance in oral surgery/oral medicine. Alty HM. Health Trends. 1983 Aug;15(3):64-5.
112 Manpower imbalance in oral surgery. Cawood J. Br Dent J 156, 6 1984. Also see correspondence in subsequent issues.

know each other very well.

John did get a job in Chester [1979].

It was a part time job. When I arrived there were no facilities, no beds, instruments, funding or support staff. However I had good support in building it up from the local consultants and Harry Alty and it did build up. So anything is possible if you have determination and co-operation.

Brian Avery had been a senior registrar in Glasgow for four years and five months [1982].

When I came to apply for a consultant post, it was a very difficult time to get a consultant post. When I applied for the Middlesbrough job, it was the first post that had been advertised in the UK for a calendar year. It was that bad. There were about 20 fully trained senior registrars, which was just over half the senior registrars in the whole UK who were applying for the post. It was a tough time to get a job. In that field of 20, there could well have been almost half of them who were singly qualified. We'd known for some years that the writing was on the wall for only a dental qualification. So these people knew they were near the end. They were going to be last few appointees in the specialty who didn't have a medical degree. They eventually all got posts, but one or two were in post as a senior registrar for about ten years before they were appointed to consultant.

Out of about 20 applicants, six were shortlisted, as I recall. I didn't get the impression that there was any jiggery pokery. They didn't have a senior registrar at Middlesbrough so there was no local candidate and I think it was an open field. They appointed the person who performed best on the day, I suppose, I don't know. The interview was in October '82 and I took up my post in February '83.

I'd applied for a job at Charing Cross Hospital. When I went along for the interview at Charing Cross, I wasn't up to date with all the gossip in London. When I arrived and sat in the waiting room the other candidates said to me, 'Oh you're one favourite for the job'. That was news to me.

I remember we had a trial by sherry the night before whereby we'd met all the other hospital consultants, and we'd actually had an interview with them. We had sat down at a table and they'd pressed us with questions. I got an idea what was going on because I got some very hostile questions that were plainly aimed at me. I remember one anaesthetist said to me, 'Now what's the paper you've done about clomethiazole, what is clomethiazole anyway?' And I said, 'Heminevrin.' I was a bit shocked by the question and there was silence and a few titters, I mean this anaesthetist didn't actually know what the correct name for Heminevrin was. So I detected hostility towards me.

The next day I was interviewed and again quite a difficult interview, but they didn't appoint anyone. Apparently there was a huge row which went on, in the appointment committee, because there was a local candidate who applied for the job; the incumbent consultant wanted him to take up the post. These huge rows occurred and I don't know what all went on in the background, but a lot of authorities got involved. I have to say that Charing Cross failed to thrive in subsequent years.

Tony Markus was a senior registrar and looking for a consultant job at the same time as Brian [1982].

There were 28 senior registrars, and there was a terrific shortage of jobs. There'd been an expansion of consultant posts in the '70s, then a terrific number of senior registrars were appointed without a view to the future. So we got caught in it.

I had a couple of interviews. There was the one for Luton, which I didn't get, but I subconsciously didn't want it, and I made a mess of the interview. I went for one in Manchester; I was told to go for Manchester. I got up there and I got straight back on the train and rang them up and said I'm sorry I want to withdraw my application, didn't like Manchester.

I'd also gone for one on the Isle of Wight, which was horrendous really, and then didn't get shortlisted for it. It was half senior dental officer, half consultant. I remember driving back from Southampton or Portsmouth, having got the ferry back and driving back across Richmond Park to Kew where I lived and thinking what the hell do I want to live on an island like that for? I remember not being shortlisted; I was insulted.

It was a bit of a club really, 28 of us going around. And then I went for the Poole job. Winston Peters, who had been appointed as the second consultant to the unit in 1979, decided he would survey the available senior registrars. So he gave people one week locums. I did a locum in November. I arrived for my week, some people did two, but I did a week, and on the Wednesday night Winston invited me to his house for dinner and drinks. And I'm pleased to say I behaved myself.

Then the next day a patient came in who had been knocked off his bicycle, a 50-year-old man in Weymouth. He came in with a bandage around his head and an airway coming out through the bandage, with multiple panfacial injuries. This was about six o'clock in the evening. So we took him to the theatre, and I did a tracheostomy first, without extending his neck. Then I took the bandage off, at which point his left eyeball fell out onto his midface and there was basically no midface at all. The skin was intact but a complete skeletal mess up.

I called the eye surgeon in, who exenterated it, and I spent the rest of the evening trying to sort him out, putting back; not reconstructing, but at least make him liveable. Anyway, he did very well. I did my week and subsequently I was told that it may well have been that that got me the job, my management of that patient. But I got the job fortunately, because the next job up was Birmingham, which Bernie Speculand had got, and I was delighted I didn't have to go there.

Andy Brown had things easier; he was a senior registrar at East Grinstead [1981].

I was delighted that towards the end of my senior registrar career, Mike Awty and Peter Banks asked me one day after work whether I would be interested in joining them if they created a job in East Grinstead. I remember walking home slightly on cloud nine and saying to my wife, 'I think I've just been offered a job at East Grinstead!' I hadn't seen that coming because consultant expansion was very slow in those days. And my appointment was delayed by at least a year from when they intended while they were fighting with the Regional Health Authority, who held the contracts to try to create the job.

David Vaughan was a senior registrar at East Grinstead in a job that rotated with King's. He was committed to cancer surgery [1982].

I realised then that I needed to go to a place which was undeveloped in head and neck cancer surgery but had a big population. So it had to be a city, and I wasn't bothered by which, and the first job that came up was Liverpool.

I was a senior registrar at East Grinstead then I came up here, Liverpool. The reason I came here, it was the first job that was advertised, and I had seen Oldrich Pospisil[113] in action at one of the British Association of Oral Surgeons meetings. It was in Guildford, and Pospisil gave this crazy, outrageous lecture on cranio-facial trauma, and I was genuinely impressed. It was very much like what Tiger Wilson had done to me in the pub, there in Acton's Hotel many years before. I thought Christ Almighty; I didn't know maxillofacial surgeons were up to this sort of thing. Now how much of it Pospisil had done or not, I don't know. But he came up to me after the meeting, he said, 'I believe you're looking for a job.' And I said, 'Well, I will be.' And he said, 'Come to Liverpool.' I knew nothing about Liverpool, apart from the football team. But it was the first job advertised, and I applied for it and I got it.

In 1985 John Gibson, the consultant in Chepstow, retired; Adrian Sugar was the senior registrar in Cardiff and ready for a consultant job, he was appointed. He had earlier spent two years as senior registrar at Chepstow [1985].

For the last year or two as a senior registrar, I was well ready to be a consultant. I was already taking a lot of the responsibility, that wasn't a problem for me. I always warn people of the gulf, one day you're a registrar and you're operating on patients under someone else's name, and the next day you're responsible for the whole department, every patient who's treated in it, and the buck stops with you. It's a big gulf, but I didn't find it much of a gulf because I was perhaps over-ready, I even had one or two words or arguments with Russell and I realised afterwards that it was just my tetchiness. It was an indication that I'd finished my training; I needed to go. Many colleagues of our generation have commented on the paucity of consultant posts at that time and the bulge of around 20 accredited senior registrars. I believe those were the numbers when I applied for the Chepstow post after John Gibson retired.

Because I was going to Chepstow, I had a very good idea of what I needed to do there, what my targets were, and there were some fairly challenging things. I also knew that when I was appointed, Max Gregory[114] had seen one of the plastic surgeons and said, 'Adrian's appointed now and whether you like it or not, neither of us will take

---

113 Consultant in Liverpool.
114 Formerly senior registrar on the same rotation and subsequently consultant at Newport.

any nonsense anymore, and I think you should think about that.'

When I started my job in Chepstow, one thing that I missed was a father figure to go to for advice. Not because I couldn't get advice from Russell Hopkins, but the sort of cases I was treating up there were cleft and congenital deformity in children, and that was very much outside Russell's experience.

But I knew Khursheed Moos well, and when I had to ask for advice, I often would have to ring him. No matter how late I rang, it was always too early, and so if I'd ring at half-past eleven at night and ask Kate if Khursheed was at home, she would laugh and say, 'Don't be silly Adrian, you know him.' So, I would often end up speaking to him in the early hours of the morning and always got good advice, and it was really nice to have somebody that I could trust and that I could ask, even though I'd never worked for him.

The irony was that some years later I started doing cranio-facial implants for ears etc, and Khursheed came on one of the first courses that we ran, and after then I used to often get phone calls late at night asking me for advice. I felt especially privileged to be asked for it from Khursheed, for whom I have the hugest respect for everything that he's done for our specialty, and everything he's contributed to me. I remember when he was retiring, the late Barrie Evans[115] who was a good friend, saying to me he didn't think that Khursheed was valued enough in the specialty. Nobody would ever replace the fantastic advice that he gave to so many of us, and for which we were so grateful.

I had an interesting lunch about six months before I was appointed, with John Gibson and he said 'When you get your consultant post, Adrian, what are you going to do about all this huge amount of dento-alveolar surgery that we get coming in?' And of course, his question itself was quite informative because he obviously had decided that he knew what I would want to do and he knew that I would not be spending the rest of my working life treating dento-alveolar cases; he just knew that from the way I was. I said, 'Well, I think 'ninety-nine percent of dento-alveolar cases can be managed, either under local anaesthetic or a local and sedation or as day stays. And my only exceptions are normally those with major comorbidities who might

---

115 The late Barrie Evans had been a registrar in Cardiff and subsequently consultant in Southampton. Much admired and now sadly missed.

need a hospital overnight stay. And my first job as a consultant will be to make sure that I create those facilities.'

My first two years in Chepstow were spent persuading the health authorities' planning department that we had to have a major expansion to the outpatients. I won that battle, and they gave us about £50,000 to do a refurbishment.

Initially, I only had two morning lists, and that was very difficult because I couldn't get a bi-max[116] through in the morning. Now I do a bi-max in a morning, but at the time I wasn't quick enough. Nevertheless, I started doing that, and then there was the cleft stuff and I still did pre-prosthetic cases and I was doing cranio-facial implants for ears.

Ian Martin has considerable frustration applying for consultants jobs [1989 - 1993].

When I had been senior registrar at East Grinstead for eight months, a consultant job came up at Liverpool. I would really have dearly loved to have gone to Liverpool, but I'd only done about eight months as a senior registrar. That job went to James Brown. There was a vacancy at East Grinstead. I loved East Grinstead and I would have loved to have stayed there, but I wanted to do cancer, and Andy Brown wanted to do cancer.

I spent about between eighteen and twenty months as a senior registrar; I avoided going to the King's side of the rotation. Then two jobs came up, but I still wasn't accredited. One was in Stoke and one was in Sunderland. And Peter Banks was chairman of the Specialist Advisory Committee[117]. Ken Ray was the Dean of the faculty.[118] Peter Leopard was pally with Peter Banks, and they'd obviously talked and they wanted a head and neck cancer surgeon who was microvascular trained to take things forward in Stoke.

So I was invited up and wined and dined by Peter Leopard and his wife. And the interview dates were set, and Sunderland's interview date was before the Stoke one. So Peter Leopard said, 'Oh, we've got to do something about that.' So he then changed the interview date for

---

116 Bi-maxillary osteotomies.

117 The Specialist Advisory Committee in Oral and Maxillofacial Surgery, an intercollegiate committee which advised the Royal Colleges of Surgeons on training in Oral and Maxillofacial Surgery.

118 Faculty of Dental Surgery of the Royal College of Surgeons of England.

Stoke to be ahead of the Sunderland interview date as he was keen for me to go there. And he sorted out with Ken Ray that it would be all right, there would be no sanction applied by the College if I was appointed without a certificate of accreditation, they'd give me a certificate even though I'd only done eighteen months or twenty months. I think you were supposed to do four or five years as a senior registrar, or something to get your stupid accreditation. Anyway, so that was me sorted.

Come the day, it all looked like it was going to go fine. David Vaughan had been appointed as the College assessor and Peter Leopard was there. There were three of us being interviewed.

However, I was due to go on a sailing holiday in Greece, and I was the only one with a Royal Yachting Association skipper's ticket, and we were going with another couple. I was entitled to skipper this yacht, which was a forty footer around the Greek islands. But nobody else had the ticket. Peter Leopard was very keen on me going to Stoke, even though it meant I couldn't go on my holiday. So Diane, with a young baby in tow, went with this other couple. But they had to hire a skipper to sail the boat round the Greek islands because none of them were qualified to do it.

I turned up for this interview. The first candidate was interviewed and then there was a long pause, and then I was taken in and told that I couldn't be interviewed because I wasn't accredited. And Vaughany was making gestures, because I was about to explode because, I'd only gone to this because Peter Leopard had as near as you could promised the job, and made me drop my holiday and change the dates to put it ahead of Sunderland.

I'd obviously lost money out of not having my holiday. So the British Medical Association, on my behalf, took West Midlands Regional Health Authority, or threatened them with legal action. They settled out of court, and they gave me about two grand, I think in compensation for having lost my holiday, and my being refused an interview.

So then a couple of weeks later, I was interviewed for the Sunderland job. And the College advisor then was John Lowry. I said, 'Look, I just want to make things clear, if I'm appointed', and I was the only applicant, 'if I'm appointed to this post I want you to give me an absolute assurance that I will not have sanctions applied to me by the

Faculty.' And he said, 'Oh, yeah, yeah, yeah. No, it's all been sorted, we will give you a retrospective certificate of accreditation to coincide with your start date.' So I was interviewed in October of '92 and appointed. But the agreement was, so it looked vaguely respectable, that I'd do twenty months as a senior registrar.

Ian Martin took up his consultant post in Sunderland in April 1993

And it was just Leo Stassen and me, so it was one in two on call. The deal was I was going to do all the cancer, and he was going to do all the facial deformity, and he was still doing clefts.

The first week I got up there, there was a case that had been sent over from Carlisle that had failed radiotherapy for a tonsillar/tongue base tumour. He had a big hole in the neck, a recurrent tumour, and a necrotic mandible; it was a right mess. And this was reminiscent of my first day in East Grinstead when I'd gone in and done the lat. dorsi,[119] and it was a sort of test case for the new boy.

I'd looked at this hole in his neck, horrible tissues, recurrent tumour, radio necrotic mandible. So I did a composite radial, to play reasonably safe, and put some bone and soft tissue on the inside, and then a pectoralis major[120] on the outside. And, thank the Lord, it went well. I think those are the kind of defining moments that you either sink or swim, and if that had gone badly, and it could have easily gone badly, my life in Sunderland would have been a bit different. Because of that, I didn't have any hassle from anaesthetists and people, and I got on and did a lot of head and neck cancer, and microvascular stuff.

Peter Ward Booth[121] had done microvascular reconstruction there, but they didn't have proper equipment, I mean he was trying to do it with some crappy old ENT microscope. And the first thing I said was, 'Look, you've got to give me the tools for the job, so I want a proper set of microvascular instruments, a proper microscope, and a proper microvascular chair.' In fairness to Sunderland, they gave me that, so I had the tools for the job.

At the time there were just the two of us. There was one senior registrar on loan or whatever you'd call it, from Ireland, which was Duncan Sleeman and then a couple of housemen, and a senior house

---

119 Latissimus dorsi flap for reconstruction.
120 Pectoralis major flap for reconstruction.
121 Previous consultant in Sunderland had left to become a professor in Bristol.

officer. There were no registrars behind us. So it really was quite a shoestring operation, you were doing a lot of the stuff yourself. About nine months in from there, we were in the position of appointing a third consultant.

There was so much work in Sunderland. We had a catchment of a million with a high incidence of industrial disease and all the stuff that goes with that. A high incidence of smoke and alcohol, etc. so four times the national average of cancer; there was loads of head and neck cancer. There was an ENT guy who did the ENT head and neck stuff predominantly, and myself, and we were sub-specialising in that.

There was no plastic surgery, which was good. ENT and I worked well together. Over the years we developed a fairly strong multi-disciplinary head and neck team. We had good radiotherapists who were very pro surgery. So we created a good quality cancer team and eventually were joined by other team members and the unit expanded. It was a very stable environment. Because it was a district hospital, which didn't have cardiothoracic, it didn't have neurosurgery, so we were relatively big players covering the catchment of a million with our own dedicated operating theatres. It was a good place to work.

Chapter 15
The Battle for Cancer

'There were seven plastic surgeons in the viewing gallery'

By the 1950s, the surgical management of head and neck cancer had not progressed beyond excision, prosthetic replacement and local flap reconstruction. Most patients were primarily treated with radiotherapy. I can remember as a Houseman in the 1970s taking impressions for the dental technician to make protective lead-lined prostheses for patients to wear when they were having interstitial radiotherapy with radium needles for cancers of the tongue. Oncology as a discipline was in its infancy, and radiotherapy was given by 'radiotherapists' who had their own operating lists to insert radium needles and caesium implants.

By treating oral cancer primarily with radiotherapy, surgery might be avoided. Before antibiotics, it was considered dangerous to operate simultaneously in the mouth and neck due to the risk of spreading sepsis. Surgery was not an attractive occupation as it was usually done after radiotherapy, so soft tissues were very slow to heal, with patients often in hospital for weeks as their wounds were breaking down. Osteoradionecrosis was common and would have been even more prevalent if whole hemi-mandibles were not frequently removed.[122]

Before axial pattern flaps, particularly the delto-pectoral and forehead flaps, were used in the 1960s, tube pedicles were needed for extensive soft tissue replacement. In the 1970s, the pectoralis major myocutaneous flap replaced the delto-pectoral as it was a one stage procedure. Free tissue transfer did not take off until the late 1970s and early 1980s, when the radial forearm flap replaced the pectoralis major as the workhorse for floor of mouth reconstruction.

Furthermore, the 'dentists' were not involved in the surgery. Indeed, Terence Ward at East Grinstead wrote:

'In my opinion, the definitive treatment of malignancy is not in the

---

122 For an historical review of the early management of head and neck cancer see: Head and neck cancer and its treatment: historical review. M McGurk, NM Goodger. British Journal of Oral and Maxillofacial Surgery 2000 38. 209 - 220.

field of the dental surgeon.'[123]

John Bradley was a senior house officer at the Westminster Hospital in 1959 and later as a registrar soon after the department merged with that at Roehampton and subsequently as senior registrar until he left to take up his consultant job in Burnley and Bury. He described the role of the 'Dental Department' in the management of cancer [1959-69].

Mostly cancer was dealt with by doing a biopsy, then they went to the radiotherapists. The rationale was that they had radiotherapy, then an operation to remove the tumour as best you could. We made shields and appliances to carry radium needles, which we implanted into them wearing rubber lead-lined gloves and standing behind lead blocks.

Westminster was a major cancer hospital and the top surgeon was Sir Stanford Cade, a man full of energy and enthusiasm.[124] *He was quite small in stature but had a commanding presence. I used to assist Cade when he was resecting part of an upper jaw for a malignant tumour, and my job was to fit a prosthesis to cover or fill the hole left.*

Looking back on it, it wasn't terribly successful. Mind you, the survival rate of oral cancer is still pretty grim. The main difference is that the quality of life these poor people have is vastly improved from what they had 40 years ago. Basically, they were left with a big hole and then we at the dental department came in and made them a prosthesis. We were making obturators frequently.

Russell Hopkins was a senior house officer in Nottingham [1969].

In those days we'd make a diagnosis, do the biopsy, and then we'd refer it to ENT. Tom Battersby would chop off various superficial cancers; we used to excise precancerous lesions. I don't remember Tom doing resections for cancer.

Gordon Fordyce was a senior registrar at Hill End and at Mount Vernon when the unit moved there in 1953. He became a consultant there in 1958. Mount Vernon was the regional radiotherapy unit.

As far as cancer was concerned, when we got to Mount Vernon, we were the junior people. The radiotherapy department was linked with

---

123 See: Annals of the Royal College of Surgeons of England. 1967 Summer; 41(Suppl): 128–131.

124 Sir Stanford Cade was a pioneer in the combination of surgery and radium for cancer management. See his Wikipedia page.

the Middlesex Hospital staff-wise and was seeing a lot. I became friendly with the senior chap, Paul Strickland. Paul would ring me up and say, 'Come and see this,' and I would go and see what he had and we discussed cases. I knew more about oral pathology than Paul did, which he found interesting and was helpful to both of us. We had a joint clinic for years, once every two months or so; students and others would come along and we would discuss oral malignancy.

I only operated on two or three patients for oro-facial malignancy by myself, as being the principal operator. Dick Dawson[125] would come and do a bit. Because of Mount Vernon, its name meant that we were being sent patients with oral malignancies. Nobody wanted it; it wasn't a popular thing to do from the point of view of the operator.

We were interested in osteoradionecrosis because Mowlem ended up with people with half a mandible left and he would use his skin grafting techniques to reconstruct them.[126]

Mike Davidson was a resident house surgeon at the London Hospital [1976]. What cancer was being done in oral surgery?

I saw little or none. Gordon Seward would do some things such as a resection, a radical neck dissection, and if a reconstruction was done, a delto-pectoral flap or pectoralis flap. Sometimes they would use split skin grafts for partial glossectomies. Patrick James did the odd one, but not Hugh Cannell or Terry English.

There was some done there when I was a houseman because John Langdon was a senior registrar there. That was when he got into all the trouble about publishing the results and not getting full permission, and that really upset Gordon Seward. But I was very junior, so it was only something I was vaguely aware of.[127]

John Langdon confirmed the paper wasn't appreciated.

There was a big row. The paper was written by me, Alexis Rapidis and Newell Johnson. It was a retrospective study; we traced 200 of Gordon Seward's patients and we analysed this and wrote the paper.

---

125 Plastic surgeon.

126 Rainsford Mowlem had been the senior plastic surgeon at Hill End and after the unit moved to Mount Vernon in 1953. Dickie Dawson had been his senior registrar.

127 Oral Cancer: The Behaviour and Response to Treatment of 194 Cases. J D Langdon, P W Harvey, A D Rapidis, M F Patel, N W Johnson, R Hopps. J Maxillofacial Surgery 1977 Nov;5(4):221-37.

We, rather naively, didn't really consult Gordon Seward very much about it. He took exception to it when it was published because he thought it showed him in a bad light. In fact, it didn't in the least. The figures aren't that different to what they are today. 50% get recurrence and 50% survive five years.

The overall five-year survival, not corrected for age and sex, was 32.8% and the overall uncorrected five years survival for females was 42.1%. John:

Well, remember the papers you read these days are all corrected figures Kaplan-Meier calculations, these were all raw figures. Anyway nearly all Gordon Seward's cases were after failed radiotherapy.

Were there joint clinics with radiotherapists? Mike:

As a resident you weren't part of that, so I don't know, we didn't go to any; I think it was almost on an as need basis. So, at the London there may have been something, but at my low place down the pecking order, you weren't involved. When I got to Brighton, there was a joint cancer clinic, and Richard Juniper encouraged the senior house officer to go. ENT were at that clinic with the oncologists, but the plastics weren't.

ENT surgeons were doing the cancer surgery, but again it was a pectoralis major if they did anything. They did the odd maxillectomy, the obturator was often asked for after the event. They would just let you know, 'oh, by the way'. That was just poor, the way any prosthesis wasn't thought about, they would just put something in a hole and let you know.

Most of the cancer surgery was done by ENT surgeons as they had a presence in most hospitals. Plastic surgeons were fewer and in a limited number of hospitals. The standard operation for an oral cancer was the 'commando' operation, so called because the tumour was attacked from two directions, the mouth and the neck. Crile had described the neck dissection at the beginning of the century.[128]

Ian Martin graduated at King's College Dental school and after a house

---

128 For the account of how George Washington Crile observed that mouth cancers recurred in the neck and devised the radical neck dissection (after clamping the carotid artery!) see: George Crile: an autobiography with sidelights by Grace Crile. 2 volumes. Lippincott 1947 (in Royal Society Medicine library).

job became a senior house officer in oral surgery [1981].

All the head and neck cancer at King's was done by ENT; we did nothing like that. It made me realise just how bloody awful some surgical procedures for head and neck cancer were. Essentially, if you had a cancer of your tongue or floor of mouth, your average ENT operation was the commando procedure. They did a radical neck dissection, took the jawbone out, half the tongue, stuck it in the bin and stitched it together. And then you probably had radiotherapy as well. And the patients had dry mouths, half their tongues stitched to their cheek over no jaw with a chin point way over here, and a scrawny neck, and it was bloody awful and difficult.

We made these very odd acrylic dentures. If you were lucky, you might get a canine on one side, and the rest of it would just be a sort of flange that sat on a groove of soft tissue, bouncing up and down. Retention was poor because there was no saliva. And we made obturators for maxillary defects, which were all horrible and gungy, and nasty.

I saw no pectoralis major flaps at King's. They were just, essentially, chopping stuff out. Some delto-pectoral flaps were done, but I don't recall ever seeing a one used inside the mouth. They just stitched stuff together. But if they had to take a bit of skin off as well, they would use a delto-pectoral flap.

Adrian Sugar was a registrar in Teesside [1972 - 76].

We would go to the joint head and neck cancer clinic which was held in another hospital which had the radiotherapy department; we'd do a joint clinic with ENT and with radiotherapy.

We sometimes got involved in some of the surgery, but not very often. Often ENT would do the major resections, though of course, as with most ENT setups, they had not much of an understanding about reconstruction. Resections yes, but reconstructions no; and I'm talking about soft tissues as well as hard tissues. In the '70s and the '80s there really were no hard tissue flaps that had a blood supply. I suppose, in some places, what would they have been using in the '70s? Forehead flaps maybe, maybe delto-pectorals, but I never saw those when I was in that job in Teesside.

By the 1970s there was some limited involvement of the 'oral surgeons' in surgery for cancer, other than biopsies and getting their juniors to do prosthetics. Like most advances in the specialty this occurred in smaller district hospitals. Khursheed Moos became a consultant in Warwick [1969].

The general surgeons there would ask me what I thought, or could I help with doing their cancer cases? I said I had no experience of doing 'necks' or anything like that, but I would be reasonably happy to do resections and that type of surgery. I did some of those with them for the first time.

Laurence Oldham was the single consultant in Taunton for 11 years before he was joined by a colleague, John Hamlyn [1975].

Then we increased the scope, and we used to treat our own malignancy patients, which was quite a breakthrough. Then we decided we needed a multi-disciplinary clinic with ENT and oral surgery and we'd got to do it properly; so radiotherapy came down from Bristol and we had a tripartite arrangement, oral surgery, ENT and radiotherapy.

Russell Hopkins became a consultant in Cardiff [1968].

I started doing tongues, soft tissue tumours, alveolar cancers, maxillary resections, and putting obturators in.

John Bowerman at Roehampton described a kit of titanium metal, which they used to put in to replace the gap.[129] I gave a paper in which I described a series of 12, where I'd put in 12 implants and taken 12 out as they had ulcerated through the skin. I pointed out that this was an appliance that didn't work. It strained our friendship for a bit, but I think we got over it. It was being sold as the kit. I said at best it's a temporary space holding thing before you put the bone in. So then I started putting ribs and iliac crests in. I did three types of bone grafts for resections. Some which worked very well, some which didn't.

At this time, which would have been the late 1960s, early 1970s, did your patients have radiotherapy first?

No, I used to get them first and send them for radiotherapy afterwards. I did combined clinics with the ENT people, so I used to turn up for the clinic and bring my patients to see Mike Henk, who was a radiotherapist. I didn't bring them for the ENT boys, unless they

---

129 See: A universal kit in titanium for immediate replacement of the resected mandible. Bowerman J and Conroy B. British Journal of Oral Surgery 1968 6, 223 - 228

needed a full block, I kept out of full blocks. I didn't feel I was competent; I hadn't had the training, so I didn't do that. A friend of mine, Iloa Griffiths did them, and supra-hyoid blocks when I couldn't feel any nodes anywhere else. I'm not aware that they've developed nodes lower down in the chain with the supra-hyoid block, but I didn't follow them up for 50 years.

We put the obturators in with skin on, I always grafted the cavity for the maxilla. Then they went to Derek Stafford, who made the obturator.[130] He did all the facial obturation.

There was a lot of oral cancer around, because people smoked and drank a lot. But it mostly went to ENT people and the plastics. I don't think they made such a great job of it. Quite often they'd let the jaw swing, and they'd end up with disfigurement. They wouldn't end up with a sulcus that enabled them to wear dentures; they couldn't wear anything. They'd fill the hole, but the quality of life afterwards was not much good. Now, I don't claim that what I did compared with what goes on today was great, but it was better than what was going on then. And patients were rehabilitated, I think, much more so at that stage.

I did tongues, and I used to swing the frontal forehead flap down over the zygomatic arch or under it, into the mouth to line the tongue. I used to swing the naso-labial flap into there. I did local flaps rather than graft the forehead, in the approved manner, and I did that all on my own because there was no assistance from elsewhere. But later that got taken over by microvascular repairs, which was good.

Mike Bromige became a consultant in Nottingham at around the same time [from 1968 and early 1970s].

I did a lot because I had a good relationship for most of the time with the plastic surgeon who was appointed, Malcolm Dean. We had a combined list where we used to operate together. And by together I mean that by and large I would share the soft tissue work, both the approach and the repair, and do most of the hard tissue work on resections. There was another consultant appointed later in about 1980, I guess, who brought microvascular surgery and free flaps, and I used to work with them in the early stages of doing free flap work. The microscope work was done by this new consultant and Malcolm

---

130 Honorary consultant and senior lecturer and subsequently professor of prosthetic dentistry at Cardiff dental hospital.

and I used to do the excision and then hand over and he'd do the repair.[131] So I did a fair amount, but I got fairly disenchanted with it and from the mid '80s onwards I did less and less.

Why did you become disenchanted?

I saw a lot of major resections not working in terms of survival afterwards and being left pretty moribund. But it improved of course once the free flaps came in. And also my senior registrar got deeply involved, and I let him work with Malcolm Dean rather than me. Then a certain amount was done by the new consultants, Sheila Fisher, to begin with and then Mark McGurk. That's been continued of course by the present consultants in Nottingham, McVicar and Rowson.

John Williams participated in cancer surgery as a registrar at Roehampton and Westminster Hospitals and a year later as senior registrar. The cancer was mostly done at the Westminster. John described how he got involved [1969].

Stanley Lee was the senior of the surgeons, and Charlie Westbury was the junior of the two. Stanley Lee, when he was doing private work, would almost always come to one of us on the max-fax side because we were prepared to help him, and so you did one-to-one work with him. He was doing the work because it was private patients, but you were learning huge amounts by working with him, and then working with Gerald Westbury; but he was always known as Charlie.

We had these joint operating sessions on a Monday morning and I would get in there early and almost always get the skin grafts whipped off with the plastic boy who was there; we would work as a pair. There wasn't a permanent plastic surgeon. Ian Wilson, who was there was only there by invitation for these occasions. He wasn't on the staff at the Westminster, so he didn't have a senior registrar; so when he went, the only person left behind with any experience would be ourselves.

---

131 Free radial forearm flaps were developed in China in the 1970s and were used initially for burn contractures in the neck. They were subsequently used for cancer reconstruction. The plastic surgeons at Glasgow pioneered their use in the UK in the 1980s. See: A brief history of vascularized free flaps in the oral and maxillofacial region. Steel BJ., Cope MR. Journal of Oral and Maxillofacial Surgery 2015 April 73(4) 786 e1-e10 and: Soutar DS, Scheker LR, Tanner NS, McGregor IA: The radial forearm flap: A versatile method for intraoral reconstruction. Br J Plast Surg 36:1, 1983 and Soutar DS, McGregor IA: The radial forearm flap for intraoral reconstruction: The experience of 60 consecutive cases. Plastic and Reconstructive Surgery. 78:1, 1986.

By getting in early, we would actually get all that lot done before the actual operation started.

So I got used to sewing skin back onto the forehead, forehead grafts because that's the type of grafts we were using, transposition flaps, underneath the flailing elbows of Ian Wilson. I got on with him all right; he actually came to my leaving party when I left as senior registrar. But it was a tremendous experience. I learnt a lot, and I was taught a lot and I did a lot on that unit.

Khursheed Moos moved from Coventry to a consultant post in Canniesburn, Glasgow [1974].

When Amir El-Attar retired, Graham Wood was appointed. He had had more experience in head and neck tumour surgery; he was very competent to do that. When he started, there was a significant battle with plastic surgery. Unfortunately, there was little I could do for him. He said he had done it competently with good results in North Wales before coming to Canniesburn and had been doing it regularly, but our plastic surgery colleagues would not have it and would not bring him into their team in any form. They had moved on to do regular microvascular work. Even though he was happy to pass that on, they were not prepared to accept it. Unfortunately, he did not continue with malignancy surgery until the unit moved to the Southern General Hospital, but that was after I had retired.

Gordon McDonald, was an oral pathologist in the Glasgow Dental Hospital, who did an audit of the pathology undertaken by him and compared it with that done by one of the principal plastic surgeons. His clearance success rate was definitely better than that from the plastic surgery side. That was an interesting discovery, and we knew the results were accurate, as the same pathologist was seeing all the cases. That was just about the time I retired, so I left the battles for others to undertake before they moved to the Southern General Hospital.

On moving from Canniesburn to the Southern General:

I struggled to get the unit split and for maxillofacial surgery to go to the Southern General where we were welcomed by the neurosurgeons and administration. That was completely opposed by plastic surgery because they thought we should join them in the Royal Infirmary. They only offered us a smaller department and no hope of increasing the number of consultants there. After talking to our neurosurgical colleagues and the administration at the Southern General, we had the full backing from them to join them. They had a powerful administrator there who was very senior, and he backed us completely, but the actual move did not occur till after I had retired.

The move was hugely beneficial for maxillofacial surgery, and I think to patients in general. The results now are brilliant for head and neck cancer compared with what they were, particularly in the reconstructive field with John Devine and Jeremy McMahon, one of our past trainees. They are doing great work in that field.

When John Williams became a consultant in Chichester, he found his former senior colleagues were supportive of him doing cancer surgery [1973].

One attraction of Chichester was this huge amount of malignancy to do. I didn't appreciate until I came here that there was a huge amount of soft tissue malignancy too. Quite early on I started doing a joint clinic with a dermatologist, incidentally because he was in the next consulting room to me.

Our soft tissue malignancy work built up until David McPherson was doing a routine clinic every week with a dermatologist. This big build-up of soft tissue malignancies was very good for teaching, because the boys got a lot of experience with it.

John Langdon was a senior registrar at the London. Cancer surgery was being done there [1974-76].

Gordon Seward and Patrick James were doing cancer. A lot of the cases in those days were failed radiotherapy, so we had a lot of flaps breakdown. Neck dissections often broke down. I can remember having to do Thiersch grafts on the ward to cover exposed carotids. I never witnessed a blow-out. But they were exciting times.

The move into cancer surgery by oral and maxillofacial surgeons was sometimes done by the trainees. This was so at King's and was supported by Professor Sowray. Ian Martin was there as a house surgeon and subsequently senior house officer [1980 - 81].

I remember Malcolm Harris operated on a case at the Ospedale

Italiano.[132] *I can't remember whether he was still at King's or he had moved to the Eastman by then, but still had some sort of teaching relationship with King's. We trekked off to the Ospedale Italiano and did a pectoralis major. That was the first one I ever saw, so that would have been about 1980. The first pectoralis major I saw at King's was when Bob Ord came from Canniesburn, where he'd been a registrar. He became the King's/East Grinstead senior registrar; I was a houseman.*

And while I was a houseman and senior house officer, David Vaughan came and Nasser came later while I was a medical student.[133] *And gradually they started doing pectoralis majors with John Sowray giving flack cover. He didn't do it himself, and didn't profess to do it himself,*[134] *but he was happy to let senior registrars like Bob Ord, David Vaughan, and Nasser, do stuff.*

Before about 1980 the only reconstructive stuff that they did in oral surgery, that I can recall, was Geoff Forman for, essentially, benign disease, so ameloblastomas and stuff like that. Geoff Forman would do a rib graft, maybe. Malcolm Harris, I seem to remember, did a free iliac crest bone graft for an aneurysmal bone cyst, which bled everywhere. But that was all fairly traditional, dead bone grafting.

Then Bob Ord and David Vaughan started doing neck dissections and all that sort of stuff. There were no flaps until about 1980 when senior registrars came in who'd had a bit of surgical training, well in David Vaughan's case, a lot of surgical training. It was quite an exciting time. And the ENT guys weren't happy about it because that had been their preserve, but John Sowray just stood his ground and said, 'I'm a professor of surgery in the University of London; clear off.'

As housemen and senior house officers, one thing you all had to do was service on primary dental care. So anything that came in that looked vaguely suspicious we would organise the work up and get biopsies done and instead of, as in the old days, sending it off to ENT we would then send it to Bob Ord or David Vaughan, so they were then

---

132 The Italian Hospital was in Queens Square. At one stage it had beds used by the Eastman Dental Hospital. It closed in 1990 and the building was acquired by the Hospital for Sick Children

133 Nasser Nasser was a senior registrar at King's and subsequently a consultant oral and maxillofacial surgeon at Barnet and lately Whipps Cross hospitals.

134 Professor of oral and maxillofacial surgery.

kept in house. And that was a big change.

John Langdon returned to King's as a senior lecturer/consultant in February 1983

John Sowray was incredibly loyal to his department. And, as you say, the combination of David Vaughan, Bob Ord and myself, we were a bit maverick. Once we got to theatre many interesting things happened and there would be occasional complaints about how senior house officers had behaved, or not turning up when they were called to the A&E department, that sort of thing. John Sowray would always defend people from whatever they had done to his colleagues. And then bollock them on the quiet.

When I went back to King's as senior lecturer consultant, David Vaughan and Bob Ord were on the King's/ East Grinstead rotation. David Vaughan rotated back to East Grinstead soon after.

When I arrived, there was no cancer surgery. Malcolm Harris had left by then to go to the Eastman. He was the only one doing cancer surgery. So it was me that started the cancer presence at King's. David Vaughan had been at King's before I got there and soon after I arrived rotated back to East Grinstead and Bob Ord came as his replacement.

Were Bob Ord and David Vaughan not getting cases in and doing them?

I wasn't there, so I don't know. But if they were, I don't know what happened to the patients because I never saw them. Knowing John Sowray, it wouldn't have surprised me if they had done some on his lists in his name. But how those patients were subsequently managed or where I have no idea.

When I went to King's there was a plastic surgeon who did sessions at King's but who was based at East Grinstead, but wanted to withdraw from his King's sessions and base himself full-time at East Grinstead, which he did. He contacted me one day and explained that he was giving up his sessions at King's. He said, 'I've got a handful of head and neck patients. Can I hand them over to you?'

One of them was a middle-aged woman for whom he had done a premaxillary resection including her upper lip and lower nose. He presented her to me with the resection defect and the first stage of the tube pedicle that he'd raised from the abdomen which he was waltzing up the body from her umbilicus up to her left breast, to carry on from there. So it's the only tube pedicle I ever managed myself. She ended up with an upper lip that she could seal against her lower lip, and a sort of nose. So that was good fun.

Then we had two ENT surgeons who basically did tonsils and adenoids and the odd larynx. But they were doing a joint clinic with one of the radiotherapy consultants at King's. So I barged into that. I didn't ask if I could join it; I just turned up. Then I started booking my own patients into that joint clinic and rather took over. And first one retired, he'd had enough of it and then the other, who was quite young, went off sick for a few months and never really came back. So I was the sole head and neck cancer person, which in a way, was my own undoing.

Once I'd appointed Martin Danford to the unit, we could manage all the free flap reconstructions between us. We always worked together. Typically, I did the resections and the neck with a registrar and Martin would come in and do the free flap.

But, of course, when it came to all the rejigging of cancer and joint clinics and all the rest, working in isolation without ENT and plastics was frowned on. Martin Danford had left by then. We had Andrew Lyons, and that's when they moved it all to Guy's.

Andy Brown had been inspired by David Vaughan, who was a fellow senior registrar at East Grinstead, but he had previously been inspired as an ENT senior house officer [1974].

I worked first for six months as a house surgeon in ENT surgery, which was a fairly well known way to proceed. Many of the ENT surgeons at Guy's were very happy to have the dentally qualified house surgeons working with them. And I worked for an absolutely superb surgeon called Omar Shaheen, one of the early surgical oncologists in ENT surgery in the UK. He came from that generation who, in the in the '50s and early '60s, had taken themselves off to America to learn quite a lot of surgical oncology, because the Americans were leading the way in head and neck surgery. He was the first slick dissective surgeon I had seen. You could see exactly what he was doing when he was doing a neck dissection or a parotidectomy.

Later, as senior registrar at East Grinstead [1979].

David Vaughan came to us and I think he was the first senior registrar in our specialty I had met who had done an accredited, proper, surgical rotation training. The first thing that I had to do was to teach him some orthognathic surgery because he had never seen any. In return, he taught me two things. He refined some of my skills in dissective surgery, such as they were, but what he really brought was a view of the specialty that opened my eyes as to where we should be going.

We were sitting in a specialty where we had gained more proficiency in things like osteotomies. We were also doing a lot more extraoral approaches for our facial trauma because the mini-plating systems were arriving and we were plating more zygomas, and we were already doing lower border approaches to the mandible.

We were doing all these things, and we suddenly realised that there was more to oral surgery than just surgery of the mouth. We should think of surgery of the whole maxillofacial area. I can remember sitting around with David, chewing the fat and having a drink, and going out for curries, and he was the one who made it quite clear to me it was crazy that we were treating the benign diseases of our area but we weren't treating the malignant diseases. And I was challenged to think 'Is that true of any other surgical specialty?' Yet here we were with patients with cancer of the mouth and jaws, and as soon as that happened we were sending them off to another specialty, and yet we were seeing the patients in our clinics. It was our area of pathology.

So towards the end of my training I realised that if we were to get into this area, particularly at East Grinstead, but I think also as a specialty as a whole, there were two operations that I knew I needed to get under my belt fairly quickly once I was appointed as a consultant. One was a parotidectomy since, although we were doing submandibular gland surgery, we weren't doing parotid surgery, even though it was still salivary gland surgery. And the second thing was a neck dissection. I realised you couldn't do anything in head and neck cancer unless you could address the neck in order to deal with involved lymph nodes, or to control haemorrhage. So I needed to get proficiency in neck surgery. Those two things I hadn't done as a senior registrar.

What influenced me was thinking that we should naturally do the cancer surgery. What David Vaughan did was to cement that opinion and enthuse me to realise that's where we needed to go.

Andy was appointed as a consultant and described the first cancer operation at East Grinstead by an oral surgery consultant [1981].

Within the second or third week of my being appointed an elderly lady came into my clinic with a squamous-cell carcinoma on the mandibular alveolus, invading the edentulous mandible with a palpable node in the neck. Now this was before the days of head and neck tumour panels and boards, and all the other ways in which we manage head and neck now. Everybody and anybody were dabbling in head and neck surgery. So I realised this was a case that needed a hemi-mandibulectomy and a neck dissection. In those days we didn't always restore the mandible so it was quite in order to remove, particularly with an older patient, part of the mandible and carry out a neck dissection.

I was appointed just ahead of David Vaughan going to Liverpool and he was at that stage working at King's as a senior registrar with Professor John Sowray. So I rang up Professor Sowray and asked whether it would be possible for David to come and assist me on a patient at East Grinstead and John Sowray, bless his socks, said 'No problem at all, old boy!'

David, who was still living in East Grinstead, was quite happy not to travel up to King's on that day. So, I put on the list, since the operating lists were published and printed and circulated around the hospital, 'removal of intraoral lesion and associated neck lump', or something like that, so it wouldn't be a red rag to everybody!

David joined me and off we went, and to give credit to him he was patient to stand on the other side of the operating table and more or less guide me and say 'Cut here, do that, do this'.

I had read up neck dissection in every single book I could find. I hadn't seen one since the days as a house surgeon in 1973 when I was working with Omar Shaheen at Guy's. So I read it up like nobody's business and he took me through it. We took the hemi-mandible out. We didn't put any bone in, but used a lateral tongue flap to put some soft tissue in because we didn't dare start raising delto-pectoral flaps or anything else as an alternative.

And the patient did very well. Just to complete the names involved, the senior registrar was none other than Bob Ord, who is now a much respected oral and maxillofacial surgeon in the United States and who has taken on the specialty there. He was my senior registrar, and it was a good job he was because he was a very bright guy who was much more up to date with medicine.

We nearly over transfused and over hydrated this poor old lady afterwards and I think she nearly drowned, but Bob was the one who *recognised that her chest problems were because she was about six litres positive, so once we got that out she was okay. And she did very well; I can still remember the patient's name. These things stick in your memory, don't they?*

Now, as you might imagine, it soon got round the hospital and in those days Nick Breach, who was a consultant in plastic surgery, who then went on to the Marsden, used to do most of the head and neck oncology at East Grinstead. He had trained as a registrar in oral surgery and was fairly friendly to our specialty, although I'm not sure what he thought of it. But I know there was a certain amount of 'chuntering' amongst the plastic surgeons. We used to have a weekly meeting of the consultants. Nick was the chairman and the meetings were held informally on a Saturday morning because all the consultants, many of whom had West End practices, particularly the plastic surgeons, used to do a ward round on a Saturday morning before meeting for a drink in the mess bar afterwards. So a lot of the business of the hospital was done, outside of, not during, the normal working week.

Nick forewarned me. He said that one of the other plastic surgeons, who paradoxically has also ended up as quite a good friend, was intending to raise this at the consultants' committee. Namely, that we were straying into areas that we shouldn't get involved in. I subsequently found out that this particular plastic surgeon had visited Mike Awty in his office and had rather gone on a bit about what did Andy Brown think he was doing, doing a neck dissection? To his eternal credit, I know that Mike Awty said to him 'I didn't realise that any problems had occurred?' Fortunately, the case had gone alright, and the patient was fine and was sitting on the ward doing okay. So he just threw back that, 'He's done it and it's gone well and the patient's okay, so what's your problem?'

So that's the story of the first case of head and neck cancer that I did and how it was not officially stopped at that stage, which meant really that once there was a breach in the dam, if you'll excuse the pun, it was going to be very difficult to stop it again. So we went on from there and expanded.

David Vaughan [1981].

Andy had just been appointed, and the consultant oral surgeons were very much the second consultants to the plastic oligarchy. It would have been '81. Essentially, at this stage I was available for hire. So Andy rang Prof. and said, 'Can I have Vaughan to give him a hand down in EG to do this case'. I lived in East Grinstead. So I went into theatre and Andy did a neck dissection and I nudged him occasionally from time to time. He opened up the neck, he did a McFee incision, and chased the bleeders and clipped them and tied them and what have you. And between us we did a radical neck dissection and then he split the jaw open, and at that stage I looked up and there were seven plastic surgeons in the viewing gallery, looking down at him.

I said, 'Don't look now, but the opposition has come out in force.' So on we went, we resected the tumour. I think it was an alveolar carcinoma if I remember correctly, and we reconstructed it with a lateral tongue flap, which is a thing he and I had written up.[135] We closed it all up, put the drains, and there were all these sorts of looks and glances. You could have cut the atmosphere with a knife. Anyway, the patient did okay; I mean she lived, I think, a natural life. I wasn't involved any further. I was working in King's, but I used to meet Andy for a beer and he was saying, 'It's broken the ice.' And it did, and it gave him a status, which they found very difficult to say, 'Well you can't do this,' or, 'You're not competent to do this,' and it went on from there.

Andy Brown

For the first ten years of my consultant career I did a bit of everything, which was great fun. It may not have been good for the patients, but I could do orthognathic surgery and cancer surgery and salivary gland surgery. When we appointed Ken Lavery to join us at East Grinstead, we could sub-specialise proper.

I got into microvascular surgery, and it wasn't long after that that we were reading the literature and realising that you didn't need to do a full radical neck dissection in all cases. So I got into selective neck dissections quickly. And to the end of my career I still felt much more comfortable doing a selective neck dissection than a full radical neck dissection. I always felt a little less sure in the posterior triangle of the neck.

But if you ask, how many did I need to do? My feeling about surgery

---

135 The versatility of the lateral tongue flap in the reconstruction of defects of the oral cavity. Vaughan ED, Brown AE. British Journal of Oral Surgery. 1983 Mar;21(1):1-10.

is that if you know your anatomy, and if you have learnt some basic dissective skills that enable you to realise that tissue planes are important and how to work in tissue planes, if you know how to control bleeding and keep the area tidy, then it may take a bit longer, but you can learn surgery from a book. You can read an operation and do it. And that was actually the self-taught basis of my training.

The only free flap that I'd ever seen done, before I did one myself, was a radial forearm flap. Every other form of free flap I ended up doing, including the composite scapulas and fibulas and DCIAs,[136] I'd never seen one done; I just read the book and did it. I might have rung up my mate, David Vaughan, in Liverpool and chewed the fat with him the night before and asked whether he had got any tips.

I know it's scary, but that's what I did. With neck dissections, I felt confident enough in the neck after a year or so. But I firmly believe you need to have a decade or more under the belt as a consultant before you are truly confident going into an operating theatre and truly comfortable to relax over cases.

Ian Martin then became senior registrar at East Grinstead [1991].

I went to East Grinstead as senior registrar, and that was because Andy Brown has always revered David Vaughan and Andy was doing the same sort of thing in East Grinstead, but of course, he was surrounded by ten plastic surgeons. He was doing his own stuff and doing microvascular surgery and all the rest of it. Paul Johnson was the senior registrar there. He was due to rotate to King's, I think.

I had only done twenty months as a registrar by the time I finished on Merseyside. Paul Johnson, when he was registrar at Stoke, had created a very good relationship with a consultant ENT surgeon and they had gone off and done the Northwick Park microvascular course together.[137] And with Peter Leopard's blessing, Paul and the ENT guy did quite a lot of cancers that came in to Peter Leopard's service. So he'd gone down to East Grinstead as a senior registrar with already some experience of microvascular reconstructive stuff where Andy was

---

136 Deep circumflex iliac artery flap.
137 Northwick Park Hospital in North London had a medical research centre attached which was doing research into rejection of organ transplants. The research technicians who did the animal transplants used to run a course twice yearly to give instruction and practical experience in vascular anastomoses in live rats. Most senior oral and maxillofacial surgery trainees went on the course, as I did, which ran for several years.

doing it.

He'd started off doing it with the plastics guys, but the main guy he was doing it with was Brent Tanner, who was a nice guy. He wasn't bothered about boundaries, he was perfectly happy to collaborate. But most of his colleagues weren't. There was one particularly nasty piece of work who particularly didn't like the dentists doing anything like this.

The set up in East Grinstead was these open plan theatres. There were four theatres with balconies and lots of glass, and in the centre was the anaesthetic area. So anybody could see what anybody was getting up to all the time, and of course, it was literally like being in a goldfish bowl, so anything you did wrong people were going to know about. So Andy was very much under scrutiny.

I think the reason I got the job was because he and David had been best pals, and David must have been on the phone to him and Banksy[138] saying, 'Look, he can do microvascular. If you need somebody to come and help you do it this is the guy to do it.'

Brian Avery started doing cancer surgery after he was appointed as a consultant in Middleborough [1983].

There was a plastic surgeon cutting out tumours, usually in bits. I was doing one or two tumour operations, the odd wedge resection for lip cancer or something like that; I wasn't doing any other oncology.

I'd been there about six months and I came out of the operating theatres one evening. It was about 8 o'clock at night, and the senior pathologist of the hospital was waiting outside. He said, 'I've come to talk to you about the head and neck cancer.' I said, 'Okay,' and I wasn't sure what was going on here.

He said to me 'I've got to tell you I would say at least 80 percent of the tumours currently cut out by the plastic surgery service do not have clear margins and I've noticed you've done one or two and you've had clear margins and I'd like to ask you if you'd take on the head and neck oncology.' I said, 'Well, I'd love to do it but I haven't got much experience.' My total experience as a senior registrar had been one neck dissection with Peter Ward Booth and I think we'd both agree that we hadn't done it very well.

---

138 Peter Banks. Oral and maxillofacial surgery consultant.

I thought I would have to take this on. Now Peter Ward Booth had been appointed about a year ahead of me up the road in Sunderland, and he was in a similar situation. He'd done very little oncology. He was just sort of working around the edges of oncology, and he didn't have experience either. We decided to work together, so we began racing up and down the A19 between Sunderland and Middlesbrough. I'd go and help him, he'd come and help me as we were gaining experience.

Then Peter appointed a colleague, Bob Ord, and Bob was a real inspiration. He'd had quite a bit of oncology training, working with John Langdon at King's in London. He joined in going up and down the A19. I was doing three resections a week, some weeks, two of my own patients and then going up to help him in Sunderland. It was exhausting. We were not quick, so we were finishing late, but we were doing them properly I don't think there's much doubt about that. We took on some very big cases and some of these patients were living for many years. We hardly had any perioperative deaths, certainly none on the table. Suddenly the cases started pouring in and I ended up 75-80 percent of my time dealing with cancer. By the end of my career, I had treated 1,000 plus cases. When you're doing three cases a week, it doesn't take long to develop the skills and start doing more and more.

The most common flap of course was the good old pectoralis major, but within a few years we were doing free flaps. I never got good at them because I started doing them two or three years after I'd become a consultant, but I did them. And then I got a new colleague, Colin Edge, and he was very interested in the free flaps, so from then on I'd usually do the resection and he'd do the reconstruction. Then the link between Sunderland and Middlesbrough started to fade. Although we were still in close touch, we didn't have to go up and down the A19 to help each other any longer. Colin had been trained at King's and East Grinstead with John Langdon and Andy Brown.

Tony Markus was senior registrar at Mount Vernon Hospital. He described how free tissue transfer started there [1979].

We did our first free flap, forearm, radial forearm flap, Chinese flap, in 1979. And we'd imported a Belgian gynaecologist called Wiley Boeckx. He had a lovely wife who was a dentist, and they came for a year to show everybody how to do the first microvascular surgical procedures. Then we rapidly moved on to horrible things like the dorsalis pedis, which of course had awful post-op comorbidities. We did some deep circumflex iliac artery flaps, but the forearm flap became standard, very quickly. We would start at 8.00 am and we'd be finished by 2.00 or 3.00 pm., as opposed to what goes on nowadays, which seems to be 12 or more hours. Dick Dawson[139] was a very fine surgeon and shared his experience across the board. It was a great opportunity.

---

139 Dick Dawson was the senior plastic surgeon at the time at Mount Vernon. He had been a senior registrar at Hill End and Mount Vernon with Gordon Fordyce and they had been close friends.

Chapter 16

Liverpool - The First Super Unit

'We all had a vision of how we wanted to practise'

John Cawood left his registrar job in Edinburgh to take up a senior registrar post in Liverpool [1978].

I was in Liverpool from '78 to 1983, five years. There were two main hospitals we worked in; curiously they were two regional units. One was Liverpool Royal Infirmary, where the only consultant was Lawrie Finch. The other hospital was Broadgreen and the consultant there was Harry Alty. For a short time whilst I was in Broadgreen, Paul Bradley was the senior lecturer/consultant, oral surgeon, before he went to North Wales.

Lawrie Finch was based in the dental hospital for his clinics, and the only operating that he could get at the Royal Infirmary was on a Saturday, so we'd do an all-day list on a Saturday, and Monday to Friday was all spent at the dental hospital.

In those days Liverpool had a very strong head and neck unit at the Royal Infirmary led by Philip Stell, one of the leading head and neck surgeons of his day.[140] So both Lawrie and Harry had a good relationship with Philip Stell and so all the oral cancer was referred to him.

Otherwise we practised the full range including temporo-mandibular joint, some orthognathic surgery, not done in large numbers but it was done when necessary. We had a reasonably good working relationship with the orthodontic department in Liverpool. I didn't get involved in neurosurgery because that was based at another hospital, Walton. Oral and maxillofacial surgery was fairly low key at Walton until Oldrich Pospisil and later David Vaughan arrived and then things changed very rapidly, very dramatically.

So Liverpool was a fairly middle-of-the-road maxillofacial unit. It had a bit of a profile because of the work of Paul Bradley, but I found

---

140 ENT surgeon in Liverpool whose specialism was head and neck cancer. He wrote 'Head and Neck Surgery' which was published in 1972 and was the standard textbook at the time.

personally, I was not really moving forward. But I had a great respect for both Harry and Lawrie. Eventually Lawrie and I got very close, mainly because of our involvement with the College in Edinburgh. He was Dean of the dental faculty in Edinburgh.[141]

When David Vaughan was appointed as a consultant oral surgeon at Walton Hospital, Liverpool, he intended to establish a head and neck cancer practice. He was to become the first oral and maxillofacial surgeon in the UK to use vascularised free tissue transfer. Taking over the cancer surgery from other specialities required organisation and co-operation from colleagues, as well as learning and improving on the techniques.

David [1982]:

There was rival activity taking place in Whiston Hospital, which was where the regional plastic unit was in east Liverpool. There were two plastic surgeons who had aspirations to do head and neck cancer work. Martin Littlewood was one, and Len something or other was the other. But Littlewood was the prime, so-called head and neck surgeon. He was, if you wish, Liverpool's answer to Ian McGregor.[142]

But Philip Stell was based at the Royal Infirmary, and he was the scientific one. Stell could speak fluent German; he used to translate textbooks from German into English. He had a vast relationship with the continent of Europe in the ENT fraternity. And the one thing that Stell had over everybody else, he was a bean counter; he actually did audit, which was unheard of. When I got up here, Stell was the dominant individual in managing head and neck cancer, no question.

The guy who saved my life here, in terms of clinical cancer practice, was Bill Tyldesley.[143] I had a day in the dental school and Bill was doing oral medicine. And I got on well with Bill and I said, 'Look, I know that the Royal Infirmary and Broadgreen units are throwing all their mouth cancers to the ENT people.' They went to Philip Stell.

Right from the beginning, Bill Tyldesley sent me all the mouth cancers from the oral medicine clinic. So I threw the hospital dentist out of his list on Monday afternoon. And three weeks into my job I said to the anaesthetist, 'I'm going to do a cancer case next week and it'll

---

141 Royal College of Surgeons of Edinburgh.
142 Plastic surgeon in Glasgow whose specialism was head and neck cancer.
143 Oral medicine specialist at the Liverpool dental hospital and school.

involve a tracheostomy, a neck dissection, a splitting of the jaw and a resection of the tongue. Are you comfortable anaesthetising that?' And he said, 'Yeah, we'll have him.'

So I cracked on, did the trachy, started the neck, and somebody came in and said, 'The senior general surgical consultant is pacing up and down outside the theatre door wondering whether you need a hand.' And I said, 'I don't need a hand, I'm fine, but he's very welcome to come in if he wants to.'

So we did the job, and there was no intensive care because the attitude was, 'The dentist putting a patient in intensive care? How dare you?' So I stuck it on the ward and I went into intensive care and said, 'Look, I've just spent ten hours operating, the bloke has got a trachy, he's had five units of blood, I think it'll be a good idea if he was stuck in ITU overnight.' And the bloke who was running ITU was a physician, and he said, 'Do you really think it's necessary?' and I said, 'Absolutely.' So in we went. And I said, 'I'll stay here,' so we're all happy. And from that it just went on.

Anyway, Bill kept me afloat with cases and we gradually eroded into all the fortifications within the hospital over a period of several years. They came to accept that we were here to stay, and we were doing the appropriate surgery.

I was using pedicle flaps, delto-pectoral, pectoralis major and forehead flaps. Those were the standard ones. But by the time I had finished my formal surgical training as a vascular surgery registrar, I was quite familiar with embolectomies and putting Dacron grafts into patients. And in the literature, there were sporadic case reports of microvascular surgery being done. I realised the pedicle flap situation was limited, but I needed to have some expertise or some training.

At the time in neurosurgery there was a girl in Manchester who was drilling holes in the side of the head and using the superficial temporal artery and anastomosing it to the middle cerebral to try to vascularise the brain. It was a bag of shit, but the neurosurgeons had a lab downstairs in the basement. They had microscopes, and they had micro instruments. And I used to go down there and fiddle with them. I read the articles by Soutar[144] in the journal, where they'd done a

---

144 David Soutar was a plastic surgeon in Glasgow.

radial forearm free flap.[145] And I was pally with the pathology people, and so I got a cadaver, and I did the forearm dissection. I did a couple of them and then I thought, I'm up for this.

I had micro instruments borrowed from the neurosurgeons, but I'd no microscope. So we stole one of the ENT microscopes, but I understood nothing about microscopes, and I didn't realise that the objective lens had different focal heads. And the ENT microscopes were set up to look in ears, so your hands were out like that. So the first free flap I ever did, I did with my arms outstretched because that was the only way I could see down it.

There were no training courses, but I had seen large vessels being stuck together, doing vascular surgery, so I assumed it was the same principle. We used to heparinise the patients in vascular surgery, so we heparinised the first patient because nobody had given me any guidelines and there weren't any around. But I raised a radial, and I stuck it in and it worked. That was January '85, so I'd been a consultant, what, three years?

Then I stole the ophthalmic microscope which was a Leica. I chatted up the Leica people, and we ended up in the space of a year converting the ophthalmology microscope into a double microscope, an operator/assistant microscope.

Then things took off. We got money to buy proper ones; we bought the first Leica that was in main theatres, and I was doing two flaps a week. I started in January '82 doing cancer with pedicle flaps and started doing free flaps in '85. I was well under way about '87/'88. The patients were coming from everywhere because it was the dental school; it was based in the centre of town and Stell started to feel the draught.

I was introduced to Philip Stell seven times on different occasions. What I mean is, Lawrie Finch said, 'This is David Vaughan, David works at Walton. This is Philip Stell.' 'Hi, how do you do, Philip, nice to meet you.' We'd chat away for a bit, and then maybe six months would go by, nine months would go by, and Harry Alty would come along from Broadgreen and say, 'David, have you met Philip Stell? This is David Vaughan, David Vaughan, Philip Stell.' 'I think we've

---

145 Soutar DS, Scheker LR, Tanner NS, McGregor IA: The radial forearm flap: A versatile method for intraoral reconstruction. British Journal of Plastic Surgery 36:1, 1983.

met before,' 'Oh no,' and away he'd go.

And then, in 1989 or 1990, Stell rang me. I'd been introduced seven times, and he says, 'I'd like you to come to the Artists' Club,' as he was a member there. It's a social club in Liverpool. We had lunch or dinner or whatever, and drinks and he said, 'I have a proposition to make.' And I said, 'What's that?' He said, 'I'd like you to come down and do the reconstruction work for my cases, and I'd like you to bring your cases down there as well.' And I said, 'Well, I can't commit myself to that, I'd have to discuss it with my colleagues.'

So I spoke to Pospisil and I spoke to Cawood, who was now sending me cases. There was a contretemps between Lawrie Finch and Harry Alty and me. We used to have a specialty meeting every three months to discuss business related to the specialty. And Pospisil and I decided it was unacceptable that Alty and Finch were referring their cases to Stell. Alty was at Broadgreen. and Lawrie was at the Royal Infirmary. And they had the two regional units, and they had the two senior registrars.

At that stage we were getting doubly qualified registrars, not senior registrars. We were getting guys who had done medicine, and they were coming back into the game. And we were getting people from Australia, good lads and competent lads. But we needed a rotation for the senior registrars to come through to our unit as well as Broadgreen and the Royal Infirmary. More importantly, we needed the two so-called senior units to stop referring to ENT.

So we had a meeting, and it was the only really contentious confrontational meeting I ever had with my colleagues, and I said, 'Look, we have a situation here. I'm seeing X number of cases a year. There are Y number of cases coming in or being diagnosed and roughly half of them are being treated by ENT, or maybe more than half.' And I said, 'It's unacceptable because essentially what you're doing indirectly is dropping bombs on us.'

There was a lot of huffing and puffing. And I said, 'If you guys are not prepared to co-operate, then there is no future for the specialty in this region. We either all sing from the same hymn sheet or we go our separate ways, and if that's the case, we will never amount to a can of beans.' So they agreed to send their cases. The only person who didn't send cases was Geoff Wood at the Royal and Arrow Park. So Chester, Southport, Ormskirk, Whiston (John Cooper was at Whiston),

Broadgreen and the dental school and Lawrie Finch at the Royal, all started to send cases. And we started to get inundated.

They had the senior registrars; we had a registrar and senior house officers and associate specialist. So on the back of that we negotiated with them about fusing the three units together. At that stage we still had a Regional Health Authority, and through the Chief Executive of our Trust, we had meetings and discussions and then eventually with the Medical Director of the Regional Health Authority, and we said we would wish, on the retirement of both Harry Alty and Lawrie Finch, we would wish to bring all oral and maxillofacial surgery under one roof.[146]

Before that, they agreed to share the senior registrar, so we had two senior registrars. So in three years, one year we would be fallow, but for the other two years we had a senior registrar at Walton. When Harry and Lawrie then retired, we felt that this was the time to go to the Regional Health Authority, and we negotiated that the discipline would be transferred to Aintree, and we formed one single regional unit. Broadgreen and the Royal Infirmary ceased as oral and maxillofacial units. There was a transfer of money, we lost out on it but at least we were under the one roof.

John Cawood was appointed as a consultant in Chester in 1983. He came from being senior registrar in Liverpool and he joined the Liverpool conglomerate.

Oldrich Pospisil was established in Walton Hospital,[147] and then David Vaughan was appointed, and that was the year before I was appointed in Chester. Oldrich and David were very driven. We had an unofficial monthly meeting with all the consultants in the region which was Oldrich, David, myself, John Cooper, Lawrie Finch, and Harry Alty. Geoff Wood has never been part of the regional unit, he'd never been involved, he'd always been on his own.

Oldrich was very keen to develop cleft palate repair, and he was bold enough to take on the plastics. David was very keen to promote head and neck surgery. He had a big task on his hands because Philip Stell was so established and so respected. Anyway, David, just by pure ability, demonstrated what he could offer, and quickly impressed,

---

146 The 14 Regional Health Authorities which were formed in 1974 were abolished in 1996.
147 He had been appointed in 1978.

because hitherto the management of head and neck cases, oral cancers, pharyngeal cancers, was mainly ablation. There was never any serious attempt at reconstruction. The patients' quality of life was impaired, to say the least, and there wasn't much interest in the reconstruction, so the patient would be referred back to the oral surgeons to do something. They could use an obturator or whatever they could, but the foundation was invariably poor because there was no attempt to reconstruct anatomically.

David's impact was reconstruction, particularly with microvascular anastomosis. Lawrie and Harry had not yet retired, but they started to refer cases to David. They were not unhappy with Stell in terms of his surgery; it was just the fact that the patients were far better off having benefited from reconstruction, so it was a no-brainer.

Philip Stell obviously knew this was going on, and he was a charming man, I had a great regard for Philip. He attempted to bring David on board into ENT because of his reconstructive skills, but David said, 'No, I'm not interested. I'm a maxillofacial surgeon. I'm staying where I am, thank you very much.' So David was building up his practice very successfully, being well supported and respected. Oldrich made inroads and managed to get onto a rota with the plastic surgeons, so he broke the mould and got us involved in cleft surgery.

We had formed this informal committee. We called ourselves a regional committee and with the retirement of Finch and Alty, the Regional Health Authority itself thought it was time for a reorganisation. We had many discussions with them and what they proposed was a new build unit together with plastic surgery. That was turned down as a prospect. As a group, we decided we didn't want to go down that route. So in the end when Harry retired first, Broadgreen was closed and was transferred to Walton, and the same thing happened when Lawrie Finch retired. Unfortunately, there was a bit of a hiccup because there was a bit of politicking going on behind the scenes about funding for re-establishing a chair in oral surgery which was vacant following the retirement of Paul Bradley, the senior lecturer. They wanted to make a chair of oral surgery and for that they would use the monies from Lawrie Finch's position.

But it was resolved, and Lawrie retired, and he was replaced by James Brown at Walton. So in effect, the Royal Liverpool Hospital unit closed. So what historically were the two regional units ceased to exist and then the regional unit was established at Walton, although not adequately funded. But really that didn't make any great difference because the amount of work that was going on at Walton justified the expense of more staff. So it built up very successfully, and we worked on the basis that to get this regional concept going we had an informal agreement between David, Oldrich and myself, that we'd cross-refer as tertiary referrals. So we all built up our own clinical practice in the areas of interest on the back of support and tertiary referrals. Then gradually more and more came in to be centralised, and a hub-and-spoke concept was set up.

Once the move from Walton had taken place, each of us covered a small region or district hospital where we ran our outpatient clinics and did most of our operating. But major operating was always done at Walton and later Aintree. I used to go over to Aintree for the oral rehabilitation of cancer cases. So it kind of evolved, all based round this idea of teamwork. We didn't have to like each other; it was nothing to do with that. We all had a vision and an idea of how we wanted to practise and what galvanised us superbly was the quality of the senior registrars. We had some super senior registrars, and they were enthusiastic and hard-working, and the unit became very buoyant.

John Cooper had a very strong practice at Alder Hey/Broadgreen and was very respected, and he also worked at Whiston, which is where the plastic surgeons were based. Apart from his day-to-day oral surgery, his sub-specialty interest was temporomandibular joint, both non-surgical and surgical management. He fully integrated because he moved from Broadgreen and moved all his surgery to Aintree with the regional maxillofacial laboratory which had always been at Broadgreen, and that all moved over to Aintree with all the staff. My rehabilitation for the cancer cases were all done at Walton and later at Aintree.

I think we had the first integrated regional unit where all consultants attended and politically and clinically were united. We had regional meetings all within the department, tutorials, lectures, clinics and operating. The hub-and-spoke concept started, I think, in Liverpool. So the senior registrars were all based in Liverpool but would go out to the spokes. I had a senior registrar in Chester. He came down for three months. I was still doing most of my operating in Chester, so they did a lot of orthognathic surgery in Chester. I didn't do all my operating at Aintree, but we had all the sub-specialty expertise based there.

216

The major trauma was treated at Aintree because invariably it involved neurosurgery or some neurosurgical input. Aintree has become a head and neck unit per se with close involvement with ENT who have also very much sub-specialised, so there's a lot of combined operating. And the university side has built up very strongly with Simon Rogers, Richard Shaw and James Brown spearheading the academic wing of the specialty. Now we have professors and oral maxillofacial surgery and faculty. So it's evolved much more like a German unit which has always been round that academic/research/training model with a service part of it. Liverpool has achieved a similar sort of structure and impact nationally and internationally because people have genuinely reached a level of expertise by focussing on a particular area of interest.

But there must have been good interpersonal relationships between you all. Is that so?

I think there was mutual respect. There might be some small personal wrangles, but overall the co-operation and the realisation that the unit was much more important than the individual. There wasn't open antagonism at all, there was great co-operation amongst the colleagues for the better good. We had our own ward and theatre staff, and it became a big unit and there was no time for personalities. Personalities were secondary.

Ian Martin became a registrar on Merseyside after medical and surgical jobs. David Vaughan was now a consultant there [1989].

Walton was a nothing hospital when David went there. But Oldrich Pospisil had started and was a bit of a maverick surgeon doing major cranio-facial stuff, David must have gone there in about 1983.

When I was doing medicine, I did pop up and see David Vaughan, and he was starting to do microvascular stuff in Walton. He was doing it then in a day case type theatre in A&E. He didn't have access to proper inpatient theatres, so he was really pushing the boundaries even then. But, I think he would probably admit that he was doing quite a lot of fairly small tumours that if it went wrong, it would not be the end of the world, while he got the techniques of microvascular surgery sorted out. But he'd pretty well got it by then.

Before I went to Liverpool as registrar he had said to me that the thing you must do is you must do a microvascular course. So very early on I went off to do the microvascular course at Northwick Park[148] because everybody said that was the best hands-on course. So by the time I got to Liverpool, I had done it.

How did he sort of coalesce the units into the Liverpool Regional Oral and Maxillofacial service and bring the work in?

Somehow he brought it together and got, not all, but most of the regional units together. So he got Broadgreen, which had been the centre in Liverpool, highly prestigious because Harry Alty, who had been a past president of the British Association of Oral Surgeons, worked there. He got John Cawood on side who was out in Chester. And John had been quite influential because he'd been a pioneer in mini plating and implants.

John Cooper was the clinical director when I was there. John was a very nice man, as well as a good surgeon, but he was also singly qualified. And I think that was quite important because it took some threat away from those who might have been potentially threatened by the big boys with the double qualification and doing their major surgery and stuff. John Cawood was brought on board and did a lot of work reconstructing David Vaughan's cancer cases with implants. So he was important as part of this developing regional team.

When I was in Liverpool as a registrar, there were two camps. You still had the traditional relationship between oral surgery and ENT at the Royal Infirmary, and Arrowe Park. But then you had the coming together of Broadgreen, Walton, and Chester, and between them they really created a very significant collaborative empire where everybody started to subspecialise. And that was the first time I really saw subspecialisation within the specialty where you got people cross referring. So Poppy[149] wouldn't touch cancer. He would send it all to Vaughany, and Vaughany wouldn't touch any orthognathic. He sent it all to Poppy. And then you had John Cooper doing orthognathic and temporo-mandibular joint, and you had John Cawood doing the implants and the reconstruction and rehabilitation of the cancer cases, as well as being the king of mini plate osteosynthesis. So it worked, probably because of the range of talents that were there, and probably because they chose John Cooper as the clinical lead, who was non-threatening to everybody and a very nice chap and a good surgeon.

---

148 See previous chapter.
149 Oldrich Pospisil.

I asked Ian what did he think David Vaughan's legacy to the specialty was?

I don't think without David Vaughan having gone out on a limb to do head and neck cancer with modern reconstruction at the time he did it, that traditional relationship with oral and maxillofacial surgery, being essentially diagnostic and doing simple resections, but handing anything else on to either ENT or plastics, would have changed.

I think his drive was the same as mine really, that we had seen terrible reconstructions or no reconstructions by ENT at King's where you had to do these ridiculous prosthetic dentures and stuff to overcome thoughtless resections and reconstructions.

And so, I think that although some of those things were being done outside of the UK, there were really very few places in the UK. There was Soutar in Glasgow doing some reconstruction stuff. I don't think at East Grinstead they were still doing very much. So there was probably Soutar in plastics, and David Vaughan in max-fax, who really applied microvascular techniques to reconstruction of face, mouth, and jaws.

I'll give you an example. When I was a surgical senior house officer, there was a chap who was a good surgeon, a plastic surgeon. His main interest was cleft lip and palate, and hypospadias, so kids' stuff. He was a very meticulous surgeon but once he got inside the mouth all the stuff that we knew about the mouth, he didn't. So, for example, if he was raising a flap around the alveolus he wouldn't do a muco-periosteal flap; he'd raise a mucosal flap and then a periosteal flap as a separate thing. All sorts of very odd stuff.

I remember he did a pectoralis major for a tongue cancer, and on about day two he came round on the ward round and he looked at me. He said, 'This flap's dead. It's white.' I said, 'It's white because it's got keratin, which has been soaked in saliva for a while.' I mean, he was all for taking the thing out. He thought it was dead. So I, (and he hated me for it), got a gauze swab and I wiped off the keratin on the flap, and of course, underneath was pink. I said, 'It's not, it's alive.' And he stormed off.

You could get some technically very good surgeon, but his experience once he got inside the mouth was negligible. And it was one of the many things that taught me that actually, if you're going to work inside the mouth, you need to have done more than just a bit of plastic surgery because it is different working inside the mouth.

So David Vaughan brought the expertise of dentistry and medicine together to revolutionise the management of head and neck cancer, in the UK anyway. Without him, I don't think oral and maxillofacial surgery would have become the predominant force in the management of head and neck cancer, oral cancer in particular.

John Langdon:

What he achieved was extraordinarily impressive. Through sheer strength of personality he established himself in Liverpool, notwithstanding Stell's strangle lock when he went there. He assembled around him a superb supportive team of surgeons. And managed, I guess it was politically through various tiers of management, to get all head and neck cancer referred to Liverpool. In his day they had a huge referral base, big numbers.

From the start he kept proper records, so they were able to churn out very impressive research papers based on significant numbers of cases, for years and years and trained a whole generation of head and neck surgeons.

John Cawood.

Vision. Securing a solid training in surgery and then his vision on the role of maxillofacial surgery to be the champions of the head and neck, not something that it had been. He achieved that vision by establishing a unit that could cope with everything to do with the head and neck, electively, traumatically, and ablatively. And being able to reconstruct and rehabilitate, but vision is his greatest strength. Determination, second to none, focus, preparation, and achievement. He could be a difficult man, but I think that's to his own advantage.

Andy Brown.

I have all my professional life been in awe about what he achieved in his own unit in Liverpool; taking that philosophy on and moving into an area where there was an established ENT head and neck unit and ending up at the end of his career with the premier head and neck surgical unit in the UK, and possibly in Europe.

Chapter 17
Facial Trauma

'He arrested in the recovery room, and we had a devil's own job to release the fixation'

In the 1950s and '60s, the commonest facial injuries were caused by road traffic accidents. This changed after seat belts, crash helmets and air bags were introduced. It became compulsory for front seat belts to be fitted to new cars from 1968, and compulsory to wear them from 1983. Rear seat belts had to be fitted from 1986 and had to be worn from 1991. It became compulsory for motorcycle helmets to be worn from 1973. Air bags were fitted to new cars registered in the UK from the late 1980s, and most new cars had them from the early 1990s. Safety came to be the priority in vehicle design, which included crumple zones, improved tyres and engines that didn't leak oil over the roads.

Multiple severe injuries were common before these changes, and the hospital dental surgeon's role was often limited to fixing jaw fractures with wires and splints on the teeth. Gordon Fordyce was a registrar and a year later senior registrar at Hill End hospital. Rainsford Mowlem the plastic surgeon was in charge [1949-1953].

Gordon:

It was the height of the motorcycle accident period, so there was a lot of work. Our catchment area was not clearly defined, but it extended from north of the Thames up to Peterborough, out to the North Sea and west to Oxford. So if we got calls from anywhere near Oxford or outside Peterborough, or as far as Southend, we would accept them. If necessary, we would go out to them.

The way we had looked after patients at Hill End was a team system. We had plastic surgeons, full-time registrars and senior registrars, and we would team up with them to look after patients. The plastic registrar would look after the patients' health, head injuries, broken legs, that side of things, and we would look after the maxillofacial side. If there were multiple facial injuries, they would stitch them up.

If we had to go to Southend or other places -- there were three or four other places, we would go to -- we would do what we could and if necessary have them transferred to where we could look after them afterwards. It meant complete treatment, one stop, we didn't mess about and this fell in line with Mowlem's belief about the treatment of facial injuries the day it happens, the day it should be treated. This was his dictum, and he visited the hospital twice a week and we daren't have a patient lying on a bed who wasn't treated; it had to be done.

Mike Awty was a house surgeon at East Grinstead [1954].

In those days silver cap splints were made, so you took impressions for the fractures. The technician came in and made the splints and they went on whatever time of the day or night they were ready, so you were often working into the night. They were cemented on with black copper cement; you became quite good at it. The technicians were excellent and they would tell you if the impression was no good and you would have to do another one until they were satisfied, and then they'd make the splints.

There was a lot of trauma. Remember, this was before helmets for motorcyclists, so we used to see quite a lot of horrendous facial injuries because people came off the bikes with no protection at all. We did a lot of joint work with plastic surgeons then, we would shake a maxilla free, but malars were done by the plastic surgeons. We would do simple maxillas with a cap splint and a plaster head cap. It's difficult to remember just how primitive it all was then. I don't think there were any small plates used. The finger plates were quite big and all the orthopaedic plates were much too big.

All the fractured mandibles were wired, and the bones were wired. It's a long time ago, this is '53/'54. I don't think there was a Halo frame[150] in the place. We used to make a frame with pins in the skull or a plaster head cap. We used lion forceps for impacted maxillae for gross fractures. You pulled it all forward with a lion forceps, it was quite rough stuff. Lion forceps were great big claw things you put down the nose and into the palate. I doubt that there were any Rowe's forceps in the place.[151]

Silver cap splints took some hours to construct and a skilled technician was needed to make them. This posed a problem for Paul Bramley when

---

150 See: A Halo Frame for Facial Fractures. T. C. Crewe British Journal of Oral Surgery 4. 1966 147-149

151 For a history of the development of these early techniques for the fixation of facial fractures see: The History of the Treatment of Maxillo-Facial Trauma. N L Rowe. Annals of the Royal College of Surgeons of England 1971 49; 329-349.

he started as a consultant in Plymouth [1954].

I had a real problem because I inherited not a very good technician who had been there for years, long before my time, and you couldn't go into the place and fire him because he was incompetent, you couldn't do it. He couldn't make cap splints, or he made them badly; thickness and that sort of thing. I sent him away for training but he didn't pick up. So that we couldn't use cap splints for fixation.

I got down to treating fractures by internal direct wiring, a lot of stuff was hung from pinholes, through the mouth and supporting arch bars. I had to do a lot with an open operation, which we had to get on with really much earlier than happened elsewhere. With no Champy plates or anything like that, it was direct wiring, because we had to. And I had to do a number of these bi-coronal flaps, and pretty much for the same reason. It's a wonderful exposure for the top end and you can cobble it together pretty well. I did a lot of stuff with Moule[152] pins as well.

Mike Awty became a consultant at East Grinstead in 1965. The plastic surgeons operated on all the fractures malars. Until..

I decided a bit later on that malars were no great problem, really. And so I chose one that we didn't pass on. I was about to do it when one of the more timid plastic surgeons came along and said, 'Oh, this boy's GP has rung me up to say that he'd like me to be there for the operation.' I thought hmm, all right. So I did an eyebrow incision and wired it and pulled it up, with this chap waving a sucker at me all the time.

Russell Hopkins was a senior house officer in Nottingham [1958].

The plastic unit was at the City Hospital, the oral surgery unit was in the General where the accident unit was and we drained the facial injuries into Nottingham General from Derby, Grantham, Nottingham and Mansfield. So we drained over two million people into one consultant and one SHO, and I was in my element. This was 1958, before seat belts and before crash helmets, so people went through windscreens on a daily basis.

The plastic surgery unit at the City Hospital was spitting mad at the stuff that we were doing, because they thought they should do the

---

152 Alan Moule was a consultant in Bolton.

facial trauma. That was my introduction to the antagonism between the two disciplines and Tom Battersby made absolutely certain that he kept the trauma away from the plastic surgeons. Even though they grumbled and moaned, they had no presence in the accident and emergency department. I was there.

One of the other things about Tom was that he was, I believe, the first person in the UK, if not anywhere else, to use metatarsal plates to plate mandibular fractures. Wilfred Roberts was a consultant and a friend of Tom's, and Tom had told him about using these metacarpal plates, and Roberts wrote them up when he'd done five cases. Tom had done over a hundred, but he hadn't written them up. So there's a moral there for people if you want to get known for something, you've got to write it up fairly quickly before you tell people about it.[153]

But in those days we didn't dare put a plate on through the mouth, because everybody was worried about infection, so we used to plate fractures of the mandible through a submandibular incision, which I loved doing, and then of course we didn't wire them up. Or we wired them for 24 hours and let them go, so that was my introduction, in 1958/59, to plating of fractures.

We used to wire cheekbones, we didn't put plates on cheekbones then; it was purely for mandibular fractures. For middle third fractures we used to use plaster of Paris head caps, with external steel frames. There was no Halo frame then, so it was all plaster and I used to put the plaster and the frames on. We used silver cap splints to fix the teeth together in the right place and then have extension bars attached to the fixation on the plaster of Paris head cap. It was all primitive, but it worked, and we got good results.

John Bradley Registrar Salisbury [1961-62].

At Salisbury, the registrars treated a very large number of facial injuries. The trauma load was significant and probably accounted for half of the work of the unit. Remember, there were no seat belts, the

---

153 Wilfred Roberts of Worcester had written up plating of mandibular fractures in 1963 reporting a dozen cases treated over 5 years. The term 'Roberts plates' became common parlance for the technique. However Tom Battersby had treated 350 cases over 10 years and published 3 years later. See: The Case for Mandibular Plating. Roberts W.R. British Journal of Oral Surgery 1963 1, 200-204 and Plating of Mandibular Fractures: Experiences over a twelve-year Period. Battersby T.G. British Journal of Oral Surgery 1966, 4, 194-201.

performance of cars was increasing significantly and the roads and tyres were not up to it. There were no motorways and only a few dual carriageways such as the Winchester by-pass. The summer of 1961 was hot and long and in the September it rained. The leaves fell on the long straight but narrow roads with a layer of accumulated oil on them; cars leaked oil. The result was disastrous. The unit admitted around fifty fractures over one long weekend; we nearly ran out of stainless steel wire.

After Nottingham Russell Hopkins became a registrar at Chertsey [1959-60].

I was at Chertsey for about two years and it was a great place because it had a wonderful mess, so we lived well, we worked hard and played hard. Chertsey had large motorcycle gangs, and they'd go off in 20s, 30s and 40s; they'd go at speed around Surrey, and if one came off, a lot came off and they didn't wear helmets. So we'd maybe get 20 or more facial injuries in en masse. And so the workload could be absolutely quiet or you could be off your feet, working all the time. But it was a wonderful experience.

John Langdon became a registrar at the London Hospital [1967].

All the trauma was done out-of-hours. It was never allowed to disrupt the booked lists. I never, in all the time I was at the London, either as a registrar or a senior registrar, ever saw a consultant in theatre for a trauma case, or any other emergency, abscess, whatever. I very well remember operating with Killey and Rowe's textbook open on the radiator in the operating theatre. I mean, my first lower border wire, for example, I did from Killey and Rowe with no supervision.

John Cawood was a registrar in Edinburgh. The consultant was William MacLennan [1974 - 1978].

Trauma was a huge part of the workload. He did lots and contributed lots to our understanding of the cause and treatment of fractures, particularly in children.

Trauma was managed very much in the traditional way. We worked very closely with maxillofacial technicians, they were skilful. If the fracture involved any of the tooth-bearing portion of the skeleton, the basis of it was inter-maxillary fixation using arch bars or eyelet wiring with extraoral fixation, mainly involving the plaster of Paris bandage holding an external frame to which we attached the intraoral components. That would then involve the use of silver cap splints, so models were made of the dentition with the fracture. These were then refashioned in the dental laboratory such that they could then apply silver cap splints to the teeth. The models were articulated, the silver cap splints were cast and fitted, and locking bars connecting the various parts of the splints.

The principle was that if the teeth were in the correct anatomical position, then the underlying fractures, having been reduced, would then be aligned in reasonable skeletal position spatially. In those days there was very little intraoral bone surgery, particularly in the maxilla. We did do some in the mandible. We would do some wiring of the jaws if they were fairly linear fractures, but obviously if there was any comminution then we relied more on the silver cap splints to secure the fracture.

Andy Brown had been a Registrar at the Eastman when he became a senior registrar at East Grinstead [1976].

I had seen a few fractured mandibles, both at Guy's and at the Eastman, all treated as they were in those days by just wiring the teeth together, or fixing the teeth together in some way. I hadn't seen a lower border wire or any extraoral approach to the mandible taken in my oral surgery training thus far, apart from when I was in ENT. I think I had seen one fractured zygoma elevated by one of the Eastman consultants on a private patient. I went specially to the Harley Street Clinic to watch an incision made in the hairline and elevator inserted for the old Gillies approach to reduce a fractured zygoma!

Mike Davidson was senior house officer in Brighton [1978].

Richard Juniper was the only consultant, so he was on a one-in-one rota except for the weekends where he shared the on call with a consultant at Eastbourne who I never met, despite working at Brighton for a year; I spoke to her on the phone. She had been a school dental officer and then became a consultant at Eastbourne. She was singly qualified. I don't know what she did, but all I know is that she didn't do it in Brighton when I was on call. So if I had a trauma case, and couldn't manage it myself, I had to keep it warm for Richard on Monday. Having said that, I managed most things; that was what we did.

Mike became a senior registrar at Leeds [1988].

I did a moderate amount of trauma, but you were totally on your own. It was very much self-taught and whatever you did was criticised the next morning.

As time passed, there was a gradual divorce from plastic surgeons in the management of facial injuries. Russell Hopkins became a consultant in Cardiff in 1968. The plastic surgeons were nearby in Chepstow; their hospital was due to close.

They were going to close Chepstow because it was an old war hospital, and it was antiquated, and the whole thing was a disaster. Anyway, the big day came when the proposals came out that Chepstow was going to come into Cardiff to go to Sully Hospital, which was a TB hospital which had run out of patients. The plastic unit was to go there, and that was to be where the facial injuries were going to be looked after, according to the plastics.

Professor Pat Forrest, who was the professor of surgery at the medical school, called a meeting between me and the senior plastic surgeon. There were three of us and Professor Forrest said to me, 'Well Mr Hopkins, would you like to make an opening statement?' And I said 'Well no, not really because I've come here, at your request, and I'd like to hear why I'm here.'

So he asked the plastic surgeon who said, 'Well Mr Hopkins, as you know, we're coming into Cardiff and we have heard that you have been doing very good work with facial trauma for some two, three or four years. We'd like you to continue as part of the team. What our proposals are is that we're going to admit all the patients under our care, and all of those patients we believe that you could do and look after, we will pass onto you.'

And I said to Professor Forrest, 'Well, Professor Forrest, I've been here for two, three, or however many years it is, and we've provided a service which has been found acceptable to all of my colleagues in the area. I'm a registered practitioner, I'm a consultant, I've been doing this work for several years, and I will continue to do any work that is referred to me, and if that's the proposal from the plastic surgeons, I see no point in continuing this meeting.' So I got up and walked out.

Tony Markus started as a senior registrar at Mount Vernon in 1979.

I think on my first day the plastic senior registrar came up to me to say hello. And he said, 'Now I must tell you we do all the fractured malars.' I just looked, and I said, 'thank you for letting me know, let *me just correct you, you <u>did</u> all the fractured malars.' And that was the end of it and we got on very well. He didn't do any fractured malars because he was much more interested in hand surgery, anyway. That set it right from the beginning. There was a good atmosphere.*

Before Professor Champy introduced his stainless steel and subsequently titanium plates for facial fractures and standard techniques involved inter-maxillary fixation by one method or another, anaesthetists were getting concerned about the jaws being fixed together. This compromised access to the airways post-operatively. One way of appeasing them was for the patient to spend a night in intensive care post-op.

Most of us had no problems, although I did 'hear of' a couple of fatalities on the grapevine, which made me somewhat nervous. Gordon Fordyce had no such qualms about the airway.

I can't remember an occasion when the anaesthetist said sorry, we don't want to anaesthetise this patient. I was extremely fortunate in having excellent anaesthetists, young chaps, same age as we were, and keen in what they were doing. If there was any doubt about the airway being dodgy but the patient was conscious, the anaesthetist would do a lavage where he took a big syringe with warm saline into the nostril, squirted it all and immediately there was one huge cough and anything that was in the way was up and out, finished. They did this as if it was totally routine, and it worked beautifully. So that made it easy for us to carry on when the wiring was finished, the patient was allowed to come up and we patted them on the head and that was done.

Was there never any concern about the airway with the patients' jaws wired together?

Never.

Whilst I was there, I insisted that the patient with inter-maxillary fixation was safe; safer than they were without. And I was prepared to argue the toss about this. For example, I was advisor to the aeroplane people BOAC, before they became British Airways.[154] They were frequently asked about transporting patients from abroad back to England, having had their jaws fixed. Was it safe for them to travel? My answer to them was, and it will be to you now, perfectly safe if the

---

154 The British Overseas Air Corporation merged with British European Airways to form British Airways in 1974.

fixation has not been interfered with and is okay; anything that they have swallowed or drunk since the fixation was put on, they can vomit out. And that's the end of the story. Put them on the plane. And I still hold that that's a perfectly reasonable and sensible thing to do, and much more sensible than sending them home unfixed.

Was there ever any concern by the anaesthetists not being able to get access to the airway during the recovery time when they were in theatre?

Not to my knowledge. They were fixed. They can suck them out, they can do what they like. I used to go to see patients elsewhere, where they said oh no, no we couldn't anaesthetise them, not with their teeth tied together, no, no, no. But they hadn't enough experience of it.

What about sending people to intensive care or high dependency after having their jaws wired?

We didn't have such a thing. The nursing staff were experienced, and they were happy about it. After I'd left Mount Vernon, I was up visiting somebody and they'd got a new night sister who demanded that scissors had to be kept at the bedside so she could clip them open if she had to. I said if I were in your shoes, I would give them to the oral surgery registrar but not to the nurse looking after them because they could do more damage trying to undo them than it was worth.

John Cawood had a different opinion, he spent a year in Seattle when he was a senior registrar [1979].

I became aware of mini plates just as I was leaving Seattle. I was uncomfortable with intermaxillary fixation, this arose particularly from one very narrow escape when a patient arrested; this fortunately was in the anaesthetic room. The nurse had forgotten the wire cutters and despite having reasonable light it was very difficult to release the fixation. That left a big impression.

I got interested in the concept of mini plates and visited Champy in Strasbourg who was charming, and I did a study which was funded by the company that produced the plates. I was able to do a prospective study using mini plates for mandibular fractures. And we did it randomly because we had so many trauma patients in Liverpool, it was an easy study to set up.

We randomly assigned them to the mini plates or to inter-maxillary fixation and then measured or looked at the differences in the recovery period, mouth opening, weight loss, and any complications. I presented that paper at the British Association of Oral Surgeons and that didn't go down terribly well with the old guard who said, 'Oh, we've tried plates in the past, they don't really work,' so I went back to Liverpool feeling a bit miffed. I published it in the British Journal in 1985.[155]

Anyway, I had a friend who was a respiratory physician, John Williams. I was talking to him about jaw wiring and some complications I'd personally experienced. I felt we now had a technique to treat fractures and avoid inter-maxillary fixation in the post-operative recovery period. I said, 'Is there any way you can measure the respiratory efficiency?' He said, 'Dead easy.'

So he got a group of us to go up to the respiratory lab and did flow-volume loops. We had about twenty people and they all went through the same measurements with their mouth breathing normally, and then we did the same measures with their teeth clenched together. And the differences were quite significant. The loop showed a big difference between respiratory function with breathing normally with your teeth apart, and with teeth clenched together. We looked at trauma and orthognathic cases, who still had inter-maxillary fixation, and that showed the same changes.

We presented this to the British Association of Oral Surgeons, and that went down well; we won the President's prize. And John Williams, the respiratory physician, also presented a paper. So I think that helped popularise mini plates. And then I ran several courses in Chester under the auspices of Maxime Champy and Dieter Pape.

In the beginning we used stainless steel plates and we took the plates out afterwards. Ultimately, we moved to titanium. Plate fixation came into general use somewhere about the mid '80s. I don't think there was a defining moment, it just evolved. I think by '85 it was being used in the north-west region, routinely. And I think probably by the late '80s it was pretty standard practice.

Putting a plate onto a simple fracture of the mandible requires some skill, whereas if you're just wiring the jaws together, any recently appointed senior house officer could do that. Perhaps the old guard weren't enthusiastic because they would have to come in to do it themselves

---

155 Small Plate Osteosynthesis of Mandibular Fractures. John Cawood. British Journal of Oral and Maxillofacial Surgery. 1985 23, 77-91.

rather than leaving it to the houseman. Is that a reasonable opinion?

Yes, obviously there's a bit more skill involved putting in a plate than it takes to put on inter-maxillary fixation. I'd turn that up on its head and say what's safer for the patients as compared convenient for you as a surgeon? And in the early days of mini plates we went step-by-step, and we were very specific that you were really using the plates for linear fractures, not comminuted fractures. And the protocol was that you put the patient into inter-maxillary fixation to stabilise the dentition and therefore having reduced and stabilised the fracture, then you could place the plates across the fracture line. It took a little bit of manipulation to get it passive.

I think people realised that this was a good technique, and it was a logical way of managing fractures. Time has supported that, in as much they've made micro plates, mini plates, macro plates, etc. Using biocompatible materials I think was an important step in the predictability and safety of the management of patients. That was my view about it, and my take on it was not is it simpler or easier? I felt far more comfortable when my patients' jaws were not wired together post-operatively. That was where I came from.

Chapter 18
Orthognathic Surgery

'And the angle of the mandible exploded into several pieces'

Although orthognathic surgery was being carried out for jaw deformity before the 1970s, it was not until the Obwegeser intraoral sagittal split and the Le Fort I down fracture maxillary osteotomies that it became mainstream in many hospitals.[156] [157] Probably the biggest advance was fixed band orthodontics. Before that many operations involved complicated segmental procedures with the segments fixed with silver caps splints. I can well remember, as a houseman at Mount Vernon in the 1970s, having to adjust occlusions post-operatively with a diamond wheel in a straight handpiece, after the splints were removed .

Mike Awty was a house surgeon at East Grinstead [1953].

> *Corrective work was mainly mandibular prognathism and advance of the mandible done via an external lower border approach. It was thought it was likely to become infected if you did any of that sort of bone surgery intraorally; we did vertical sub-sigmoids, or an L-shaped sigmoid. I don't remember any maxillary surgery.*

Khursheed Moos was an undergraduate dental student at Guy's from where he went to New Cross hospital [1955-57].

> *Mr McDonald did orthognathic surgery there. We went out several times to watch him. He was then doing horizontal ramus osteotomies for prognathism and mandibular setbacks.*

John Bradley was a registrar at Roehampton [1963].

> *It was all done with cap splints. The orthodontic side of all this has of course transformed that, but in those days we were doing quite complex osteotomies to the premaxilla and mandible, and segmental*

---

156 For a good history of early orthognathic surgery see: Origins of Orthognathic Surgery. Moos K.F. Dental Historian May 2000 37. 5-18.

157 For a description of the introduction of the intraoral sagittal split, the Le Fort I and the genioplasty see: Orthognathic Surgery and a Tale of How Three Procedures Came to Be: A Letter to the Next Generations of Surgeons. Obwegeser H. Clinics in Plastic Surgery 2007 331-355. Hugo Obwegeser describes his early cases, how they came to be done, even the instruments he used.

osteotomies. All this was worked out at Roehampton with Brian Conroy, the chief technician there. Brian was superb at all these things and he would produce a model of the patient's jaw and we'd think 'well this operation might work', so we'd do it on the model and if it didn't work, we'd go back to the drawing board again instead of finding out on the operating table.

For all types of deformity, unilateral ones in particular, this model business was quite important. If it was a unilateral thing which was involving the maxilla as well, we would do a segmental osteotomy on the alveolar segment of the upper jaw and put a small bone graft in, on the floor of the sinus. We'd do premaxillary osteotomies as well. That was not a problem.

An example was the Wassmund osteotomy. It was a segmental osteotomy of the premaxilla, the first premolar was removed on each side and the maxilla divided with a drill by tunnelling from a buccal approach, and the premaxilla was divided into two segments and positioned backwards. I had assisted Gordon Fordyce do this at Mount Vernon in 1975, an operation he did against the clock. It took 50 minutes. When I interviewed him, I reminded him of it.

Gordon:

At the time that they opened the M1 and stopped the motorbikes and the fast road to Southend, the trauma side was disappearing. Then we became more interested in orthognathic surgery.

When I started my consultant job, we had a case and my colleague did one, and I came along and this was something we'd not been trained to do. Denis Wedgewood used the step ostectomy for prognathism, where you took out a section on a step and slid it back and wired it.[158]

Russell Hopkins was a registrar at St Peter's, Chertsey, and Holy Cross, Haslemere, then an outreach from Roehampton [1959].

Norman Rowe did his first body ostectomy there. We used to cut a piece out of the body, take a tooth out, remove the alveolar bone down to the inferior dental bundle and sew it up. Six weeks later, we'd go through the skin and cut the lower bit out and then put the lower jaw

---

158 See: Experience with an intraoral step-ostectomy of the mandible for prognathism. Manstein G. Fordyce, G. L.; Wedgewood, D. L. Plastic and Reconstructive Surgery 1977 59. 768.

back.

Body ostectomies were the first mandibular procedure that I'd ever heard about, seen or done. It was a time-consuming, laborious business. You had to get X-rays taken with the X-ray machine at a distance so that the magnification of the patient was minimised. We made a template, cut out and measured the jaws, made an X-ray copy of this, and cut that out.

You worked out the amount of lower jaw you were going to excise, the technician would then make a metal plate the same size, and you'd cut the alveolar bone of the same width that you needed to go back Then you'd do the second stage six weeks later, using the same template so you got it right. It was a fussy, time-consuming, silly thing and we only did the lower jaw, so if you did the right operation in the right jaw, you had a good result. If it wasn't the lower jaw that was at fault, you gave them a bird face and we didn't realise at that stage that the maxilla could be moved. Sagittal splits had not come in either, that came later.

John Hovell was an innovator in British orthognathic surgery. He had an appointment as consultant orthodontist at the Royal Dental Hospital in Leicester Square and was also a consultant at St Thomas' where he carried out surgery. Gordon Fordyce was sent by his chief Ben Fickling to John Hovell's orthodontic clinics at the Royal Dental Hospital to help him pass his FDS exam [1950].[159]

Ben Fickling said, 'Look, Gordon, to pass this exam you really must get some more work on orthodontics,' because to be a consultant dental surgeon you were meant to cover all those topics. So I had an arrangement to go to the Royal Dental, and that's where I met John Hovell and I used to sit in on his clinics and he taught me quite a lot about orthodontics. And I'm always most grateful to him for having done it. He'd admit the orthognathic cases to St Thomas'. He introduced me to the interest of doing the surgical stuff on prognathism.

The sagittal split mandibular osteotomy for mandibular prognathism was first described by Obwegeser and Trauner in 1953 and he reported the

---

159 For an flavour of this colourful man, his innovation, personality interests and wives see: John Herbert Hovell 1910-1988, TD, MRCS, LRCP, FRCS, FDSRCS (Eng), FFD (Ire), D Orth. Gelbier S. Journal of Medical Biography. 2016;24(2):145-157.

first bi-maxillary surgery with combined Le Fort I maxilla and sagittal split of the mandible as 1969. In 1962 Hugo Obwegeser gave a paper on the intraoral technique to the British Association of Oral Surgeons meeting. There have been several modifications since then.[160]

John Bradley applied for a house surgeon job at St Thomas' [1958].

I went to have an interview with a man called John Hovell. He was a consultant orthodontist at the Royal Dental Hospital, north of the river, and if he couldn't do it with springs and wires and things, he shipped them south of the river to St Thomas', where he corrected the deformity surgically. I was with John Hovell and I think I'm correct in saying this; he was the first one in this country to do an Obwegeser sagittal split osteotomy of the mandible.

It was John Hovell that fired my enthusiasm; he did a mid-facial osteotomy after I'd been there about four months, with Mr Richard Battle, who was the plastic surgeon there. They took a bone graft from the iliac crest because it was a case of hemi-facial deformity. Part of the face hadn't grown properly. He did a Le Fort osteotomy and did a sagittal split on the mandible and with the gap in the maxilla; they put an inter-positional bone graft in. And so he was ahead of his time. He did this sagittal split in November or early December of '58, I think.

Donald Winstock was the senior registrar. When Hovell went away in January 1959, Donald decided he would get another problematic mandible. He wanted to have a go at doing this sagittal split. So in came the patient, and he did his side, and I was assisting, I was standing on the patient's left of course, and he did the right side and he said, 'Right you do your side.' I was only the houseman, and I was only on the dental register from mid-November, so I must have been probably one of the first housemen in the UK to do a sagittal split, well at least one half of it. I'd seen what Hovell and Winstock had done, so I just got on and did it and it went beautifully. No problem. Tickety tock, and that was it.

Later he was senior registrar at Roehampton [1963].

It was the period when correction of facial deformity was developing and Rowe, with his innovative developing skills and mind,

---

160 see: The Indications for Surgical Correction of Mandibular Deformity by the Sagittal Splitting Technique Obwegeser H. British Journal of Oral Surgery 1964 April.1. 157-171

came into full flow. When we started with all this, they were only just about beginning to do sagittal split osteotomies, which I think is a superb operation for correcting relatively minor deformities on faces.

John Williams was senior registrar at Roehampton [1970].

Obwegeser was really the person who opened up mandibular osteotomies in a big way. It was body ostectomies before that, the sagittal split revolutionised things. We were the first unit, I think, to do bi-maxillary osteotomies in the same procedure, because it had always been done in two stages before.

John Langdon visited Obwegeser's unit in Zurich [1971].

When I was a medical undergraduate, Gordon Seward arranged for me to go to Zurich for six weeks. And on the first day you presented yourself to the Herr Doctor Professor, Hugo Obwegeser, and he walked into his office, and he handed me his CV, which was about as thick as a telephone directory, and said, 'Do you know Mr Hovell?' And I said, 'Yes, I did. I've worked with him at St Thomas' hospital and previously at the Royal Dental Hospital.' And he showed me a telegram that was lying on his desk. Apparently, John Hovell had been out to Zurich to watch Obwegeser do a Tessier procedure for hypertelorism. John Hovell had gone back to London, found himself a case and did it. And this telegram just said, 'Done first Tessier, four and a half hours. John.' And Hugo Obwegeser thought this was terribly hilarious.

What was Obwegeser like?

Very difficult, very pompous, the big I am. It was a huge department with lots of oberarzts, which I suppose were a hybrid between a senior lecturer and a senior registrar. It was all big showmanship, but they were first class at orthognathic surgery. Well planned, beautiful operators, good results.

But their management of pathology was poor. But their orthognathic was immaculate and way in advance of what we were doing in the UK.

Orthognathic surgery seemed to move forward from complicated sectional osteotomies planned to get the occlusion right by people like Brian Conroy with silver cap splints, to fixed band orthodontics with practically every case a Le Fort I and a sagittal split that anybody could do in any district hospital. in your opinion, what was the biggest change?

John:

I think it was Obwegeser's modified sagittal split. And then the down fracture. I remember it vividly in about 1977-'78 because I read the paper when I was at Roehampton.[161] I think that I probably became more aware of the procedure after hearing Bruce Epker lecture in London in about 1978.

In Ashford there was a student nurse attached to my department who had maxillary hypoplasia, and I explained to her we could advance her mid-face when I'd read the article. And that was the first down fracture I ever did. That was about '79, '80.

What about fixed band orthodontics?

When I was in Zurich, the fixation wasn't orthodontics, but the oral surgeons would make their own bands and cement them on the teeth and bend up their own arch bars for fixation. It wasn't until I went to Roehampton, working with Brian Conroy and the orthodontist Glyn Wreakes, that we really got into orthodontic fixation big time.

And I think it was the confidence to do full arched maxillary procedures and to understanding the blood supply from the greater palatine and the maxillary artery. At the London, the department, when I was there, was very isolated. It had nothing much to do with orthodontics. So everything was cap splints, even the Wassmund's and Wunderer's. When I was at Roehampton, [1977] we started doing orthodontic fixation and intermediate wafers and all that. It was the first time I became aware of the concept of orthodontic decompensation prior to doing the surgery. It was the beginning of precision orthognathics.

Russell Hopkins

John Hovell was a unique individual. He was a swashbuckler; he would have been a pirate if he hadn't been born three or four hundred years later. His surgical technique was described as swashbuckling, whether he was the first to do the sagittal split. after Obwegeser described it, or not, I don't know, I wouldn't be at all surprised. I never remember Norman Rowe doing a sagittal split, and subsequently Ian Heslop, who was appointed to be the other consultant.

---

161 Le Fort I osteotomy for correction of maxillary deformities. 1975 Bell W F 1975 Journal of Oral Surgery. 33:412-426

Mike Awty returned to East Grinstead as a consultant in 1965, but Sir Terence Ward was still the boss.

Quite early on Obwegeser was all the talk, and I knew Ian Heslop at Roehampton had been doing sagittal splits, so I thought well we must have this. So I waited for Terry to go away, then I went over there and scrubbed with Ian Heslop to learn how to do it. I was surprised, because Peebles was the senior registrar, and it seemed he wasn't allowed to do very much at Roehampton. It wasn't like Grinstead, where they were often chucked in at the deep end. Anyway, that's a digression.

Terry knew everything that went on. He said, 'Oh, how did you get on with Heslop?' And I said, 'Well, it's quite good.' He said, 'I thought you would.' He said, 'I've got a patient for you to do.' So he found a very slim Vietnamese who had a very prominent jaw. So my first Obwegeser was done on this chap. And it went very well. Luckily it all split beautifully and there was no problem with it. The chap was delighted, and I followed him up for quite a long time. So that was the beginning of doing more stuff.

And you fixed it with inter-maxillary fixation, presumably?.

Yes. I might have used wires. I can't remember, I probably did because I was dead keen to get the occlusion just right because there'd been no orthodontic preparation. But his models fitted all right, so I thought we were okay.

Mike designed a retractor to use for the operation.

I had to get some tools, and I showed Ralph Sharp. He was our superb senior technician who could make anything, he was old school. I told him what I wanted to do, and he said, 'Oh, all right then, lad.' And he got a dinner fork, chopped the two prongs out of the middle, bent the handle back and I had the Awty's retractor, which went round the back. That was turned out in no time at all, and he said, 'Try that, boy, try that.' It is still made and used as a posterior limit for the ramus.[162]

Laurence Oldham was a consultant at Taunton [1968].

I think at the time the Obwegeser split was just being publicised.

---

162 A Google search for 'Awty retractor' reveals it in several surgical instrument catalogues.

Nobody had ever done anything until Switzerland came up with Obwegeser. Obwegeser was the talisman for the whole remit and so I thought, right, we better get into osteotomies next, because we'd never done any, and I thought, well I can't do them on my own.

The first thing I did was to get Colin Brady down from Birmingham. Colin Brady was very good on sub-condylar osteotomies, external approach, Risdon incision,[163] vertical sub-sigmoid cut, slide the jaw back for a prognathism.

So I got him down and we put cap splints on with black copper cement. The first chap we got was a latent acromegalic teacher. He said, 'I'm finding this prognathism worrying because it puts the students off, they don't like it, I look aggressive.' So I said, 'Right, we'll put your jaw back. I got Colin Brady down and we did a bilateral sub-condylar, got it back and it healed by secondary intention, and that was quite successful so I was pleased about that. So then I was able to do sub-condylar displacements back.

Then I thought, we'd better get into the Obwegeser, so I said, 'I better get some.' And Jack Ross came down from Bristol and Jack Ross went through an Obwegeser with me, a girl patient we had who was rather fussy about her appearance, again a prognathism. I did one side and Jack did the other, Jack Ross was a good teacher. He came with his own kit and retractors, Obwegeser retractors, and was very helpful. So then I was into Obwegeser osteotomies. It would be 1976, I think.

So then we were able to do sub-condylars, vertical sub-sigmoids, Obwegeser and then, when John Hamlyn came as the second consultant at Taunton, I said, 'Right, we better start doing maxillas,' the Le Fort I down fractures, so we did that.

Then we had a girl who was teed up for an osteotomy because her face was wrong, she also was a prognathic and by strange coincidence Khursheed Moos, who I'd known for years, was coming down to see his sister who lives in Taunton and I invited Khursheed around and he came to see us. I said, 'Oh Khursheed, I'm about to do this case next week and would you have a look at it?' and I got all the photographs,

---

163 Submandibular incision described by Risdon who used it for access for temporo-mandibular joint ankylosis surgery. See: Risdon F. Ankylosis of the Temporomandibular Joint. Journal of the American Dental Association. 1934; 21: 1933-7.

cephs. and the tracings, because in the meantime we'd worked up an orthodontic department here; we had no orthodontics when I came.

Moos came to see this girl, and he said, 'Oh this is not right, you've got malar deficiency, there's a weakness in the malars; you've got to bring them forward or graft them.' So I said, 'Well, will you come and help me?' I invited him down to operate, which he did. And that caused one tremendous uproar because we had a theatre for the whole day, never done before. We did a full scalp flap, pulled the face off and worked on the facial skeleton with bone grafts, the full one, two and three. I was tickled pink with this because it created quite a stir in the hospital.

After Moos had got back on the train and I was left with this post-operative treatment schedule I thought, 'Am I really up to this?' because Moos was used to doing these every week. I mean totally different character. I always enjoyed Moos, he was very good, he was way beyond my league. I was left with this, so I had to learn quickly how to cope with any post-operative complications. Well, luckily he was such a good surgeon, and I was doing my bit and we didn't get any problem and the girl came out very well in the end. It revolutionised her life, she lost her angst, typical of orthognathic patient, and became a normal active member of society, and the parents were delighted.

In the meantime, I'd gone to Oxford to Peter Barton and Hayton Williams; he did the Halo. Hayton Williams was the senior doyen, a very big noise in Oxford, and Barton was his number two. Barton taught us some osteotomy work as well, and I came home and did some of Barton's ideas.

Khursheed Moos had been a registrar at Mount Vernon [1966].

Certain things were done jointly between plastics and maxillofacial surgeons. I saw my first osteotomy of the maxilla, a Le Fort I osteotomy, done by Gordon Fordyce with plastics around, but he did the surgery and that was useful to me later. We saw and were involved with other osteotomy surgery stabilised with cast silver cap splints. Essentially, it was mandibular, body ostectomies and things like that which one enjoyed doing together with bone grafting procedures.

Gordon Fordyce:

I did sagittal splits, and I did Le Fort Is. Jimmy Leitch, the Barnet consultant, used to come and assist me doing Le Fort Is because he'd quite often sent the patient in the first place. I can remember us down fracturing the maxilla and cutting it from above and putting it all together and taking ages over it. I would have thought that was between '66 and '70, about then.

But looking back on it, doing the Le Fort Is, how I did it, I wouldn't sleep at night now, worrying about doing it again. It was pretty serious stuff because we were meddling in parts of the upper jaw we couldn't access. It meant putting chisels in between the pterygoid plates and trying to snap them off at the right level. That's the sort of stroke that now I would be a little bit worried about doing.

Later, Khursheed was senior registrar in Cardiff, where he was disappointed with the surgical experience, but then Russell Hopkins arrived as the new consultant [1968].

We were showing each other certain things which we had done, such as a Le Fort I osteotomy and body ostectomies from my side, and from his side sagittal splitting of the mandible, salivary gland surgery and more pre-prosthetic surgery.

I remember looking at the sagittal split paper, the Obwegeser one which told one very little, but it was the only one in English and we had it propped up in theatre.[164]

When it came to the practical details, we really did not have any proper information. Both of us were slightly uncertain of ourselves, but between us we got things more or less right and it was also very useful to have a colleague that came to do some major trauma.

And the Le Fort I you had been taught by Gordon Fordyce at Mount Vernon?

Yes exactly, I had been there, so that was fine and we could do a number of operations between us. Russell Hopkins taught me to do submandibular gland removals, which I had never done before. I think I had possibly seen only one at Mount Vernon, but I could remember little about it. I had seen a number of surgical procedures but sometimes only transiently when I was a registrar and could pop into theatre when it was not my turn to operate. So with Russell I got on well and we were in a sense teaching each other what to do and that

---

164 The Indications for Surgical Correction of Mandibular Deformity by the Sagittal Splitting Technique Obwegeser H. British Journal of Oral Surgery. 1964 Apr;1:157-71.

was great. Particularly from the trauma point of view because we had different points of view, such as for me putting pins in and that sort of thing, whereas he knew a little about bone plates.

Khursheed became a consultant in Warwick [1969].

I had a great advantage in that Oxford was not too far away, and I used to ask advice about more complex orthognathic surgery and cranio-facial problems there. I went across to Oxford to get advice from Peter Barton.[165] He was one of the few persons who had written significantly about segmental osteotomy surgery in the British Dental Journal, and I knew he himself did quite a bit.[166] I used to go over to Oxford to consult him from time to time, and I think he enjoyed having someone like me coming to discuss problem areas.

Did you ever operate with him or was it just for advice?

I didn't really have time. It was very difficult to get away because all my sessions were filled and there was no-one to replace me, so one would have to cancel sessions, and we were really too busy for that in South Warwickshire as it was an underdeveloped area. I had cases sent from other parts coming to us from much further south, from Worcestershire, Gloucestershire and the Oxford borders.

I went up to visit Canniesburn with Russell Hopkins and Gordon Hardman, surgeons from South and North Wales. I had suggested going up to see Derek Henderson because I knew him well and because of my previous knowledge of his work. I knew he was doing major mid face surgery, the Le Fort II and III level osteotomies. I think I saw the first publication of the Le Fort II osteotomy around that time in 1973.[167] The three of us went up together and saw what was going on there, and I was impressed.

I thought this was an incredible advance in the range of surgery that one could now see and become involved in as well as other changes and ideas about trauma.

---

165 Peter Barton was a consultant in Oxford from 1965-1983 and President of the British Association of Oral Surgeons 1976. He had spent some time with Hugh Obwegeser in Zurich. See: Obituary Peter Richard Barton 1921-2010. British Journal of Oral and Maxillofacial Surgery. 2010 48; 566-567.
166 The role of alveolar surgery in the treatment of malocclusion. Barton PR, Rayne J. British Dental Journal. 1969 Jan 7;126 (1):11-27.
167 Henderson D, Jackson IT. Naso-maxillary hypoplasia - the Le Fort II osteotomy. British Journal of Oral Surgery. 1973;11 (2):77-93.

Russell Hopkins [1968].

For the osteotomy work, Khursheed Moos and I used to take the books into theatre, and use them to make certain we knew what we were doing. We started to do the sagittal osteotomies; got the kit in, but we did all these operations reading the books. I mean, we trained ourselves. Khursheed hadn't done them, I hadn't done them. But we did them together, fortunately with good anaesthesia, and we didn't have disasters.

The first sagittal split osteotomy I did looked very simple. The ramus was so thin that you could almost see through it; and I didn't realise the significance of this. I did the cuts with the burr, then I put in the chisel, then I knocked the chisel and I knocked it through. And the angle of the mandible exploded into several pieces and the inferior dental bundle was separated and bleeding. I thought, oh my God, I'm in trouble.

So I did the other side twice as carefully; did the cuts, did the split, and that exploded. And I'd got both sides with the inferior dental bundle severed, and the angle in pieces, and I thought, oh, I'm going to be sacked for incompetence, negligence and everything else like that. Anyway, we wired the chap together for a bit longer than usual, and he got a very good aesthetic result, but his lip was numb.

I watched him, and cared for him, and nurtured him, as you do when things go wrong. Consultants have got to look after their patients. I did that. And a year later, he came back again. I'd seen him in the meantime, and I said, 'Well, how's the lip?' and he said 'fine, it's normal.' I thought, this can't be normal, and I did the usual tests, and it was normal. And I said, 'well, I have to tell you, I really didn't believe it would recover.' 'Oh,' he said, 'I had no doubts it would recover.' I said 'why?' 'Well', he said, 'I'm a member of Apostle Church,' or something, an evangelical church and, he said, 'every Sunday night we prayed for my lip recovery, so I knew it would get better, and it did.'

And I thought to myself, well if I've got God on my side I can do well in Cardiff. I think I sewed the nerves, the bundles together, but without a microscope and with no great skill or belief that it would work. But enough regenerated to supply the lip, or it picked up ancillary supply from somewhere else or whatever; but he got lip sensation back again, and he had a very nice result and was delighted.

I thought I'll never do an Obwegeser again, and it was probably two or three months before I did, and then found I could do them quite quickly and did them as routine.

I don't know when I started doing Le Fort Is, but I did them. In the earliest stages, I'd been brought to believe you only did mandibles. The other thing I did in Cardiff, I formed with my orthodontic colleague, Derek Seel, and with the prosthetists, combined clinics. One was for pre-prosthetic surgery, and the other for orthognathic surgery. Derek Seel did great work sorting out the occlusions for me and making certain that I got the right assessment of which jaw was wrong and how much they were wrong.

Then he'd align the teeth beforehand so I could put them into a decent position, and then he could tidy it up after we'd got the bits together. So, that was a great help. Derek and I needed each other. We were the only two non-academic consultants in Cardiff, and we were both being badly abused by the academia and by Professor Cooke in particular. We needed each other for support to withstand this.

Adrian Sugar had been a registrar on Teesside and Leeds [1972 - 76].

I knew that the world of oral and maxillofacial surgery was much wider than trauma, but what little orthognathic surgery I'd been exposed to, was insufficient for me to be trained and it was mostly mandibular osteotomies.

In Teesside it was almost none. In Leeds Alex MacGregor did quite a lot of mandibular osteotomies, mostly sagittal splits. He was quite reasonable at doing them. The other senior registrars were trained in that as well, but I don't recall anything more complicated than a single mandible. Fixation was with upper border wires, no plates. I can't remember orthodontics, I never went to a joint clinic in Leeds but the orthodontists in Leeds were quite good. My senior registrar time in Cardiff a year or two later was totally different.

Mike Bromige was a senior registrar at Wordsley Hospital, Stourbridge [1963].

I did a few osteotomies at Wordsley, but I did my first sagittal split as a consultant from the book, as they say. Before all major operations, planned elective operations, it was my habit to spend the previous evening going through and typing out a sequence of events, a programme if you like. I mean minutiae because you tend to forget things when you're operating, so each stage of the operation was put down in tabulated form and that was put on the X-ray viewer so I could turn around and look.

In 1990, when Peter Selwyn retired and Donald Gould the orthodontist retired Bob Nashed came in as orthodontist and things altered considerably in how things were treated. There was good liaison, but bad liaison between the orthodontics and the plastic surgeons. The plastic surgery unit in Nottingham suffered from a lack of good leadership. The kind of things that happened was you'd have an ongoing cleft case, being treated pre-surgically, but it would then be taken off the list and admitted and operated on before the orthodontics was complete. And that happened regularly, and that upset the orthodontist, and so relationships between the orthodontists and plastic surgeons deteriorated badly.

When maxillary surgery at the Le Fort I level was started, a concern was the blood supply. It wasn't until later that it was realised that there was an adequate blood supply through the palate. Tony Markus was registrar at Guys [1976].

We were doing the vertical midline incision and two lateral incisions in the region of the malar buttress. And then we undermined and did the cuts through the tunnels, and smashed off the pterygoid plates with the pterygoid chisel, and then just advanced.

And did you adjust the occlusion with a diamond wheel?

Yes, you had to get this black copper off first. Wasn't it horrendous? It was the most awful thing, but they worked. And for segmental osteotomies we had all the little locking plates and screws, it worked very well.

With Dick Haskell I learnt the Sowray-Haskell technique, of course.[168] Doing essentially an anterior segmental but taking out a piece beneath that in the midline of the mandible so you could narrow the mandibular arch and you took out the premolars and then the upper segment would fit in nicely. I probably did a few with Pat O'Driscoll but I can't remember so much. He was quite a difficult chap to work with.

---

168 Used for the surgical treatment of a prognathic mandible with cross bite by a subapical osteotomy and ostectomy at the mandibular symphysis. See: Ostectomy at the mandibular symphysis. Sowray J.H., Haskell R. British Journal of Oral Surgery 1968 6; (2) 97-102

Tony became senior registrar at University College Hospital [1977].

That was the beginnings of my exposure to some serious surgery, lots of orthognathic surgery. Bi-maxillary procedures, segmental procedures, old-fashioned vertical sub-sigmoids, the C-shaped osteotomy of the body, Schuchardt, Wassmund's and so on. That was terrific.

Most of the orthognathic surgery was at UCH and then the correction of the secondary deformities at Great Ormond Street and some of the cranio-facial deformities. We used to see some hemi-facial microsomia, some Treacher Collins, do bone grafts and procedures on the mandibular condyle.

There'd been a plastic surgeon who had done a lot of primary bone grafting for the anterior palate in a way that actually caused a lot of restriction of facial growth. So David James did lots of mid-face osteotomies on these people. We used to see them at Great Ormond Street, but if they were over 16, then they came to UCH. That was the beginning of my exposure to clefts in quite a big way, working with Brian Morgan,[169] who was at UCH and at Mount Vernon.

I did the first down fracture at Mount Vernon, when senior registrar, on my own. Gordon Fordyce thought it would compromise the blood supply too much and wouldn't support me. But I had already been influenced by Derek Henderson, who I was going to work for anyway, I'd been on the major anatomy course that he and Derek Wilson ran, and when I did my first down fracture at Mount Vernon, Jimmy Leach, came to me and said, 'I know it's not my patient, but I will cover you; I'll be behind you if anything goes wrong.'

Brian Avery was able to see some cranio-facial surgery as senior registrar in Glasgow [1978-83].

Yes, I saw it. The surgery was done at the Southern General Hospital, which was the nearest neurosurgery centre, and it was predominantly the neurosurgeons and plastic surgeons, Ian Jackson, working together. Khursheed Moos did a certain amount. He worked with Ian Jackson to reconstruct the skull. The senior registrar in max-fax surgery very rarely got to the front line in the operating theatre; the theatre was usually crowded and I was second or third row back

---

169 Plastic surgeon.

for much of the surgery.

After starting at Middlesbrough as consultant, I took on orthognathic surgery and salivary gland surgery immediately. I then took on the oncology. And then by the time I'd been in post four years I got friendly with a newly arrived neurosurgeon called Sid Marks.

Sid Marks had had some training in cranio-facial surgery at Oxford. We got on well and did some trauma cases together. I don't know how we came to start, but we started doing cranio-facial surgery on the babies. So in '87 I took on the cranio-facial surgery.

They were coming in to see the neurosurgeons, but once they were being identified as cranio-facial problems they were being sent to Glasgow or occasionally to London to be operated on. The neurosurgeons realised that they were sending these kids halfway across the UK to get treatment, and I asked them, 'Well, have you seen any of the results?' They said, 'We've never seen a case that's been operated on.' And for whatever reason, these kids in Teesside were being referred were never getting their surgery. Extraordinary.

Now I'd been in Glasgow and I knew jolly well what happened to many of these patients. I can remember one time a family, from Middlesbrough who were walking up the corridor in the ward in Canniesburn in Glasgow. There was mum, dad, the baby and two tiny siblings wearily walking up the ward in the early evening. They told us they had spent all day travelling from Middlesbrough and they'd come to see my boss Professor Moos for assessment. It was now the evening, and the ward said, 'Well we haven't got a bed, but we can find you a bed, but there's a problem, the boss in on holiday so you'll have to go home tomorrow and come back in a couple of weeks.' I realised that one of the big problems undoubtedly was this problem of travelling.

The nature of cranio-facial babies is often they've got siblings, and it also seems to be more prevalent in socially deprived families. Getting treatment was nigh on impossible for them. And so Sid and I started treating these patients. There weren't a huge number. We had a catchment population of a million, but we were treating about a case a month. We treated them for 19 years as a team, just the two of us. There weren't many syndromal patients, they were mainly patients with scaphocephaly, turricephaly, plagiocephalies, and we selected the cases well. We did whatever we had to do, whether it was partial or total skull reconstructions.

In the 19 years that we treated them, we had no deaths and no major complications, causing any sort of loss to the patient. We had intra-operative problems occasionally, like excessive bleeding or whatever, but no deaths.

Did you have orthodontics at Middlesbrough?

Custom made arch bars were usual. I had them for my osteotomies, particularly in the early days I didn't have orthodontic back up, which made life difficult. I would have to do things like multi-segment, Le Fort I maxillary procedures. So I'd chop the maxilla into three or four bits to move the teeth into the correct occlusion.

There were orthodontists there, but they weren't doing this type of work. I kept going and pestering them and saying, 'How about taking this case on and what I want you to do is correct them so they'll go into a good occlusion after surgery and if they're Class III correct the incisor angle so I could get good results.'

But eventually you got the orthodontics and the incisor decompensation and everything?

Yes, and yes, that worked out well, and the orthodontists treated also the clefts when Alastair Smyth[170] was there. I think the orthodontists enjoyed it. Instead of just dealing with practitioners, they were using fixed appliances, and they were dealing with the orthognathic surgery and with the cleft cases.

Andy Brown spent six weeks in the USA when he was a senior registrar [1978].

I was fortunate to be awarded a travelling scholarship by the British Association of Oral Surgeons, the so called Leverhulme scholarship. I spent about six weeks visiting units on the East Coast of America, taking in Dallas and Fort Worth.

Around that time, although the sagittal split osteotomy of the mandible was well established, at East Grinstead we were still doing low-level osteotomies of the maxilla through what's called a 'tunnelled' approach, preserving some blood supply from the buccal side of the maxilla. But around that time papers appeared about the so called 'down fracture' technique, and papers were also appearing

---

170 Oral and Maxillofacial Surgeon with interest in cleft surgery – see chapter 20.

from America about bi-maxillary surgery, doing both jaw operations at the same time.

I ended up going to Dallas and Fort Worth, where one of the leading lights was Bruce Epker,[171] who was working with William Bell,[172] who had done a lot of the research work in this area. It was an eye opener to me as well to see how they planned their cases, how they assessed them clinically, because one thing that I think had bedevilled the treatment of orthognathic problems by oral surgeons was that we were always dentally focused. I also think that bedevilled a lot of our treatment of facial trauma, because to us restoring the occlusion was the most important thing that we could do, and we sometimes disregarded some of the cosmetic effects.

Similarly in osteotomies, we were so concerned about restoring the occlusion from these jaw disproportions we didn't really think about the effect on the face as a whole. What was happening in Dallas was the whole aesthetic approach, looking at what the soft tissues did when you moved jaws around. That all happened in the late '70s and early '80s. So it was a great influence to spend some time in Dallas and, although I was still a senior registrar, I came back from America and I think helped to enthuse both Mike Awty and Peter Banks to think that way as well.

Really, my expertise in the final years as a senior registrar was to help develop, even though I was only a registrar, the surgery of facial deformity at East Grinstead, which I think we took forward quite a lot. We were doing a lot of osteotomy and facial deformity surgery. So that was a big influence.

Adrian Sugar became senior registrar in Cardiff [1980].

Russell Hopkins and Derek Seel had been carrying out regular joint oral surgery/orthodontic clinics for years. But it was not an orthognathic clinic in the way we would do them now, but it was a very well-established clinic. It was ninety percent orthognathic surgery.

---

171 Bruce Epker was an oral and maxillofacial surgeon in Texas with a high profile in research. He authored Esthetic Maxillofacial Surgery and co-authored Integrated Orthodontic and Surgical Correction (1995).

172 William Bell, American oral and maxillofacial surgeon and professor of surgery in Dallas. He did early work on the Le Fort I osteotomy and the blood supply and later on distraction osteogenesis. He co-authored Surgical Correction of Dentofacial Deformities (1980).

There were occasional ectopic canines, but mostly they were deformity cases. But they rarely did orthodontics before the orthognathic surgery. If I remember rightly when I started in Cardiff in '80, I think there were about sixty to seventy orthognathic cases on Russell's waiting list for surgery.

Some had orthodontics afterwards, but we never did the surgery with fixed orthodontic brackets or bands on; they were always cap splints. When we did multi-piece osteotomies, sometimes they weren't with cap splints on because they were more challenging to do if you had cap splints on. I used to do all the planning for those cases, and the planning was most heavily influenced by Derek Henderson and by Canniesburn, and I went on the Canniesburn course in '79/'80.

I kind of made my name as a senior registrar for orthognathic planning. But it was mostly done in that cut-and-paste way, and it was only later when I took up my consultant post that one of the first things I did was to buy a cheap IBM compatible computer, that was assembled by a company in Morriston, and computerised it. So, we had the British COG software,[173] and I used to do all my planning on those cases with that. And then we upgraded it over a period of time.

I went to the United States in 1982, where we did at least six orthognathic cases a week on top of everything else that we were doing. Even though this was still long before the plating era, all the cases were done with the fixed orthodontics in place, all of them had had pre-operative orthodontics. The fixation was all with internal suspension and inter-maxillary fixation, mostly inter-maxillary fixation wires.

When I came back I persuaded Derek Seel and Russell Hopkins that we should change the way we did orthognathic surgery and every case would have orthodontics and every case would be done with the fixed bands on. It was quite challenging to do that and persuading Derek Seel was quite difficult.

A few months after I had this discussion with them, Derek went off to a meeting where Bruce Epker was talking and so was Proffit,[174] the orthodontist from Chapel Hill, and obviously they were talking about

---

173 Orthognathic planning software produced by the Consultant Orthodontic Group of the British Orthodontic Society.
174 William Proffit. Orthodontist and professor at the University of Carolina, Chapel Hill and co-author of Surgical Correction of Dentofacial Deformity.

the same things that I was talking about. He came back, and he said, 'This is the way we've got to do it,' as if I hadn't talked to him about it at all. But we changed the way things were done from that point, and besides that we also started to use plates and screws.

In '83 I had a fellowship in Basel and so I started using internal fixation for pretty well everything, orthognathic, trauma, everything. Even though I took a bit of flak, especially at national meetings where people used to joke about, 'Adrian will put plates and screws on everything.'

But people like John Cawood, myself and one or two others, we were pioneers because we were introducing this at about the same time, John did that kind of thing in Liverpool when I was doing it in Cardiff.

Later Mike Davidson was resident house surgeon at the London Hospital, in 1986, and describes the orthognathic surgery.

The vast majority was mandibular, but we did bi-maxillary surgery as well. It was very much the era of cap splints, so the day before surgery patients would have the cap splints put on with black copper cement. The resident's duty was to put those on.

I never got to go to the orthognathic clinics, and they weren't as formalised as they were in later years. The patients just arrived in a clinic, 'oh, this patient's coming in for orthognathic surgery, this is the procedure we're going to do'. The planning was very much done by the oral surgery registrar and the boss to some extent.

The osteotomies were predominantly single jaw but some segmental osteotomies were done and I remember one private case turned up, and I just got a message from Patrick James, 'This patient's coming in, take some models and do some segmental surgery on them.' So I had the textbook in one hand and was trying to work it out. He was closing an open bite on a private patient with no orthodontics, and it was just an upper and lower segmental procedure to close it. It was very strange, and that was probably the worst example of lack of planning that I've ever come across in orthognathic surgery.

John Langdon had been a registrar at the London [1967] and later senior registrar [1974-76].

They were doing mandibular surgery, I can't remember ever doing any maxillary surgery at the London. It may have been going on, but I can't remember. They were fixed with cap splints at that time. There was segmental surgery. I can remember Gordon Seward doing Wunderer's when you used a tunnel to do the trans-palatal cuts and supra-apical cuts. Gordon Seward, in particular, was doing a reasonable amount. Because it was obviously through him, I got to spend time in Zurich with Hugo Obwegeser in about 1972.

Mike Davidson.

The kit was quite antique by modern standards. The drills were big, there were heavy air-driven saws, and the osteotomies were held with wires of course, because the plating wasn't being used at this time, certainly not at the London, and patients were put in cap splints.

For me, although the surgical techniques were important, the biggest advance was the much better planning and the collaboration to achieve a planned occlusion that negated the need for segmental osteotomy.

I saw more segmental surgery when I was in the states than anywhere else and part of that was that if you couldn't afford orthodontics or could only afford partial orthodontics people ended up compromising to achieving a final result and often people were on the waiting list for orthognathic surgery but their progress was being delayed until they got money together to finish off the orthodontics.

I would say that the biggest game changer was top-notch planned orthodontics to give you an occlusion whereby you didn't have to do segmental procedures. The number of segmental procedures I saw in Yorkshire I could count on the fingers of one hand. Whereas I saw quite a few in the three months I was in Cleveland and planned a few more.

In some units the orthodontist more or less planned the entire treatment and then you just did a bi-max. I can't remember the last time I discussed a segmental procedure. All my surgery was bi-maxes, occasionally we would do a single jaw and occasionally a vertical sub-sigmoid. John Hamlyn quite liked those via an intraoral approach using a reciprocating saw.

Adrian Sugar described the onset of distraction and 3D planning.

When we moved in '94 from Chepstow to Morriston, we did the first case of distraction osteogenesis in the head and neck on a young man with hemifacial microsomia. Many of the patients coming to the Chepstow unit with congenital deformities as children were misdiagnosed and not treated. One thing that I set out to do was correct that, to diagnose and treat them properly. And I started to do that and continued to do that, and part of that process was reconstructing them for their ears, for hearing, working with my colleagues in Cardiff. Distraction was part of that process, and I did my first case in September '94 and continued to do a significant series.

We actually reviewed some of our early cases jointly with our colleagues from Great Ormond Street who came to Morriston and we held a private joint seminar discussing their cases and ours and commenting on them and making suggestions. So, it was very nice to have that sort of professional collaboration and in a similar sort of period of time towards the end of the '90s and the beginning of the 21ˢᵗ century I suppose we got involved in 3D planning initially with models, and we also developed a collaboration with our design engineer colleagues in Cardiff Metropolitan University.

And we've continued to extend that. We now employ and have employed I think the first dedicated person doing 3D planning on these cases fully employed by the National Health Service, not a max-fax technician, not a surgeon, but a person purely with degree qualifications in this area of work. And that's been extremely successful, and we now have about four or five people who are capable within that unit of doing that level of planning, but one person working full time for whom it is their sole duty.

Chapter 19
Dento-alveolar Surgery

'And why the hell I was taking it out I have no idea'

My earlier interviewees didn't talk about dento-alveolar surgery. It may have been that there had been little change in how they were managed before they retired from clinical practice. For most of the second half of the twentieth century there appeared to be a consensus within the specialty about how they were managed. This was described to me by my later subjects.

Adrian Sugar was a registrar in Teesside [1972-1975].

A few patients would be treated for wisdom teeth under local anaesthetic, but the vast majority were admitted, usually for at least two nights, maybe three, and treated as an inpatient under general anaesthetic. That was the norm.

Mike Davidson described dento-alveolar surgery at the London Hospital a decade later in 1986.

Virtually every operating list would have third molars on. It was in the days where if you had a third molar that was giving you trouble, all four would be taken out almost no matter where they were. All four would be done at once, and therefore you had a general anaesthetic. General anaesthetics were done on inpatients, and so the patient would come in the day before, would be worked up and then they would hang about overnight, and the following day they would have their surgery.

Drills were available, but the burrs were stainless steel, often blunt, and you really had to lean on them. You did sometimes have air-driven drills which were faster, but you had to be incredibly careful of the soft tissue because you could easily cut lips and damage people. So third molars were nearly always removed using the split bone technique using chisels, and teeth were often divided with osteotomes.[175] so you raised big lingual flaps and you had big retractors so you could get

---

175 The split bone technique for removal of lower third molar. Ward T. British Dental Journal. 1956 101. 297 301, 297.

your chisels in.

Often, you were chasing third molars that were entirely asymptomatic, but because they were there; that was the attitude. Well they're having a general anaesthetic, we'll get them all out. The worst ones to go chasing were the upper third molars, which often were incredibly high, and you had to raise a lot of mucosa to find the thing and remove a lot of bone. The patients were incredibly swollen, and often they would stay in a day at least after their procedure.

As a resident, your main duty was to protect the beds for the next list later in the week; you almost hot-bedded the patients. You would allow one out and one in. If you left it fallow for a night it would vanish, and you would be in real trouble. 'Why haven't you protected the beds?' The boss was just interested in getting their patients in, even if they weren't there for the list. That was your duty.

Then there were apicectomies being done, again often under general anaesthetic. There was a lot of dento-alveolar surgery that nowadays people would wonder a) why was it being done, and b) why was it being done under general anaesthesia? Why was it being done under general anaesthesia as an inpatient? It was a different world.

They were done under local anaesthetic as well. John Langdon was at the London Hospital [1974-76].

Most of the inpatient operating lists were dento-alveolar, wisdom teeth, apicectomy and cysts. But equally the outpatient department was busy. There were six chairs in minor oral surgery, of which two were manned by registrars and senior house officers full-time, knocking through cases. There was quite a lot done under local. But, like most oral surgery in those days, the inpatient lists were predominantly dento-alveolar too. And of course there were the outpatient general anaesthetic sessions.

Ian Martin describes dento-alveolar surgery at King's in the early 1980s.

We did quite a lot in local anaesthetics and quite a lot of intravenous sedation. As dental students we were taught to give conscious sedation with, originally, intravenous diazepam. That was all taught as part of the undergraduate curriculum for minor oral surgery.

But there was still a culture for wisdom teeth; if a patient wanted they would be offered a general anaesthetic and there were long waiting lists. At King's the oral surgeons, as they would have been then, shared the ward with ENT, and there were five or six lists a week of inpatient general anaesthetic stuff, which was predominantly dento-alveolar surgery.

If we say the working week started on the Sunday, the patients were brought in on Sunday for their wisdom teeth to be taken out on Monday. They wouldn't be discharged, probably, until the Thursday. And part of the reason for not discharging them until the Thursday was if you did then your bed would have been nicked by somebody else and you wouldn't have a bed for the patients coming in for the Thursday lists. So they were in for nearly a week quite often, having had just wisdom teeth out.

This was really before decent drills. It was nearly all done with lingual splits, and so they got pretty swollen and uncomfortable. It was black silk sutures. We had got into the era of giving high-dose dexamethasone to reduce the swelling; I think it was 8 milligrams, which was quite a big dose, but they still got massively swollen. They also had big doses of benzyl penicillin as Triplopen, three different versions of penicillin that had different release time and a massive pre-med of omnopon and scopolamine; so they would not be jumping up and down after their operation. And it wasn't uncommon for you to have to be faffing around in the middle of the night stopping the bleeding, trying to put another stitch in somewhere.

When I was a senior house officer, we were doing lists out in Lewisham and Hither Green. King's was expanding its empire. Hither Green was predominantly an infection control hospital but there was one of those porta cabin operating theatres that had been just shoved in a car park and David Vaughan was supposed to do that. But he hated it; so although it was really his list, I was sent off to go and do this.

It was all big West Indians with teeth that probably didn't need to come out. I can remember one guy who I struggled with for hours in this theatre; taking a buried premolar that was somewhere near the lower border out of this ivory hard bone. And why the hell I was taking it out, I have no idea. Oh god, I was digging around with no drill. It was all chisels with the lingual flap, buccal flap, trying to find this thing down at the lower border of the mandible. A bloody nightmare.

There was another case on John Sowray's list in theatre 4 at King's, which was just a simple dento-alveolar list. I was a senior house officer, doing it with a houseman, and it was a really high palatal canine, rammed up against the apical third of the lateral. Again, all with chisels, no drills. And there was a call from the cardiac ward; somebody had a pulmonary embolus and needed an emergency pulmonary embolectomy. So, of course, they looked around at what was going on in the various theatres and decided, oh, there's just a tooth on in theatre 4 so we'll send this case to theatre 4, cos he'll have this tooth out soon.

So the cardiothoracic surgeon then was a chap called Angus McArthur, and I was told that they were going to break my list of teeth after this case for Angus McArthur to come in and do this pulmonary embolectomy. So the patient was brought round from the cardiac ward into the anaesthetic room, put off to sleep ready. Meanwhile, I'm still struggling up this deep dark hole in the palate with my chisels trying to get some bone out from around the tooth without taking the roots off the incisors, and trying to find a point of application on this thing, and struggling like hell. It took me about an hour to get it out, and meanwhile, in the anaesthetic room Angus McArthur had opened the chest, done the emergency pulmonary embolectomy and sent the patient back to the cardiac ward. And I still hadn't got the tooth out. Oh dear!

After his medical training and jobs, Ian returned to oral and maxillofacial surgery as a registrar on Merseyside [1989].

By then things had changed. Drills had improved dramatically, and it was very rare to use chisels. Most of the dento-alveolar surgery by then, in Liverpool, was being done as day case stuff under local or local and sedation, and not a lot being done on inpatients or if it was done under general anaesthetic, it was often being done as a day case. That was a fairly big change that had happened over that period of time. We used mainly Aesculap drills actually because there were some very high speed ones which were the air driven, and Stryker drills.

The first time I came across that different approach was when I did locums at Addenbrookes Hospital, Cambridge. Bill Lamb always used these very high-powered air motors, which were very good at cutting bone, but they didn't have any irrigation. So you had to have another pair of hands to squeeze water on, otherwise you rapidly burnt the bone. Ted Varley had used Aesculap drills, which were self-irrigating, so I was always quite impressed with the fact it was much easier to know that you were drilling bone rather than tooth. With the very high powered Stryker thing, it was quite difficult to know what the hell you were drilling.

Of course, there was no need for these patients to come to hospital at all. Many of us used to do this surgery in dental practice, particularly when we were at medical school.[176] Adrian Sugar spent several months working in a dental practice after his senior house officer job and before starting his registrar job in Leeds [1976].

The practice had a consultant anaesthetist who used to do a session there once a week. Before I started, I had a chat with him and asked how he would feel about doing some eights and things like that. And he said, 'Yes, why not?' So, this was a practice in a big old house, as I think a lot of dental practices were in those days, and they had about three or four surgeries upstairs. We would do a list of eights, about twice as many as I could ever get through in the hospital. He would induce them with methohexitone through the external jugular vein. He would stand behind them and before they knew what had happened, they were out, and then he'd intubate them, and put a pack down and I'd take the eights out. If he thought I was struggling at all, he'd put a laryngoscope and act as my retractor and nurse at the same time.

And we also did a lot of kids for dental extractions as well. He even carried around a pair of eagle beak forceps. It was the first time I'd ever seen them. He pulled one out of his pocket when I seemed to be struggling with a six, and he said, 'Try one of these,' and of course it popped out straightway.

We got through quite a lot of work. We would leave the patient recovering from the anaesthetic with one of the nurses, and then we would wheel the anaesthetic machine into the next room. We went from one room to the next, and eventually we'd go through four rooms and when we were doing kids, we'd be back fairly quickly to the beginning by which time most of the patients had recovered and were close to being well enough to go home.

That went very well, very safely, and I earned good money doing that. Mostly because the Dental Estimates Board had no real idea

---

176 See my paper from 1993 favourably comparing the performance of a dentist in practice with Mount Vernon Hospital oral surgery department. The dentist concerned had no hospital training in oral surgery, he just got on and did it. Specialist practice for minor oral surgery: a comparative audit of third molar surgery. Sadler A, Davidson M, Houpis C, Watt-Smith S. British Dental Journal. 1993;174(8):273-277.

about what fee because if you were going to do a wisdom tooth you had to send in an X-ray and ask them to quote a fee for you, and they always quoted a fee far over what I thought I ought to get. So, I learned early on not to tell them how much I wanted because that's what they'd give me, and if I left it up to them to decide, I always got more than I would have asked for. It was quite enjoyable, really.

Chapter 20
Cleft Lip and Palate Surgery

'Don't you come down here telling me what I can and cannot do.'

Brian Avery became a consultant at Middlesbrough [from 1983].

I'd had no training in cleft lip and palate; this was done by the plastic surgeons, and I have to say I didn't think the standards were good. Colin Edge and I were colleagues together when our senior colleague, Richard Pratt, retired. We wanted to appoint a cleft consultant because we realised there was a big gap; the patients weren't getting a good service. I'd done some bone grafts and osteotomies on the adults, but I wasn't doing the primary clefts. So we appointed Alistair Smyth. Alistair started a cleft service, and he was good.

At first it was difficult because they were all going to one of the plastic surgeons. He went and saw the paediatricians and said, 'I have got an interest in clefts.' He really made sure he got experience and went to India several times and operated on, I think, a couple of hundred cases. He put it around that he was interested and he got the odd referral which he did using Professor Delaire's technique.[177]

He was repairing the palate, and he didn't have a single palatal breakdown the whole time he was with us. People were saying what wonderful results he was getting, and so he quickly cornered the market. And what's more, patients got to hear about him and we had, for him, the rather embarrassing situation where patients in the big city of Newcastle heard about him and wanted their kids treated down in Middlesbrough, by Alistair.

Alistair was very discreet about this and he wouldn't take them on; he felt it would cause problems and it might be difficult to manage them because of the distance involved. He was only with us for a few years and this was because the whole national cleft surgery situation was altered and there was a big battle in the north east whether the unit should be based in Leeds, where there's a huge population, or at

---

177 See: Functional primary closure of cleft lip Markus, A.F. and Delaire J. British Journal of Oral and Maxillofacial Surgery, Volume 31, Issue 5, 281 - 291

a Middlesbrough/Newcastle centre where there was a very good surgeon in Middlesbrough.

They plumped for Leeds, which I could understand. They had a catchment population of probably five million. So eventually Middlesbrough lost out, but of course they were smart enough to appoint Alistair as the cleft surgeon in Leeds and he's been there ever since doing huge numbers, still. And as far I know, working pretty well on his own but getting excellent results. Still, the patients being treated at the Newcastle end of the region wanted to go down to Leeds for treatment but were not allowed to.

Were the orthodontists involved with the cleft cases when the plastics were doing them?

Yes, but it was very rudimentary. The reason the patients were not getting a good service, in my opinion, was that they were getting their lips and their palates repaired and then nothing beyond that. They were never getting their alveolar bone grafts or any secondary surgery. They were having the old-fashioned Millard's lip repair. Millard's repair looks lovely immediately after surgery, but doesn't look very nice a year later, just the reverse of the Delaire technique which doesn't look good after surgery but a year down the road the results were wonderful.

Tony Markus was a senior registrar at Mount Vernon [1977].

We saw a lot of clefts. Brian Morgan and Roy Sanders were plastic surgery consultants there. And Roy and I got on very well, he was a very good surgeon, very fine standards. We set up a proper multi-disciplinary clinic for clefts and set up the first cleft support group. I became increasingly interested in the clefts.

In 1979 we had one of the senior registrar annual get-togethers, which were a small amount of science and then a lot of drunken socialising, in Leeds. There I met Professor Jean Delaire. He came and gave two stunning lectures, one on the physiology of the workings of the face and the other on how one assesses facial deformity. I met Delaire, and he sort of extended an open invitation. He said if anybody wants to come and see my work, you're welcome. So I went to him and I said, 'Can I come?' And he said, 'mais oui.' And so off I went in due course.

I was still a senior registrar, and I became rightly infatuated by his functional philosophy. It was absolutely right, and it was just so obvious that we needed to understand what was going on properly to get good outcomes. Just making a nice Millard incision in the skin and getting the skin together for a cleft lip was inadequate. One also had to pay attention to all the other structures, whether it was the periosteum or the muscles or all those structures of the face, if one is going to get, not just a good aesthetic outcome, but excellent facial development. So I had a few short visits, and I came back and I was quite fired up. Roy and I spoke about this quite a lot.

Tony became a consultant in Poole [1985].

I got there, and I thought this was a lovely, fabulous place to work and looking out over the harbour, not a lot to do, best fishing chalk streams in the country; this is going to be a doddle.

I was in the consultant car park one day, just about to go home, when I was cornered by two paediatricians, one who was part time at Great Ormond Street and another who was full time at Poole. They said, 'We don't like the service that we're getting and we've heard about you and we'd like you to start a cleft service here.'

They had heard that I had an interest, that I had some training. So I said, 'Well that's okay, but I need to consolidate my training and I would also need to make sure I've got everybody that we need to have a proper multi-disciplinary service.' This was 1985, people didn't talk about multi-disciplinary teams in those days.

So I said okay. The unit general manager said, 'If you want time off you can go.' Rapidly they'd put together a supporting service. Winston Peters, the other consultant, was a terrific support. I got an anaesthetist who was the only trained paediatric anaesthetist, a member of the newly formed of Association of Paediatric Anaesthetists. They found a speech therapist, had a designated developmental paediatrician, an acute paediatrician, a health visitor, a specialist nurse, ENT surgeon to do the otology, and orthodontist.

I did the first one at the end of '85, which was a cleft palate. I'd spent more time with Delaire, and as time went, it became easier because although initially the ferry from Poole to Cherbourg was just trucks, so I had to go to Portsmouth, it then became a passenger line as well. So I could just get on the boat in Poole, go to Cherbourg or St Malo, drive down to Nantes if I wanted to see something. So it was fantastic.

I learnt how to speak French. He could speak English and we spoke English and Franglais, but he said, 'When I operate I think in French,' so we spoke French. I had reasonable French beforehand. We did the first cleft palate in '85, I'm still in touch with him, a nice chap, he has done very well. Then in '86 we saw the development of significant local, regional referrals, much to the annoyance of the plastic surgeons. They insisted that we only had six patients a year.

So where were you getting the referrals from?

The ones that were going to Salisbury were all local. There were local postcodes plus South West Hants, North Dorset, South West Dorset, East Devon, quite a large area.

And who were sending you the patients? Presumably the paediatricians?

Yes, from Poole and Bournemouth and South Hants, mainly from Poole and Bournemouth. Everything came to Poole for the obstetrics, so that's pretty straightforward. And there was quite a lot of sympathy from South West Hants. The Dorchester paediatricians were a little more reluctant, but we got patients from there as well.

So presumably the paediatricians were liaising with each other at their meetings and it was getting about?

Yes, they were hugely instrumental. And of course bad news spreads like fire and we started coming in for quite severe criticism from plastic surgeons who were saying, 'Well they better only have six a year.' At the end of '86 we were getting 20 new referrals just from Dorset alone, so God knows what happened to the other ones, but they were verified by the Health Authority. The plastic surgeons complained to the regional medical officer, and he said, 'Well if you're worried about six cases then clearly you haven't got enough work to do, so let me know what work you are doing.' So they didn't like that. And then they complained to the Medical Defence and to the General Medical Council and they were told, 'Well, what's the problem? He's had the training; he's providing a service.'

The regional medical officer was very supportive. I even had a phone call whilst I was doing outpatients at the Royal Victoria Hospital in Boscombe on Thursday afternoon, from Frank Haselden who was the maxillofacial surgeon at Odstock, ringing me up and telling me I really shouldn't be doing this because it's not our territory and it upsets the relationship between our specialities. Never mind the outcomes, he was more concerned about the relationship between the specialities.

One of the plastic surgeons came down for the party that we'd put on annually for the senior nursing staff for Christmas, He approached one of the anaesthetists who he had been at medical school with, who he knew, and said, 'Where's this so and so dentist who's taking all the clefts away from us?' And so he pointed to my anaesthetist, and he said, 'You want to talk to that anaesthetist and he'll tell you more.'

We were pretty well back to back, and there was this great big commotion and I turned round, as did everybody else, and the anaesthetist had got this chap by his jacket lapels and was bouncing him out; he pushed him out through the double doors of this lounge. And said, 'Don't you come down here telling me what I can and cannot do.' And it was only afterwards that I knew what was going on. So they tried every way possible to stop me. And so it just went on and on. And we built up the service. It was consolidated; it was the only truly comprehensive service available for cleft children in this country.

I had had nothing like this before, because I'd worked in an environment where we'd all worked together on these things. So I was quite surprised by the vehemence, but it wasn't totally unexpected. I suppose in retrospect it was provocative, but I hadn't done it to be provocative. I had done it because we'd been able to establish a first class centre, and I'd been asked. I hadn't gone in there and asked to do it.

But this is how things were in those days. When it came ultimately to the CSAG, Clinical Standards Advisory Group, review of cleft lip and palate services,[178] there were 57 centres, 87 surgeons doing, I can't remember exactly, 600 cases a year in the UK. And it was quite uncoordinated. And it was assumed that the plastic surgeons would do the primary cleft work.

So they were upset because you weren't a plastic surgeon?

That's right, it was a turf war, and I was a dentist. Just like the outburst when John Langdon wrote his editorial for the Annals of the Royal College of Surgeons, what are the dentists doing head and neck

---

178 Report of the Clinical Standards Advisory Group Cleft lip and/or Palate. HMSO 1998.

cancer for?[179]

We've only just got over it now because now post CSAG we're probably seeing slightly more maxillofacial surgeons than plastic surgeons doing primary cleft work in this country. But it's taken that long to get there.

We had 20 new cases a year, locally, from Dorset and the adjacent environs. And then I was getting several from around the country, because we'd had articles. We had a provocative editorial in the British Medical Journal that I wrote with Peter Ward Booth.[180] That was an editorial, saying that there was very little evidence base for the clinical practice amongst cleft surgeons in this country, and we needed to look to Europe to see how we ought to organise ourselves. That came at a pretty critical time because the CSAG, Clinical Standards Advisory Group, cleft lip and palate review committee, had just at that point been established. There'd been in the early '90s the Eurocleft study looking at six European centres, including two UK ones, which showed the results in the UK were very below the other four European ones.[181]

There were articles elsewhere as well, I think, including in the British Medical Journal. But the one that the plastic surgeons took real offence to was the September '96 editorial Peter Ward Booth and myself. They said we were completely denigrating, and yes we were, but we didn't say as much, so it was their interpretation. That was post-CSAG.[182]

In 1995 you wrote in the British Journal of Oral and Maxillofacial Surgery, 'Surgery by Numbers' you were saying that the number of cases you do a year are of less importance to the technique that you

---

179 See: Team Approach in the management of oral cancer. Annals of the Royal College of Surgeons of England. Rapidis A. Angelopolous A. Langdon J. 1980 62 116 - 119. Also see chapter 26

180 Managing Cleft Lip and Palate. Tony Markus and Peter Ward Booth. British Medical Journal. 311, Sept. 23rd 1996 765 - 766 See also letter and reply BMJ 25th November 1995.

181 The Eurocleft Project: overview. Shaw WC., et al. Journal of Cranio-Maxillofacial Surgery 2001 June 29 (1) 131-140.

182 See also: Cleft care: life after CSAG. Williams J Ll., Markus AF. British Journal of Oral and Maxillofacial Surgery 1998 36 81-83.

use? [183]

Yes. The numbers are important. But that wasn't the point. Everybody said that we could go on if we just increased the number that justified our doing the service. It didn't, unless they were prepared to support it with evidence of their outcomes. So patients might have been seen by any of the consultants and the operations might have been done by the senior registrars and they then go away, become consultants and they might have done one case. So what sort of training's that?

So that was what I was trying to say there. I don't think that 20 is the right number either. By then I was already doing a lot overseas, so my local 20 would be bolstered by probably another 40 overseas every year. But now I was involved with this big hospital in Hyderabad for example, where they do 1,600 clefts a year, plus 300 cranio-facial. 1,600 clefts between three surgeons, and they're able to train people properly. So it's a different kettle of fish. But at the time everybody was saying, 'Oh, it's just the numbers,' and we were arguing from extremities. I was saying it's not just the number; the numbers to some extent are important but you have to have a proper training, good technique and then if you are well trained, a good surgeon with a good technique the chances are that the outcomes will be pretty good.

Has the Delaire technique taken off throughout the UK?

Yes, the principles are widely used by many of the former trainees. We wrote a paper two years ago in Plastic and Reconstructive Surgery.[184] We looked at 800 unilateral cleft lip and palate patients, 400 of whom had had a Millard incision and 400 who had had a Pfeifer incision on the skin. And the outcomes were the same; there was no statistical difference. And the reason there was no statistical difference is because of what was done underneath. So it was the principles of not just closing the skin and maybe a bit of muscle, but of trying to do everything meticulously repaired so you would return as close to normality as possible. That was the principle.

Delaire would say, 'Well that's not my technique, it's what you call

---

183 Surgery by number? Editorial. Markus A. British Journal of Oral and Maxillofacial Surgery 1995 33 205-206.
184 Choice of incision for primary repair of unilateral complete cleft lip: a comparative study of outcomes in 796 patients. Reddy GS, Webb RM, Reddy RR, Reddy LV, Thomas P, Markus AF. Plastic and Reconstructive Surgery. 2008 Mar; 121 (3): 932-40

it.' And he's quite right. I mean he used the Millard, he used Pfeiffer, he used Petit, all sorts of people who influenced him, Tennyson, and so on. And he eventually got to that technique which produced very good results. In 1997 in Milan, Roberto Brusati, who had also trained in Nantes, convened a conference of the Delaire technique 25 years on. There was Roberto Brusati, Jean Claud Talmont from Nantes, David Precious from Canada, Uli Joos from Muenster and myself. And the five of us each had to give a presentation on unilateral complete cleft, a bilateral complete cleft palate, etc, the different operations.

Delaire sat like the king in the middle and wasn't just presiding there silently, but he would come in and add things. And we were all slightly different; some people were doing one stage palate repairs, some of us were doing two stage palate repairs, (but they were the exception) and it proved the point, that actually we'd all been influenced heavily by Delaire and his philosophies. And which are not just confined to cleft but to lots of other things. We saw lots; we used them in the management of things like Binder's syndrome – early treatment; don't wait for the deformity to develop.

In the management of facial asymmetries, do treatment early, get on and do it, don't wait for the deformity to develop, make the most of growth potential. And so I did what I call Delaire and Gosla Reddy in Hyderabad does Delaire and Paresh Devani does Delaire and Chris Penfold in North Wales and Liverpool does, and so on. But it's actually not Delaire, strictly, it's influenced by Delaire. And I think that's normal and I think as we become more experienced we develop our own little variations which we know, in our hands, will produce good results.

So we had CSAG. We went all over the country; we looked at 17 UK units and we looked at two units overseas, Oslo and Nantes. It was always loaded against our specialty. But we fought pretty hard; I fought pretty hard. I was pretty well a lone voice for our specialty there. It was quite difficult, with statistics coming from Bill Shaw,[185] anything to justify centralisation, which was quite right. We couldn't have 57 centres in the UK, it was absolute nonsense.

I learnt a lot in my time at the Department of Health. I learned that if you want to achieve anything, which ultimately when I became associate medical director was very helpful, you establish your own

---

185 Professor of orthodontics, Manchester.

agendas and set them very high and give yourself a bit of room to come down; but it was a good starting point.

It was very belligerent, the whole period during when we sat at the department. At the same time I was on the council of the British Association of Oral and Maxillofacial Surgeons, the medical director said, 'Do try to stay in Poole a little bit if you can.' I did, I managed. I had a wonderful PA and my wife keeping me going to the right places. We were training people overseas, India in particular, people in Eastern Europe. I'd got a grant from the UK Government to transfer knowledge with a wonderful centre in Moscow. That was extremely interesting. And so it developed into travelling around to Minsk, Bratislava, and latterly Moscow, St Petersburg, in Europe and of course developing lots of contacts in Europe.

Post-CSAG, during the implementation there was a lot of argument about where the centres would be, the definition of centres, audit and so on, huge discussions. They went on till I think 1999 and eventually the various centres were set up. Not quite in accordance with the recommendations of CSAG but they were established.

How is cleft surgery in the UK now?

I think it's probably better. Whether it will be bettered remains to be seen. The fact is, we've got over eight centres, we've got 16 centres because most of the centres are twin sites, like the Spires Cleft Centre is Oxford and Salisbury, but they don't necessarily do the same technique. They might be managed by the same manager, but they use different techniques at each centre. So we in essence probably still have got 16 centres. Now 16 centres, which are England, Wales and Northern Ireland; Scotland is the managed clinical network, and it works pretty well. 16 centres for 600 patients is still ridiculous. And we probably really ought to have just one centre for the whole of the UK. But there'd be an uproar.

There's still work to be done. But I think these arguments are now behind us. The turf wars are behind us and we've established the inter specialty working groups for cleft, cranio-facial, the head and neck cancer and for cosmetic surgery, at the Royal College of Surgeons; terrific meeting places. We've established proper training programmes, limited numbers of cleft fellowships or cranio-facial fellowships or whatever, and they're open to any specialty where the person has had the right sort of training. So in the south west it's a plastic surgeon and two maxillofacial surgeons, south Wales, two maxillofacial surgeons and one plastic surgeon as the primary surgeons. In south west Thames there are two maxillofacial surgeons, two plastic surgeons and so on. So for the specialty it's good. And it's established. And the people there now are not having these fights, they can get on and raise standards. But it was necessary to get there.

You were awarded an FRCS 'ad eundem'?

Yes. I was very chuffed about that. Just a terrific honour and I was really chuffed.

Chapter 21
Pre-prosthetic Surgery and Implantology
'Sometimes the patients are worse off'

Implantology has largely replaced the demand for pre-prosthetic surgery, which was used earlier in the twentieth century when tooth loss in early adulthood was common. The resorbed edentulous mandibular ridge was a particular problem for denture retention.

Gordon Fordyce explained the sulcoplasty or buccal inlay, which was widely used to aid lower denture retention. It was so good that patients sometimes had difficulty getting the denture out [1949 - 1988].

It took a long time. Patients had to come and go for months because the grafts would always shrink. They were also used in my time for patients with congenital deformities such as micrognathia.

A case I remember was a girl who was a dental nurse, and she had a wisdom tooth coming through. A dentist in Athens looked at it and took a biopsy, and the biopsy report came back and said malignancy behind the molar. They gave her radiotherapy and burnt her mandible and the temporo-mandibular joint, and she had radionecrosis. Then they asked me to see her. We did a bone graft and got that healed. But by this time she had no chin and it was across to one side.

She was edentulous because of the radiotherapy and extractions necessary, so a buccal inlay was used. You made an incision at the junction of the attached mucoperiosteum and the labial mucosa, freed the lip, which fortunately wasn't shrunk. By this time, we'd made some sort of splint, taken gutta percha and made a mould much bigger than we wanted, down to the lower border, avoiding if possible any nerve left. Then a skin graft was taken from the arm and skin put onto the mould. The plastic surgeon was skilled in doing it and knew how to get a graft, which was big enough. We put the graft on the mould, put it in and put the fixation on, and that was left for about three weeks.

After about three weeks they had a short anaesthetic and the mould was removed, with difficulty sometimes because what was holding it down was that join between the graft and the mucosa. It was a straight line which could do nothing but shrink into a tight band. We were quite pleased to see it. By the time six months had gone past, the graft had shrunk to the size that we wanted. And the patient had learned how to get the appliance in and out themselves and keep it beautifully clean. The grafts were miraculous.[186]

After he was appointed as a consultant in Cardiff, Russell Hopkins set up joint clinics with prosthodontics for pre-prosthetic surgery [1968].

Well, no one else did it, as far as I knew. It could only happen in a dental hospital, and I don't think it happened anywhere else initially. I think that later it became standard practice, but at that stage it was unheard of.

When I started to do pre-prosthetic surgery, I think I had to persuade Bates[187] that it had a role and I had to show him cases I'd done. I then sent him cases after I'd finished the surgery asked whether he would do the dentures. What I did was combining a sulcoplasty with deepening the alveolar ridges.

I used to put splints on to deepen them and hold them in position so they stayed down a bit and increased the whole denture bearing surface area. He found that a considerable help, and it developed from there.

And then they sent me cases, and then we had a combined clinic. Then I didn't operate on patients unless I'd sent them first to the prosthetists. They often made a new set of dentures first to see whether that would solve the problem, and if they couldn't we used the new set of dentures as part of the prosthetic splintage after we'd taken the mould out of the skin grafts. That way we had something which had the right vertical dimension and the correct occlusion.

Russell also used the sandwich osteotomy technique in the maxilla.

It was a Le Fort I with blocks of bone from the iliac crest and bone chips packed around it, and then the upper jaw put back again. I think I did the first sandwich, the first multi piece maxilla, through a Le Fort I approach in about 1973.

Adrian Sugar described prosthetics with Derek Stafford as senior

---

186 The operation had been described by a Dutch plastic surgeon in 1917. See: Studies in plastic surgery of the face: I. Use of skin from the neck to replace face defects. II. Plastic operations about the mouth. III. The epidermic inlay. Esser JF. Annals of surgery 1917; 65(3) 297-315.
187 Professor Bates. Professor of prosthetic dentistry at Cardiff dental school.

registrar in Cardiff [1980].

Long before I went to Cardiff, Hoppy[188] had established a monthly joint clinic with orthodontics and a monthly oral surgery/prosthetic clinic. The max-fax registrar used to do a session with Derek Stafford[189] on max-fax prosthodontics because that was Derek's specific remit. I don't think they ever entirely enjoyed it, but I got some wonderful stories from them about some experiences they had.

Derek Stafford was a lovely person to work with. It was out of that clinic that we did a lot of pre-prosthetic surgery, mostly vestibuloplasties, but also augmentations such as sandwich osteotomies, and I did one of my first clinical studies on all sandwich osteotomies that had been done. Derek used to tease me mercilessly when I was a senior registrar because I never came to do any prosthetics with him. And I always explained to him I had a lot of experience of doing obturators for maxillectomies, and although I thought he was very good at what he did, I didn't think I needed any more training.

I was learning how to do the pre-prosthetic techniques that Russell Hopkins had more or less single-handedly initiated in Cardiff. I'd already been introduced to those and did some with Max Gregory[190] in Newport, and so I already had some understanding of those techniques. I didn't even know, in those days, what a buccal inlay was.

I gradually learned that sulcus deepening was something that very few people in our specialty had much experience of, and nowadays it's obsolete except in some of the most difficult cancer cases because implants have overtaken and replaced most of those techniques.

But there are still cases where you put in implants and where the soft tissue is very mobile, especially in reconstructed cancer cases, and that application of sulcus deepening procedures can be very helpful and I've done some of that. Where there were vertical or lateral bone deficiencies, we did onlay augmentations. If the residual bone without the bone graft was of adequate height to retain a stable implant, we'd sometimes insert implants at the same time as the bone graft.

John Bradley consultant at Burnley and Bury [1968 - 1995].

---

188 Russell Hopkins was affectionately known as 'Hoppy'.
189 Senior Lecturer and later professor of prosthetic dentistry at Cardiff dental school.
190 Former senior registrar and later consultant in Newport.

The sulcoplasty worked. We had nothing else to offer. The Brånemark implants hadn't appeared at that point. We had other implants which were the subperiosteal ones; these were chrome cobalt frames with studs that came through the mucous membrane and on which you mounted your prosthesis on the top.

These things didn't do well because almost all of them, eventually, got infected. I didn't do them but I had to take several out and the mouth was in a dreadful mess after that and you'd have to leave it for 12 to 18 months before you could go back to do some sulcoplasties and skin grafts and then they were better. With the Brånemark implant, with titanium you get a union between the soft tissues and the hard tissues which you can't get with the chrome cobalt ones, the vast majority of them failed.

Ian Martin:

John Cawood was one forerunner in developing dental implants for pre-prosthetic surgery. Because prior to that King's pre-prosthetic surgery was the sulcoplasties and various things to augment atrophic mandibles and endosseous implants that these great big metal structures that sat under the gum on the jaw. So that was pre-prosthetic surgery, but one of the big transformations in the management of prosthetic cases was the implants, and John Cawood had been definitely at the forefront of that.

Brian Avery, was a consultant in Middlesbrough. I asked him if implants came in during his time there [From 1983]?

Yes. I negotiated it personally with the Primary Care Trust and negotiated a service that would allow us to do 12 cases a year and there was a protocol, priority given to trauma patients, cancer patients, deformity patients. And the very last patients in the priority list were the denture cripples.

I started doing implants using a visiting conservative dentist who came down a day a week. I started using the Brånemark kit, and I got that on the back of waiting list initiatives. They funded the kit for doing a few waiting list initiatives. That was a deal, and so I started inserting a few implants. But I never did many as I was just too busy, and we appointed another colleague eventually to come along and do more orthognathic surgery and the implants. I'm afraid I don't think it's taken off and I don't think implants are currently done in my old unit.

Khursheed Moos, consultant Canniesburn [1974 - 1999].

Another development which we started from scratch was the cranio-facial implant system (Brånemark). We could not get any funding for that, but I chased around a lot of different companies to help us finance this and we got a starter of £10,000 a year for three years and after that more from other sources as well.

So we started first with extraoral implant borne prostheses, ears and noses, because they were obvious to the public. They could see the change there with visible reconstructed ears, noses and orbits following cancer surgery, congenital deformity and trauma. There was no satisfactory reconstruction for ears before that time.

We added intraoral implants as soon as we could for difficult major deformity cases, raising about £100,000 from different sources to fund that. Then we ran out of funding towards the end of the 90s and then we had big troubles. We told the health board we had all these patients there who were in the middle of treatment and we could not raise any more funds to help them and so eventually they gave in.

Initially, we started doing bone anchored hearing aids for the ENT department and then they did that themselves and now have developed that field further but we were the initiators of it.

When Adrian Sugar became a consultant in Chepstow Derek Stafford went there to do a clinic with him [1985].

Out of that we started to do cranio-facial implants for ears and eyes and noses, etc. I'd observed in Chepstow, when I'd taken up my consultant post, that there was quite a lot of that work around, but nobody did it or hardly anyone.

I found out about these guys in Sweden who were doing this work in ENT. Derek knew everybody, especially in Sweden, and the two of us went out in January '86 to Gothenburg and we met Brånemark and a lot of his team. And out of that we started doing this work in '87.

The first patient was referred by one of the plastic surgeons, and that became quite an important part of our work. I was very fortunate to have worked with two first-rate maxillofacial prosthesis technologists. I started doing facial implants for ears and eyes and noses years before I started doing dental implants, but the techniques are very similar, but the anatomical situations are completely different.

John Cawood spent 3 months in Arnhem in 1980, just before he started his consultant job in Chester. He had just spent 9 months in Seattle.

I probably learnt more from Hans de Koomen the prosthodontist than from the surgeons. Because Hans, who subsequently wrote his PhD on the subject and latterly became professor at the Free University in Amsterdam, said pre-prosthetic surgery doesn't really work. It looks good on X-ray, but bone grafts usually shrink, and sometimes the patients are worse off than before, because of comorbidity. My interest in pre-prosthetic surgery was developed from Arnhem, and I was very interested in jaw atrophy, and Hans was also interested in jaw atrophy.

In the early days, pre-prosthetic surgery all came from Germany and Switzerland; Obwegeser was a very strong component. It was all about vestibuloplasty and skin grafting to improve the denture bearing area. Then it followed on from that with bone grafting, and they devised procedures such as visor osteotomies and onlay grafts. But it looked very good on X-ray but generally the bone just resorbed. Arnhem did a lot of this type of surgery and published. Hans was having to treat these patients, and he said it was a nightmare because often they came with mental anaesthesia and paraesthesia; they just found it difficult to cope.

Nevertheless, they were tackling a problem that was a challenge which hadn't been solved. The arrival of endosteal implants made a huge difference, and I was just lucky enough to get in at the beginning, partly from visiting Seattle and then when I was in Arnhem, which was a big milestone in my career.

Within eighteen months the bone grafts resorbed, and Hans highlighted the problems of pre-prosthetic surgery for the patient and for the prosthodontist. So they had a symposium on pre-prosthetic surgery, and surgeons with an interest were invited to attend and to bring their prosthodontist. So Paul Stoelinga and Hans appeared, Bill Terry and Dick Grecius from North Carolina came. Russell Hopkins and his prosthodontist Derek Stafford came, and one or two others.[191]

They had a consensus meeting and out of that came the conclusions that bone grafting didn't really help. Some mucosal grafts were useful. So it was really going nowhere as a solution to the problem of the

---

191 See: Arnhem Consensus on pre-prosthetic surgery. Cawood J. International Journal of Oral and Maxillofacial Surgery. 1990: 19. 10-11.

atrophic jaw, particularly the mandible.

Endosteal implants, as developed by Brånemark, transformed outcomes in the management of the atrophic jaw. Prior to that there was a chap in America who had a staple implant which he put through the lower border with two prongs in the canine area. They bolted onto the lower denture and that seemed to have some success and was quite popular in the States.

So Branemark put a scientific basis onto why titanium was biocompatible, then demonstrated some pretty impressive results. So endosteal implants suddenly became kosher again.

A patient with very severe atrophy didn't have enough bone to accommodate implants predictably, so pre-implant surgery supplanted pre-prosthetic surgery; pre-prosthetic surgery suddenly became pre-implant surgery. So a lot of the techniques of pre-prosthetic surgery had relevance again, particularly because of grafting. The results were predictable and sustainable because the bone wasn't shrinking because it was stimulated by the internal tensile stresses from implants. So that's how that area opened up.

I did a study in Edinburgh with Bob Howell. I'd been stimulated by Hans de Koomen to look into it further and came up with this descriptive classification of the jaws, and we backed that up statistically with a study at the Royal College of Surgeons of Edinburgh measuring dry skulls. We had 300 skulls we looked at and made measurements and found that there were very much clearly identifiable stages of atrophy which were descriptive, and you could see and diagnose. And that was all backed up statistically, so this jaw classification then became fairly widely used by clinicians and by insurance companies and various others.

That was another milestone in my career because I built a sub-specialty interest around that, from the jaw form or which stage of jaw atrophy we were dealing with, we worked out different operative procedures and bone grafting techniques to provide the bony support for implants, and also restore facial form. So it kind of grew more into rehabilitation than just pure reconstruction, because then we could improve the patient's ultimate wellbeing because they could not only chew better, but they could look better. And then that spilled over into rehabilitation of the cancer cases.

My interest latterly has been the International Academy for Oral

276

and Facial Rehabilitation beginning from a meeting in Berlin about relative augmentation of the atrophic jaw which was evolved into pre-implant surgery, which then evolved into rehabilitation.[192] And what is rehabilitation? I've always used three prongs. There's reconstruction, there is restoration of function, restoration of form, and hopefully restoration of wellbeing.

And Simon Roger's work[193] in health-related quality of life has been very interesting and very significant, measuring outcome from the various treatments that we perform. So this group, the OFR, has involved surgeons and prosthodontists, and then now it's involving material scientists, bio-engineers, immunologists, all sorts, because of the expertise that's growing.

---

192 See: International Academy for Oral and Facial Rehabilitation - Consensus Report. International Journal of Oral and Maxillofacial Surgey. 35 (3): 195-8.
193 Professor Simon Rogers, Consultant oral and maxillofacial surgeon at Aintree.

Chapter 22

Temporomandibular Joint Disorders

'Of course everybody sued everybody else'

The hospital based oral and maxillofacial service has been the usual destination for patients complaining of pain, discomfort, and clicking in the temporomandibular joint and, or limitation of mouth opening. The limited enthusiasm for dealing with this affliction I saw among many of my colleagues was reflected among my interview subjects to talk about it, although opinions were more forthcoming when it came to surgery.

Rob Hensher was a senior house officer at Whipps Cross. He describes the management of temporomandibular joint dysfunction, as it was called [1980].

The first thing was, they were listened to. I'm not sure whether 'the old man'[194] felt it deserved quite as much science as was emerging, but he was very tolerant of these things. Management would begin with a good interview, and then we'd look at dental things. We'd use splints and physio, and all the sort of conservative measures that we still advocate today, indeed, that one overlooks at one's peril before moving onto drug treatment and so on. So, I got the chance to prescribe the accepted medication a little bit.

The local orthodontist, who was also quite a good influence, was quite keen on this and we did use some oral rehabilitation, spot grinding and balancing. I wasn't sure what I was doing as I'd not had any proper formal training in this, but the orthodontist oversaw a lot of that. And yes, we approached the dental aspect, the third joint, as we call it nowadays.[195]

Surgery to the temporomandibular joint for ankylosis and derangement had been carried out from early in the twentieth century. Russell Hopkins

---

194 Denys Brock, his consultant at Whipps Cross.
195 See: Management of temporomandibular joint disease - occlusal rehabilitation. Thomson H British Journal of Oral and Maxillofacial Surgery 1987 25; 121-124. Hamish Thompson described the symptoms of patients referred to the Eastman Dental Hospital between 1954 and 1983 and the theory of how the dental occlusion and parafunctional habits cause them and their management with splints and adjustment of the teeth.

as senior house officer Nottingham [1958].

Tom Battersby would do condylectomies because the treatment of OA joints and fractures was a condylectomy. There was no other clever stuff at that stage.

One favoured operation for derangement was the closed condylotomy carried out with a Gigli saw. Enthusiasm for this seemed to have originated from East Grinstead as described by Sir Terence Ward in his 1960 Tomes lecture at the Royal College of Surgeons of England.[196] I can remember doing this several times when I was a registrar in Norwich in 1980-81 under instruction from Geoff Cheney, who had trained at East Grinstead. It was a quick and easy operation, but the patients were very sore and swollen afterwards and had permanent deviation on opening afterwards. But they didn't seem to complain about their symptoms again, perhaps because they thought we might do it again?

By the late 1980s, news of more sophisticated techniques was coming from the United States. Imaging of the meniscus with arthrography, computerised tomography and magnetic resonance imaging. Open surgery was being used by some, and arthroscopy had started.

In 1989 there was a seminar held in Newcastle and many of the forward thinking surgeons in the country attended to learn about arthroscopy from friends from the USA.[197]

One of those attending the symposium was Laurence Oldham, consultant in Taunton [1990].

Arthroscopy suddenly came on the horizon, everybody was talking about arthroscopy, I said, 'We've got to do arthroscopies.' So Hugh Walters, Torquay consultant, and I both went to Newcastle where they flew over the American bigwig, can't remember his name, but he was the leading American figure for arthroscopy. And he went through all his lecture slides and technique and equipment and kit, the whole gamut.

We came back, and Hugh started doing them in Torquay, and I started doing them in Taunton. This was a preliminary to any joint

---

196 See text of lecture: Surgery of the mandibular joint. Ward TG. Annals of the Royal College of Surgeons of England. 1961 Mar; 28 (3): 139-52.
197 See the report of the symposium with a photograph of the attendees: The first temporomandibular joint arthroscopy symposium. K Jones. British Journal of Oral and Maxillofacial Surgery 1990 28, 63-64.

surgery that we did. I'd been doing some temporo-mandibular joint surgery, and it just came in as I was more or less coming to the end of my period of consultancy really, so I just did some but I didn't get it very far, just some.

By the 1980s surgery was still used sparingly for internal derangements, but surgery to the meniscus was in the ascendancy. Some used it frequently and took tertiary referrals. Tony Markus was a consultant in Poole. Apart from the cleft surgery, his main clinical interest as a consultant was temporomandibular joints [from 1985].

I did lots and lots of arthroplasties; I don't know how many arthrocentesis. We did some arthroscopy for a while but didn't find it really was of any great benefit.

Winston Peters, the other Poole consultant and I were supported by a fantastic radiologist who allowed us to see what was going on inside the joints initially with intra-articular arthrograms and latterly with MRI scanning, so we could develop a really good algorithm of care. We were the only people doing them on the south coast, so we got quite a lot sent to us. That's partly because of Winston's interest; we worked very closely together. It was a great partnership until he retired after 23 years together; and it was partly because of the radiologist's terrific input. But I had also been influenced by Paul Toller; he'd died by then, but was in the background of my training.[198]

We had an algorithm which we worked to with various treatment modalities, first conservative, but the scanning made a big difference. If there was an irreducible displacement from an internal derangement, or if there was a significant pathology there, then we would operate. We probably did more than most; you could argue that a lot of them would have gone away and got better. But I think a lot of the people who went away didn't get better, they just got fed up coming back repeatedly to be told well have another plate or don't eat this or don't yawn or whatever, and thinking this is a waste of time so why bother. It's difficult to know.

Peter Banks was doing post-condylar cartilage grafts, and there

---

198 Toller was a consultant at Mount Vernon hospital and had an interest and wrote about joints. Tony had been a senior registrar there but after Toller had died.

were all sorts of temporo-mandibular joint things going on.[199] We don't do arthroplasties quite so much now and arthrocentesis is very effective much of the time.

Brian Avery was not so keen; he was a consultant in Middlesbrough [from 1983].

The temporomandibular joint surgery I did tended to be dislocations and ankyloses because I got a few of those and I treated them with gap arthroplasties usually.

When I first went as a young consultant in Middlesbrough, I did a few operations on people with temporomandibular joint derangements. I had been trained to do this at Canniesburn, things like plication of the meniscus, reduction of the tubercle, and I started using these techniques.

I got excellent results for a few months but the patients virtually all returned, and it soon became apparent that surgery was not the right treatment and I stopped within a couple of years of becoming a consultant and I never carried out surgery again on these patients.

I'm sure they did better without surgery. I think we just magnified the complications and the difficulty of handling these patients if you did surgery that was invariably not successful.

Ian Martin discussed the treatment for temporomandibular joint pain and clicking in the 1980s

It was the usual conservative stuff, not tricyclics. When I was at King's many years ago, 1979-81, with Malcolm Harris, he was big into tricyclics. He worked with Charlotte Feinmann, who was a psychiatrist. He was very much on the medical side.[200]

---

199 Mandibular advancement using a retro condylar cartilage graft: a 20-year prospective study. Banks P. British Journal of Oral and Maxillofacial Surgery. 2005. 43; 484-492.

200 See: Psychogenic facial pain: presentation and treatment. Feinmann C, Harris M, Cawley R. British Medical Journal 1984 288; 436-438. Charlotte Feinmann and Malcolm Harris point out that the incidence of malocclusion is no higher in these patients than in the general population and that occlusal adjustment had been shown to be ineffective. They reported a double blind trial involving 95 patients and concluded that splint therapy was ineffective and that tricyclic medication was significantly more helpful than placebo and independent of it's antidepressant effect.

In Liverpool John Cooper[201] would always go through doing bite raising appliances, some horrendous though, hard bite raising appliances which, hardly surprising, people couldn't get on with. They then ended up, after a bit of conservative treatment with bite raising appliances or whatever, quite often having open joint surgery.

It was one of the things that convinced me that open temporo-mandibular joint surgery was not a good idea. I mean, he was a lovely man and a very meticulous surgeon. Many of these patients who had long standing temporo-mandibular joint problems, and so called meniscal displacement, got some symptomatic relief for the first few months after they'd had their surgery. His standard procedure was an eminectomy and meniscal plication, and they did okay for a few months. But then Monday morning was his review clinic; and he saw all these people, who after a few months were back to square one with their temporo-mandibular joint pain, and clicking, and miserable lives. So that put me off temporo-mandibular joint surgery for life.

While I was there, we got an arthroscope and started doing arthroscopies. I have to say though, in quite a lot of the arthroscopies, I suspect we weren't where we thought we were when we were looking at whatever we were looking at. And I suspect some of the effects of that were placebo effects of having something shoved into your temporo-mandibular joint. He would fairly rapidly progress to open surgery, which was typically eminectomy and meniscal plication.

At King's they didn't really do much open surgery for temporo-mandibular joint problems, but they did for dislocation. They seemed to have a lot of dislocation; I don't know why and they would use a Dautrey's.[202] But John Cooper very sensibly was of the view Dautrey's wasn't really necessary. So for people with recurring dislocation you would also do an eminectomy, which I thought was eminently sensible because it meant they couldn't dislocate anywhere.

In my consultant practice, the only time that I did any open temporo-mandibular joint surgery was for recurrent dislocation and I probably did it less than half a dozen times. I did eminectomies for it,

---

201 Liverpool consultant

202 First described in France by Dautrey in 1975 the operation involved fracturing the zygomatic arch down to stop the mandibular condyle from translating forward and hence dislocating. For a description of the operation. See: Recurrent dislocation of the mandible: treatment of ten cases by the Dautrey procedure. M G Lawlor. British Journal of Oral Surgery 1982 20, 14-21.

and that was by and large successful. Anyway, that was the standard treatment at the time.

Rob Hensher became a pioneer in temporo-mandibular joint replacement in the UK. When he was a registrar at Westminster and Roehampton, he spent some time in New Orleans [1983].

That's where I got interested in the jaw joint surgery and replacement. When I got to New Orleans, Jack Kent had designed and implemented a jaw joint prosthesis. I thought I quite like this and I enjoy doing practical things and this is a really good idea for those people who really have nowhere else to go. And his prosthesis, which I saw then, did a lot of good.

However, there was a cloud on the horizon which was that the company who were making these things also made an artificial temporomandibular disc and this was very unsuccessful because of fragmentation and granuloma production. The second thing was that the first series of Kent joints, which were chrome cobalt versus polyethylene, were plagued because the fossa fragmented in use and they caused a granulomatous reaction. The later, the second series of Kent joints, had much higher molecular weight polyethylene, and didn't suffer from this.

But there were many patients in the US who had had this first series of joints put in, who then developed granulomas to the fragments of plastic, which were highly aggressive. And what you don't need around the base of your skull is a highly aggressive bone eating granuloma. A lot of these joints had to be removed with reconstructive surgery.[203]

In a later visit to Kent, when I was more senior, I saw some surgery that he was doing to repair this. And of course everybody sued everybody else. The company went out of business and Dr Kent, Professor Kent now, was very much in the firing line, but withstood a lot of this and his attorney defended him vigorously. I think there was a happy ending in the sense that it wasn't his fault.

Fortunately, I never used one of these disc prostheses, and I never

---

203 See: Foreign body response around total prosthetic metal-on-metal replacements of the temporomandibular joint in the UK. Sidebottom AJ, Speculand B, Hensher R. British Journal of Oral and Maxillofacial Surgery 46 2008 288–292.

used one of the first series Kent joints. But later on, when I was a consultant, I used a series two Kent with success. Patients were very grateful. But of course, when all this happened, supply dried up, we didn't have any joints, and I found myself in the position of saying I'll do your joint replacements, but I haven't got any joints.

Later he was in private practice in London [from 2000].

Because by that time I was a jaw joint replacer, and I used to get a lot of referrals both in the National Health Service and when I was in private practice, from far afield.

Chapter 23

Becoming a Medical Specialty and the Influence of Europe

'It was by dint of being seen to do good work'

The evolution of oral and maxillofacial surgery into being considered a medical specialty was gradual. Mike Bromige was involved with politics as secretary of the British Association of Oral and Maxillofacial Surgeons and was a consultant in Nottingham. I asked him at what stage did he think that it changed from being a hospital dental surgery service to oral and maxillofacial surgery? Mike:

In Nottingham it started during late '70s, and increasingly so through the '80s and then it was finally rubberstamped in the 1990s with new people coming in. Nationally there was almost the same time span in all honesty, quicker in some units than others.

I suspect a lot of units who said, 'We are a maxillofacial unit and we do this, this and this,' were not doing it all within the maxillofacial unit, that it was spread round through other specialities. That there's an established maxillofacial unit in Nottingham and the reason it's come together is that we took over a wing of the University Hospital and therefore got all the operating, beds, outpatient time and everything else we wanted. And it could all be put into one hospital.

While all that was going on, we were battling to keep the specialty as a surgical specialty in the eyes of managers, who still saw it as the dental department. That didn't go away for a long time. If you ask me when did dentistry become oral and maxillofacial surgery, well a lot of colleagues and other people recognised us for what we were, but in the eyes of many people we remained the dental department. And there were some people who delighted in making sure we remained the dental department in name.

In terms of the evolution from the hospital dental department to oral and maxillofacial surgery, what do you think has been the most important things on bringing that forward?

In my personal experience, it was by dint of being seen to do good work. It was as simple as that. I took on things which a few people raised their eyebrows at, then they saw that it was done and accomplished well. There was never any problem of being called a maxillofacial surgeon that I can remember.

Nationally we had to establish ourselves with the same credentials as everybody else. The early FRCS in Edinburgh and then the need to have a Fellowship and everything else that went with it and the more structured training was very helpful.

The last thing which can be said of my training was it being structured. I mean right from house officer onwards it was anything but structured. So later on we were seen to be aligning ourselves with every other surgical specialty and equipping ourselves in the same way. But again, I'm sure that a lot of it is being seen to be doing what you're doing and how you do it and the care you take of your patients and the results.

There also had to be a political movement so that oral and maxillofacial surgery became a specialty within the medical profession registered with the General Medical Council. Brian Avery is a former Dean of the Faculty of Dental Surgery of the Royal College of Surgeons of England, President of the British Association of Oral and Maxillofacial Surgeons and consultant in Middleborough. Brian:

I think it happened after Professor Sir Peter Rubin with a team from the General Medical Council visited. I think they went to Sunderland, because they were invited to go there to see what oral and maxillofacial surgeons did. There had been talk about moving them out of the hospital, which was ridiculous. When they went they said, 'Right, you need a medical director and therefore you need to become a medical specialty.'

Of course the effect has been that gradually the emphasis is moving away from dentistry. For instance, I think we've probably got as many people who got a medical degree first before doing dentistry as there are now dentists who did a medical degree. So we're gradually shifting so that candidates for oral and maxillofacial surgery have medicine as their primary degree. I think there's a degree of inevitability that this will happen. There won't be a lot of dentistry in oral and maxillofacial surgery because these chaps who all started life with a medical degree, followed by a short dental degree, have had little practical experience. I think there will be a severance to some extent between dental practitioners and oral and maxillofacial surgeons because of the way they've been trained.

Is this is a good thing?

No, because I always remember that more than half the cancers that were referred to me, came from dental practitioners. So the referral basis is what's important, and I think even today most referrals, certainly the minor cases of dento-alveolar surgery come from dentists. Even most of the major referrals come from the dental practitioners still. So there's a great danger that the specialty may lose that referral base.

I asked Andy Brown if European practice had much of an influence on the development of oral and maxillofacial surgery in the United Kingdom and its practice? Andy:

In the mid '90s, the specialty flew the dental nest as its primary link and became recognised under the European guidelines as a medically based specialty, with maxillofacial surgery being the medically based specialty and oral surgery remaining as the dental specialty. I think the European Directives were a big change because we then had to make sure that our training was transportable; that we had the same parity of training quality with other European countries so that there was the ability for mobility of labour, which was all part of the wish list of the European Union.

At the end of his training John Cawood spent some time in the USA in Miami and Seattle and then Arnhem in the Netherlands [1979].

Arnhem was my introduction to European maxillofacial surgery and I started to attend European meetings. I remember going to a meeting in Hamburg and I was amazed at the extent of the surgery they were carrying out and witnessing the heavyweights from Europe who would dominate the proceedings and insist that their method was the best; there were lively discussions and I was impressed.

What I concluded from my experience in north America and Arnhem was how far behind the UK really was in oral surgery. Not only clinically but also politically and academically because we were really controlled by governments and our purpose was mainly service and we were bogged down by lots of dento-alveolar surgery.

John Williams is a former president of the European Association of Cranio-Maxillo-Facial Surgery.

Until we got involved in Europe it was pedestrian, to put it mildly. Involvement with and exposure to what the specialty did in Europe, was one of the big triggers behind the development of the dual qualification, because that was the norm in Europe. And the final crunch came of course when the Mono Specialities Group was forming the definitions on specialities when max-fax had to have a fully recognisable qualification in both medicine and dentistry to be recognised in Europe. So any sort of volitional thing before that became obligatory really from that moment onwards.

The scope of our specialty just whoomphed, and this is one of the reason that Norman Rowe got on so well in Europe, whereas Terry Ward would have nothing to do with it. First, Terry Ward was tied up with the International Association and its formation, and that very much was UK and the Americans with a few Scandinavians thrown in. Whereas the European Association had a very dynamic lead, all the professors in Germany in particular were doing things that we hadn't thought about. I mean Obwegeser was really the person who opened up mandibular osteotomies in a big way; it was body osteotomies before that, the sagittal split revolutionised things and that was entirely a European influence.

If you look at the spectrum of work that happened over that period of time when we first got involved with Europe, it was huge and it was escalating by the day. So there's no doubt that our specialty was hugely influenced. Now we've taken our own lead within that as well, and so we are one of the frontrunners in Europe now. The Scandinavians have never picked it up. The Germans have stayed very prominent, but the French have come on. Bernard Devauchelle was the first person to do a face transplant, and he succeeded me as President next but one of that Association. So we have been hugely influenced in terms of the way we have developed by our association with Europe, more than anywhere else.

If we had decided that we were going to carry on as a singly qualified specialty in dentistry, would that have been possible with us being in Europe? John:

You couldn't have become a max-fax person, no. The Dental Directives were signed before the Medical Directives and the Dental Directives included our specialty. So it was there, but they weren't specific; there was just a registered dental qualification, it was called Oral Surgery. And when the Medical Mono Specialities Treaty was signed, within it were the requirements for each specialty. And as far as max-fax was concerned it had to have a double qualification, that was an absolute requirement which is what had been the practice across the whole of the German-speaking part of Europe and the French-speaking part, the French didn't have dentistry even. So across the whole of that area of Europe and Middle Europe too, particularly going further towards the Russians where stomatology, which as a sort of medical based specialty anyway, was dominant. That dominance of medicine within it was always there and therefore it's not surprising when the Mono Specialities Treaty was signed, that we had to go along with that if we were going to be part of it.

Ian Martin:

I think that once it became a proper surgical discipline and the Specialist Advisory Committee chairs sat round the table of the Joint Committee for Higher Surgical Training, we took our place in the proper surgical community, and then subsequently we had dedicated places on the College council [204] and that sort of thing. I think that was really the recognition of it being a proper surgical specialty rather than a dental specialty which until that time it had been or had been perceived, anyway.

The European Medical and Dental Directives were in the '70s, and the whole idea of that was to provide harmonisation of training across Europe. The difficulty has always been that there were at least four specialties in Europe, which were all slightly different. So you had what was termed under the medical directives, dental, oral, and maxillofacial surgery, which is what we call oral and maxillofacial, and requires dual qualification. Then there was maxillofacial surgery, which is predominantly in southern Europe. There was oral surgery, which was what it is now in the UK, so sort of dentally based, and then there was stomatology, which was a kind of add on, which some states had when you'd done a bit of medicine and then you'd do the stomatology degree and add it on. So a very heterogeneous approach.

But there was probably a group of half a dozen countries, including the UK, Germany, Belgium which recognised oral and maxillofacial surgery as a dual qualification. And so the fact that it was recognised in Europe and we had to go one way or the other to be in line with the European directives drove us to have that specialty of oral and maxillofacial surgery, which was comparable. And we relied upon that really for mandating that acquisition of a medical qualification, which

---

204 Royal College of Surgeons of England.

was voted on by the Association back in something like 1982 or 3 with a ten-year window to achieve dual qualification as mandatory for progression in oral and maxillofacial surgery.

Later the waters became muddied with the Dental Directives and the introduction of grandfathering arrangements for the academics who are singly qualified, and whether they could get onto a list of oral and maxillofacial surgery. Answer, no they couldn't. But there was a special provision under UK statutes to allow them to hold consultant posts in oral and maxillofacial surgery based up upon the ACOMS[205] training. So that was an exception, and then the introduction of surgical dentistry and oral surgery, which really muddied the waters.

There was a big grandfathering process to sift through individuals who weren't on any of those lists. And as I was Chair of the Specialist Advisory Committee in oral maxillofacial surgery at the time, the task ultimately fell to me to chair all of those committees, which looked at, individually under the interim arrangements whether people could be grandfathered on to the various specialist lists. And that was quite a tricky process; it was quite controversial.

By the late 1980s, there was mounting disquiet over the long working hours of junior doctors. A working party was set up chaired by the Minister of Heath, Mrs Virginia Bottomley, and this led to the 'New Deal' for junior doctors which had wide support and was published in 1991.[206] It limited the number of hours of work to 72 each week by 1994 but it could be relaxed to 96 hours for doctors in 'hard pressed posts'.

Notwithstanding that, later there came the European Working Time Directive which was intended to stop employees from being exploited by limiting their hours of work unless they opted out. This was enshrined in legislation as the Working Time Regulations and was directed at all workers, not just in health. It applied to consultants and career grade staff from 1998 and juniors from 2004. Hours were limited to an average of 56 per week from 2004 to 48 from 2009. Employees had to have 11 hours of rest a day, a day off a week, a rest break if working over 6 hours, and paid leave each year. Legal ruling later, the SiMAP and Jaeger rulings said that time on call at the place of work had to be considered as work.

Ian Martin comments on the effect of the European Working Time

---

205 Academic Oral and Maxillofacial Surgery.
206 Junior doctors. The new deal. 1991 NHS Management Executive.

Directive on the way hospitals were run and on call arrangements.

People didn't start thinking about that until really late on, way after there had been technical obligations under Working Time Directives. Quite a lot of that needed to be settled by various bits of case law about how those directives applied to medicine. There were interim arrangements, but when I was appointed as a trainee it was common practice for individuals to be doing over 100 hours a week. That wasn't unusual because you were doing one in twos. Forty-eight hours then came in, and we had this whole period of transition where there were various banding arrangements with financial penalties for Trusts depending on how many hours people were working, and it was designed to be fairly punitive if you had people working significantly over fifty-six hours.

The problem for surgery wasn't just the total number of hours, it was the number of continuous hours that you could work. The restrictions that came in under European Working Time Regulations made it quite difficult for some surgical training programmes, particularly where there was a significant emergency element to those specialties, to make sure that the training was appropriate to allow people to get exposure to emergency care because if you weren't there and on call you couldn't see it. I still think that is the case, and it's become even stricter as time's gone by.

But the Royal College of Surgeons, in fairness, has always argued that there should be much more flexibility for training in surgery to overcome some of those restrictions that mean that people aren't getting exposure to stuff out of hours. I think that is still a big problem; the restriction down to forty-eight hours means by the time you've done nine to five, Monday to Friday, there aren't many hours left in the day to do emergency care.[207]

Significant amounts of care are now delivered by consultants who are exempt from European working time regulations, if they sign a disclaimer. They're not regarded as being under any duress to do it; unlike trainees who are regarded as being under duress, therefore there are limits on how much they can abdicate from that.

---

207 See: Time for training: a review of the impact of the European Working Time Directive on the quality of training. Temple J. Medical Education England , 2010.

So you've got consultants and other groups, specialist nurses, operating department practitioners, surgical assistants, first assistants etc., delivering elements of care which would previously have been delivered by junior doctors. My view is that that will come home to roost in due course because the consultants of tomorrow will not have been exposed to delivering care that we all were when we came through to be consultants. So, I think we're storing up problems for the future.

John Langdon.

I don't think the European Union has made a ha'porth of difference. Well, possibly the free transfer of personnel, but not politically. But in terms of influence, there is no doubt that orthognathic surgery developed and came to us via Germany, Austria and Switzerland.

Although they weren't maxillofacial surgeons, people like Tessier and Brånemark had a huge influence on the practice in this country, and Delaire and people like that. So there is a huge European influence on our specialty. But I don't think that's in any way politically based.

Chapter 24
The Name

'We unscrewed the 'Dental' sign and put up, 'Oral and Maxillofacial Surgery Unit', it was half past eleven at night'

In 1977, the council of the British Association of Oral Surgeons discussed whether the title of consultants in the specialty could be changed from Consultant Dental Surgeon to Consultant Oral Surgeon. It was decided that the opinion should be sought of the Chief Dental Officer of the Department of Health, the Faculty of Dental Surgery of the Royal College of Surgeons of England and the Chairman of the Central Committee for Hospital Dental Services. By 1980 there had been an agreement that new consultant posts could be advertised with the title Consultant Oral Surgeon/Oral Medicine.[208]

The British Association of Oral Surgeons became the British Association of Oral and Maxillofacial Surgeons in 1982/3 and the British Journal of Oral Surgery had become the British Journal of Oral and Maxillofacial Surgery from the first issue in 1984 along with its grey cover changing to a bright green. There had been no prior announcement of these changes in the journal.

Gordon Fordyce [1953].

> *My first consultant jobs were as a Consultant Dental Surgeon. And then, I forget how it happened, but our Association, the British Association of Oral Surgeons was set up and that was about the time when oral surgery was talked about as a topic, and jobs were advertised for Oral Surgeons.*

John Bradley was appointed as a consultant in 1968.

> *I could legally call myself only one thing, and that was Consultant Dental Surgeon. The business of being able to call yourself an Oral Surgeon legally, as far as the General Dental Council is concerned, from what I remember, was later on. It was probably early '80s before we could call ourselves Oral Surgeons, strictly speaking, although we said, 'Oh stuff it, this is what we do and we're being honest, we can't be Consultant Dental Surgeons being able to be consulted and give*

---

208 Minutes of council meetings, British Association of Oral Surgeons

opinions on the whole range of dentistry.' 'I said, 'restorative dentistry? Mine is at undergraduate level. Is that good enough? No, we're not being honest.' And this is what I argued with one or two people and they had to accept this and this is why it changed. To be expected to give an opinion on the whole gamut of dentistry wasn't very good. But Fred Monks, [209] called his department the Department of Oral and Maxillofacial Surgery and they couldn't do anything about it. This was back in the '60s, he described himself as an Oral Surgeon.

John worked for John Hovell as a house surgeon at St Thomas' and then Rupert Sutton Taylor at the Westminster Hospital [1958- 60].

Rupert Taylor was probably the first name in this country to describe himself as an Oral Surgeon. He didn't do anything else but take teeth, roots and buried teeth out, in his private practice, that sort of thing. He said, 'I'm a duffer at doing fillings and I'm not much good at making dentures but I decided I was quite good at getting them out.' This is what he did.

When did this word maxillofacial surgeon come in?

Well, it's a gradual thing. It started coming in during the 1970s, when the specialty was taking off and we had this big debate going on, whether medical training was necessary. I was chairman of the education and training committee of British Association of Oral Surgeons, as it was then, and we realised that if this specialty was to advance, it had to be trained surgically, properly in a formal manner. Given the way the world was going, it was getting much more regulated, which was quite right, I have no disagreement with that at all.

So this is where the medical bit came in and then the business of maxillofacial surgery, which was a separate medical specialty on the continent which was coming in here. And there was great rivalry with the ENT surgeons wanting to describe themselves as maxillofacial surgeons as well as head and neck surgeons. We had this big debate at the British Association of Oral Surgeons, about whether we should we change the name of the Association. And that was the seminal point of when the association became the British Association of Oral and Maxillofacial Surgeons; that was crucial.

---

209 Fred Monks was consultant in Bolton.

Khursheed Moos on appointment as a consultant in Warwick [1969].

I was appointed as a Consultant Dental Surgeon (Oral Surgery) because that was the only thing that existed at that time. Consultant Oral Surgeon was the term we used to a great extent and you were also responsible for oral medicine so there was a change to a Consultant in Oral Surgery and Oral Medicine, that was an interim one we had, then it changed and varied from place to place. There was no absolutely clear label. You did not hear about Consultant Maxillofacial Surgeons, but what you heard about was Consultant Oral and Maxillofacial Surgeons. I think that was important because we wanted to keep the 'oral' part in the specialty. We were very concerned that we weren't going into a specialist surgery which had no conventional oral surgery. We also respected our background from dentistry. Without the dental knowledge, I think we would not have become as good surgeons.

Andy Brown was a house surgeon in the dental hospital at Guy's after qualifying there [1969].

Pat O'Driscoll was appointed as a new consultant, He was actually the first consultant there appointed with the title of Consultant Oral Surgeon, or at least adopted that title. Until then all the senior consultants were called Consultant Dental Surgeons and that's exactly what they were. Most of them had Harley Street practices, and they came over to Guy's as part-time consultants the two days a week or so they were scheduled to attend. The rest of the week many of them were doing general dentistry. They were Consultant Dental Surgeons but with a broader remit in teaching; they were like the old honorary consultants pre-1948.

Laurence Oldham was appointed as consultant at Taunton in 1968. He described how his department became Oral and Maxillofacial Surgery [1973].

I was appointed to Taunton as a Consultant Dental Surgeon, because the word oral surgery never occurred to anybody. So I came as a dentist and I was received as a dentist. The department was called the Dental Department.

After four or five years on my own here, I thought, we've got to get a houseman, so I got the area health authority chief executive and the chairman of the health authority support to give me funding for a houseman.

The first houseman was Ian Burke, and so I said to him, 'Look, it's time we made a change, we're going to alter the sign in the hospital,' so I got the works department to make a sign, 'Oral and Maxillofacial Surgery Unit,' and it came back, 'Oral and Maxillofacial Sugery unit,' they missed the 'R' out of 'Surgery', so I said, 'I can't put that up,' it had to be redone. Anyway, Burke and I approached the hospital, and we unscrewed the 'Dental' sign and put up, 'Oral and Maxillofacial Surgery Unit. It was half-past eleven at night.'

The next morning in comes the ENT head of department and says, 'What's all this, what's all this?' and I said, 'Oh, well it's how we're developing sir you see, this is how we're going, we're increasing the scope,' and that was very challenging to ENT, it was an enormous inroad. It was quite a step change.

Chapter 25

Maxillofacial Fellowship of the Royal College of Surgeons of Edinburgh

'There was a sort of restlessness in the specialty'

By 1981, several of the minor surgical specialities were pushing for a specialist college of surgeons diploma examination in their own disciplines; in particular ENT and ophthalmology. When first discussed at the council meeting of the British Association of Oral Surgeons, the issue did not progress as the necessity of a medical qualification had not yet been formally established.

However, an informal overture to Sir Alan Parks the president of the English Royal College Of Surgeons was rebuffed and although by now orthopaedics and vascular surgery also wanted a specialist diploma qualification, this had been opposed by general surgeons and the conclusion was that the general FRCS was a good enough test.[210]

However, the Royal College of Surgeons of Edinburgh were comparatively swift to take this idea up. In May 1984 they instigated an FRCS in maxillofacial surgery. Candidates needed to be qualified in medicine and dentistry, have three years' experience in oral and maxillofacial surgery, and one year in another surgical discipline. It was intended to be taken by third-year registrars or first year senior registrars.

Andy Brown:

When the Edinburgh FRCS in oral and maxillofacial surgery came into the specialty, this was done as a sort of political move, and was voluntary.[211] Of course it became mandatory, as a surgical specialty, that we would have to take a basic surgical exam which was originally the FRCS, now the MRCS exam. The old final FRCS was a general surgery exam that almost everybody took in order to get into higher surgical training, rather equivalent to the FDS in oral surgery. That is now, I suppose, equivalent to the MRCS with a specialty FRCS at the

---

210 The progress was documented in the minutes of the British Association of Oral Surgeons (as the British Association of Oral and Maxillofacial Surgeons was then called).
211 But in practice, from soon after it started, there was little chance of getting shortlisted for a senior registrar job without having passed it.

end of training.

We have been pushed, willingly I think, more and more into that surgical model and away from the dental training model and that has led to some political friction between some singly qualified oral surgeons and our specialty, and between the dental schools, and their academic departments of oral surgery, and the specialty out in the district general hospitals and the specialist units.

The first examination was in January 1985. There were 18 candidates who passed.[212] They were all established senior registrars or consultants, and two were over 60 years of age. Many of the examiners went back to take the exam themselves.[213]

Khursheed Moos was on the advisory committee for the setting up of the examination and an examiner for the first sitting. What did he think was the impact of the qualification?

The oral and maxillofacial surgery FRCS of the Edinburgh Royal College of Surgeons I think came in at the right time. I was involved with Lawrie Finch over that. He was the instigator, but we talked about it a lot when he put it together. I was on the original Board of Examiners when it was set up.

We thought that in Britain we had got it right at the right time but I can remember Ian McGregor, later president of the Glasgow Royal College and a plastic surgeon, out in Singapore, saying, 'oh a new Mickey Mouse fellowship has come out called Oral and Maxillofacial Surgery'. He had no respect for that sort of thing, and that message was circulating around that the oral and maxillofacial surgeons were not proper surgeons.

I think having the Edinburgh Fellowship and making sure we had a general surgery component included in that exam was very important.

John Cawood.

Lawrie Finch was very pro-medicine and politically he was in a strong position. He was Dean of the dental faculty in Edinburgh; he

---

212 News Item. British Journal of Oral and Maxillofacial Surgery 1985 23, 231.
213 For a concise history of the setting up of the examination see: FRCS Ed (Oral and Maxillofacial Surgery): a milestone in the history of Oral and Maxillofacial Surgery in the United Kingdom. Mahmood S, MacLeod S, Lello G. British Journal of Oral and Maxillofacial Surgery 2002 40, 300–303.

was very much an Edinburgh man, having done his medicine there, and he was very interested and involved in the politics.

Lawrie was very instrumental in the FRCS supported by Paul Bradley who was in north Wales. Lawrie was able through his connections in the College in Edinburgh to propose an FRCS in maxillofacial surgery, because by this time the need for a dual degree had become much more prominent. And there was a sort of restlessness in the specialty as we wanted to move from under the wings of plastic surgery or historical surgery and be our own specialty. That was very apparent. Lawrie spearheaded the FRCS.

Khursheed:

We had several senior colleagues who came along and did the examination. They presented themselves extraordinarily well, although I had the embarrassing situation of having to examine senior colleagues such as Terry English and Patrick James from the London Hospital.

It was interesting to see how hard they had worked to make sure that the general surgery and everything else was in good order, and they did very well. The examining general surgeons were very impressed and pleasantly surprised by them and I think the fact that they were examining our consultants and senior registrars and thinking they were good and we were getting better specialty pass rates than some other specialty examinations was important, because it helped to change an attitude.

Brian Avery, one of the first candidates for the maxillofacial FRCS in Edinburgh:

Lawrence Finch from Liverpool who was a member of the Board of the Dental Faculty at the Royal College of Surgeons of Edinburgh persuaded the Board and the College to introduce an FRCS in oral and maxillofacial surgery, which of course was for those who were medically and dentally qualified. They introduced this in the teeth of opposition from other colleges like the English college, of which I was later the Dean. They arranged a first sitting of the exam about a year ahead, and then they offered training courses.

I went up with a bunch of enthusiastic individuals to the training course and we sat for the exam. There were 18 of us at the first sitting who passed. Some of us were quite senior consultants who'd been in post 20 years or more. We took the exam and passed, and it was a wonderfully happy occasion. Because I came first in the alphabetical list of candidates having a surname beginning with A, I think I can claim with some truthfulness that I was the first person ever to pass that examination.

And what affect do you think that had on the specialty?

Oh, I think it galvanised us because we were always the poor relations in terms of surgery when compared with rival specialties like plastic surgery. They had always used the fact that we didn't have an FRCS to make us the poor relations who had never been properly trained. I have to say that, even when we had all the qualifications and training that they had and more, plus all our dental qualifications and training, they still claimed that we weren't as well trained as they were, but of course that was totally untrue.

So you think it might have been a turning point for the specialty?

I do, yes. And then the English college battled away and eventually they introduced an FRCS. It came quite a few years later. You know, if Edinburgh hadn't led the way, it might have been a long time in coming at the English college.

John Langdon was also a candidate at the first exam.

We had Lawrie Finch to thank for the exam. It was largely his persuasive powers on the council at the Edinburgh College. He was a dentist who had got elected to the council of the College and he talked them into allowing it.

The regulations were published that medically qualified oral surgeons could apply to do the FRCS, and lots of us applied for the first diet of the exam, including people like John Sowray and Khursheed Moos. And the Edinburgh College suddenly realised two things, I think. One is they didn't have any examiners because there wasn't a big enough cohort of max fax surgeons with a traditional FRCS to act as examiners and, secondly, they were going to be embarrassed by people like John Sowray pitching up and not passing.

So they picked a handful of them and appointed them as examiners for the first diet. Then we sat it. Then people of my generation who had got the exam by examination, not honorary, in the first diet, were immediately invited to be examiners. So I was already an examiner for the second sitting.

Who was given an honorary one?

I know John Sowray and Gordon Seward were, and I think Khursheed Moos and Lawrie Finch. There were about six of them originally.[214]

What difference did the FRCS in Edinburgh make to the specialty?

It gave us corporate legitimacy. Until that stage, it was very much a matter of personality and ability. There were those of us without an FRCS who were obviously practising the maxillofacial side of the specialty and had earned grudging respect amongst our surgical colleagues in the hospitals we were based. But it wasn't a recognition of us as a surgical specialty, it was very much on an individual basis. Once all our trainees had the FRCS exam, then de facto we were a recognised surgical specialty the same as anybody else.

It was an odd thing, before I had the FRCS at King's I was chairman of the theatre users committee and was on the planning group that planned the new theatres that were being built. I was a bloody dental upstart at that stage without an FRCS, and yet on a personal level I gained the confidence of other people in the place. Whereas after that nobody would have raised an eyebrow about it.

Mike Davidson was not pleased when he found out he would have to do another exam.

I'd already done my FDS in 1982 and as I was going through medicine people said, 'Oh, well, you're going to need an FRCS,' because this was just as the Edinburgh FRCS was kicking off. So, I thought great I've gone back to do medicine and I've spent five years thinking that's it, I'm on the fast-track now and then they say, 'Oh, no, you're going to need to do FRCS, you're going to need some surgery under your belt,' and I was geez, I hadn't planned for that.

When I was a registrar in Chichester, the good thing was they let me go and they paid for the course at King's. I think it was about a week long. There were about 10 of us on it, and I had just been appointed as senior registrar at Leeds and I was just about to do the exam. The course was excellent with some very good teaching and I think I've still got the notes somewhere. I took the exam and passed it just after I started at Leeds, but the preparation for it was when I was in Chichester.

---

214 John Williams was an examiner for the first exam. He was already an FRCS.

The exam was written papers and viva. It was very old-fashioned in the sense that it was written. There were two papers, one was more general, and one was more max-fax, and then there were vivas which were predominantly general, bit of max-fax, and then there were clinical cases which were max-fax. I didn't find it too hard.

What did he think was the impact of the FRCS in oral maxillofacial surgery in Edinburgh?

Well, when I sat it you could do so as long as you'd done a year's surgical jobs and that included the A&E and orthopaedics. They could be anywhere of any calibre. I think it didn't really help your training except it was a rite of passage; it was evidence that you had been exposed to a wide range of things. But in many ways, it's just a form of being signed up for a Certificate of Completion of Training, but it's with an examination process.

I'm not sure it radically changed the Edinburgh college, except they got some money out of it and they got some more people signed up, some of whom have stayed with them and the odd one is on their council. I suppose it was one of the earlier specialist exams that as a discipline we were trying to get accepted as proper surgeons, so I think it helped in that extent.

I think the exam is probably much tougher now, and it's more focussed on what we need out of the training. In those days, I don't think it had that structure and it didn't have that rigour. I'd worked for two bosses who in their different ways, as a process of osmosis as much as anything else, prepared me for that exam. Everything that prepared me for that exam was from Chichester. All the other jobs, no. The orthopaedics helped me to prepare for the trauma aspects of the exam and the general surgery was pretty straightforward.

Ian Martin:

It was a good thing; I think particularly for those established consultants it provided a route to give them credibility, as surgeons, comparable with other surgical specialties.

And if you think about it, it was around the time when oral and maxillofacial surgery was recognised with the European Directives as being a medical specialty. Increasingly it was seen as a medical specialty, although up until fairly recently the administrative control of the specialty rested with the Faculty of Dental Surgery, and the Specialist Advisory Committee was responsible, primarily, to the

Faculty of Dental Surgery. Slightly anomalous because it was one of the nine original surgical specialties, which became ten under European Directives when vascular surgery joined.

The maxillofacial specialty FRCS examination in Edinburgh was the equivalent, I would say, of the ENT specialty examination. I think that was fine, but for me I always thought that general surgery FRCS was the real FRCS, this was a specialty FRCS, so I did both of them.

I didn't particularly want to do the FRCS at Edinburgh, actually. They were quite close together in terms of time; I think I did the general surgery FRCS about three or four months before the max-fax one in Edinburgh. And I remember going back to Liverpool and saying, 'Oh, well I've got an FRCS now, I'll just withdraw from the Edinburgh exam.' And David Vaughan said, 'No, no, I think you should do the Edinburgh one as well.'

I thought, I don't see what I can win out of this because I don't need two FRCSs, I've got one. And if I cock it up and don't pass, it looks pretty bad if you've got the general FRCS, but failed your specialty FRCS. When I did the specialty FRCS in Edinburgh, I can remember John Williams examining me and asking me all about the Sear's splint, which I'd never heard about, but was apparently a splint you ram up the nose for fractured noses, and was prominent in that well-known textbook of maxillofacial trauma by Williams et al.[215] But I didn't know about that. And so I thought there was a potential for me cocking things up by doing that exam. Thankfully, I passed it. But, I think it was important, particularly for the established consultants, who didn't have an FRCS to give them a degree of credibility.

John Langdon and Mo Patel wrote and edited the book Operative Maxillofacial Surgery

We wrote that specifically for the new FRCS from Edinburgh, it was blatantly directed towards that exam. It was always a multi-authored book. We were the editors but also wrote chapters in it. It took off unexpectedly well, so it ran to a second edition.

We changed the title from the second edition to the third edition to Operative Oral and Maxillofacial Surgery and included exodontia,

---

215 Rowe and Williams: Maxillofacial Injuries. Tony Sear had written up his splint idea in 1977: A method of internal splinting for unstable nasal fractures. Sear A. British Journal of Oral Surgery 14 1977 203-209.

cysts and all that sort of thing because the point we were trying to make was that it is all part of oral and maxillofacial surgery.

For the first edition the editors were myself and Mo Patel, then myself, Mo and Bob Ord for the second edition. We recruited Peter Brennan for the third; it was really because Mo Patel was running down; I was busy because of all the management issues going on, and Bob Ord was getting very busy in Baltimore. So we needed somebody young and enthusiastic, hence Peter Brennan. There won't be a fourth edition.

Chapter 26

Professional Relationships, Co-operation and Antagonism

'He shouted at me that I was not to do these sorts of operations'

It did not surprise me to find that the relationship with other surgical disciplines varied from helpful and friendly co-operation to outright antagonism. Perhaps the most important interactions were with plastic surgeons; after all at the Second World War Emergency Medical Services hospitals it was always a plastic surgeon in charge. As a junior I never experienced hostility from their juniors; it was more like patronising indifference, particularly when I was working for consultants whose main clinical interest was wisdom teeth.

In his interview Gordon Fordyce was quite clear that when he was a registrar and senior registrar at Hill End Hospital, after the war, and the dental consultants were Alex McGregor, Paul Toller and Ben Fickling, it was Rainsford Mowlem the plastic surgeon who he described as the boss. Mowlem was in charge and although he only came in twice a week, facial injuries were treated as he wanted. When Kelsey Fry wrote his book Dental Treatment of Maxillo-Facial Injuries published in 1942 in the supplement, Archibald McIndoe wrote the chapter on middle third fractures of the face and describes himself as the 'Surgeon-in-charge' East Grinstead Maxillo Facial Unit.[216] This sheds light on the culture of responsibility at the time and explains why after the war some plastic surgeons were incensed that the 'dentists' were not deferring to them and were starting to take on some work they regarded as their own.

I was particularly interested to listen to Professor Sir Paul Bramley when he told me of his time as a registrar at Rooksdown House, which had been set up as an Emergency Medical Services Hospital in the war. There his boss, and later mentor and hero, Norman Rowe gained the trust of Harold Gillies, the 'Father of Plastic Surgery' and how by his approach ended up with him doing much of the surgery. Gillies had officially retired, but he still seemed to be operating at Rooksdown House and 'in

---

216 The Dental Treatment of Maxillo-Facial Injuries (and supplement). Kelsey Fry, Shepherd, McLeod, Parfitt (1942).

charge'.

After his medical training Sir Paul had worked in Kenya with his wife. Sometime later, after returning home, he was appointed as a registrar at what was called the 'Plastic, Oral and Maxillofacial Unit' at Rooksdown House with Norman Rowe and Paddy Killey [1952-54].

We did all the medical work, and I published a paper on pemphigus vulgaris with Norman, one of my first papers,[217] we did the medical care of all our patients, there was nobody else interested. We didn't personally get to do any cutting, but we were first assistant at most of the things he was doing. You could say well why wasn't I irritated by this and wanting a go as I'd been drawing blood elsewhere. I wasn't. I knew I was there to learn as much as I could and I would take what was going to be given to me, which I was very grateful for. We did all the routine stuff, but not the progressive stuff he was doing with Gillies, we just watched. The pioneering stuff was reconstructive surgery. It was mostly WWII injuries, mainly gunshot wounds of massive proportions and complete facial burns.

Rooksdown House at Basingstoke was a big mental institution rather like Hill End at St Albans.[218] It had all sorts of other functions during the war and it acted as Harold Gillies's Emergency Medical Service centre. Maxillofacial units were set down at various places like this, and Rooksdown House Basingstoke was one of them.

A dental surgeon who had worked with Harold Gillies was in post and presumably was given a consultant job in 1948 when the NHS came in because he was specialised and had war experience. I've forgotten his name, but he retired and they made two dental surgeon appointments one after the other or maybe it was at the same time, Paddy Killey and Norman Rowe had been registrars at Hill End, St Albans with Mowlem and they were appointed and started as consultant dental surgeons; we didn't call ourselves Oral Surgeons, or very few people did.

When I came back from Africa medically qualified, generally bloodied in surgery to see what was happening. I had the opportunity

---

217 Pemphigus of Mucous Membranes Bramley P, Rowe N. Dental Practitioner 1955 5 346 - 353.
218 The hospital was Park Prewit mental hospital at Basingstoke. Rooksdown house was the part for private patients which Gillies had taken over for the plastic unit. Other parts of Park Prewit had been used for other war functions.

to go to East Grinstead or with Norman at Basingstoke. The East Grinstead job was a senior registrar, Norman's job was registrar, and I chose that because of Norman.

What Norman was doing then was what his predecessors in the post were doing, what Ben Fickling[219] and company were doing: they were the plastic surgeon's dental handmaidens, sometimes treated well and sometimes treated abominably and not given any opportunity. Norman was involved, initially assisting at the major operations, post-traumatic reconstructions of wartime injuries.

Gillies had come back by then and pottered about and did a few cases Norman was involved in. But Gillies was the controlling factor even in his retirement; an eccentric man. But here was Norman assisting, and we were assisting the assistant if you see what I mean. We were supposed to be trained by Norman, but really we were watching Gillies operating.

But Norman planned these new operations; he was involved in all that stuff with the tubed pedicle. So he worked up the cases, and he was allowed to drill the holes in the bone and pass the wire. That was about all the operative work he was allowed to do by the plastic surgeons until one day Gillies said, 'Look Norman, you know far more about this case than I do, you planned it all, why don't you do it?' So that's how he got the OK to get in, to get cracking and doing the jobs. He'd seen plenty of it done, but he's done the hard work and systematic research into the particular condition and had it all planned out. So he took over a lot of that stuff working along with Gillies as equal partners.

This was how Norman operated. He didn't go in bombastically like a Cardiff colleague of ours, apparently as he did in his book.[220] 'I can do it get out of the way,' that sort of thing. He just quietly did what he was asked to do at the beginning, worked it up, showed his worth. I followed that pattern when I went down to Plymouth.[221] They didn't know what this object coming down as the consultant dental surgeon, doubly qualified, was going to do and I thought I'll play this as Norman would play it and I'll be tactful. I called in on one occasion one of the ENT colleagues, a consultant, and he came in and I said,

---

219 Ben Fickling was one of the three consultant dental surgeons at Hill End.
220 'A Journey Through a Life' memoire by Russell Hopkins.
221 Sir Paul subsequently became consultant dental surgeon at Plymouth.

'We're going to do this chap's face and we really need a tracheostomy. Would you do it?' So he did it and he said, 'Do you mind if I watch what you do?' So two hours later in the middle of the night we had reassembled everything and got him sewn up and off the table. He said, 'This is ridiculous, if you can do that sort of thing you can jolly well do the tracheostomy.' So this was Norman's influence. And what he did after that, he started building the book of Rowe and Killey, 'Fractures of the Facial Skeleton.'

After that I should have done a senior registrar job, but I leapt that thing and went to a consultant job in Plymouth. The chances of getting any better training than I had had with anybody else but Norman's unit were nil.

Hill End Hospital at St Albans and the Queen Victoria Hospital at East Grinstead also became WWII Emergency Medical Services Hospitals. Gordon Fordyce became a registrar and subsequently senior registrar at Hill End before the department moved to Mount Vernon, where he eventually became a consultant [1949-1953].

Rainsford Mowlem was the boss. Dick Dawson was the plastic surgery senior registrar; he had been a prisoner of war in Japan, a delightful person, and he and I did most of our work together.

Dick Dawson and Gordon Fordyce both became consultants at Mount Vernon and long-time friends. Dick Dawson wrote a history of the Hill End/Mount Vernon unit.[222] I asked if there any hint of the rivalry between the oral surgeons and the plastic surgeons which was to come in the future.

None at all. At Hill End, there was none.

Mike Awty was a house surgeon at East Grinstead in 1954. He eventually was to become a consultant there. Was there any rivalry?

Not much, because we hadn't got the skills to deal with it. The consultant plastic surgeons were all very experienced wartime surgeons, and the registrars were very experienced, time expired senior registrars because there weren't many jobs so people were hanging around. They were all in their 40s. I was comparatively a

---

222 The history, antecedents and progress of the Mount Vernon Centre for Plastic Surgery and Jaw Injuries, Northwood Middlesex 1939 - 1983. Dawson R. British Journal of Plastic Surgery 1988 41 83- 91.

schoolboy.

Mike became a consultant at East Grinstead in 1965

Saturday morning was a working day and the surgeons' meeting was late on Saturday morning in Sir Archibald's[223] room, when all the problems of the week were discussed. Sir T's[224] friend was Jerry Moore, who was a very colourful plastic surgeon. He was very nice and he wouldn't let them bully me, so I was protected a bit by these very nice chaps. They were big personalities; they weren't nit-pickers. And then de rigueur you repaired to the bar in the mess after the surgeons' meeting and went home when, and if, you could still drive.

And so really you got on well with the plastic surgeons?

Well, I felt there's no place for aggro. You don't get anywhere with aggro. They were bedevilled by having not very good visiting trainees from overseas, because they didn't take any trouble over their trainees, so the people that came only wanted to get out of it what they could. I mean, this maybe scurrilous, but I got that impression.

The unit at Rooksdown House had moved to Roehampton in 1959, by which time Gillies had gone, and there was tension. John Bradley was a senior registrar at Roehampton and the Westminster hospitals. He described the relationship between the plastic and oral surgeons [1962-67].

Well, it was not very good. First, the plastic surgeons had had their noses put out of joint because of the union with Westminster Hospital.[225] The Westminster Hospital was the senior hospital and Rupert Sutton Taylor was the senior oral surgeon and he called himself a maxillofacial surgeon as well, which involved plastic surgery to some extent. So he was the senior surgeon over all the plastic surgeons at Roehampton, and he was a dentist.

Did he have any administrative superiority over them?

Yes, he did as far as the Board of Governors of the Westminster Hospital Teaching Group, as it was called then. Rupert Taylor was the senior man of the plastic and oral maxillofacial surgeons. The senior

---

223 McIndoe.
224 Sir Terence Ward.
225 The plastics and oral surgery unit at Roehampton merged with that at the Westminster in 1961.

plastic surgeon at Roehampton, didn't like that one little bit.

We come to a nice bit of high noon stuff with this, Rupert Taylor used to skin graft, I'd assisted him on many occasions and he was damn good at it. I got a phone call from him, I was a senior registrar down at Roehampton at this point. He said, 'Bradley, on Thursday of next week I'm going to do a sulcoplasty with a skin graft at Roehampton.' The day duly came and all the plastic surgeon consultants appeared. Seven of them, including their senior registrar. The senior plastic surgeon, a big man, scrubbed up. He said, 'You'll need somebody to take this skin graft, won't you?' Taylor said, 'Not necessary, perfectly capable,' and carried on scrubbing. The patient came in and the inside of the thigh was prepared for Rupert and held up properly until he got on board. And he elbowed the plastic surgeon out of the way and just put his hand out to sister and she put the razor in it and he took a perfect graft in front of these plastic surgeons.

When Rob Hensher went to the Westminster hospital as a registrar in 1980, things had improved.

I was a registrar, and this was a rotation between Westminster, Roehampton, and in my case, New Orleans. So, I started at Westminster, and there the flavour was very different. There was all the minor stuff, but there was also all the more major max-fax work, and all the cancer. So, my training then was skewed into managing patients who had really quite big head and neck operations. I was pitched into that, with guidance of course.

The consultants were John Bowerman, John Langdon and Mr Rowe. And at Westminster it was Mr Rowe and Mr Bowerman. John Langdon was another part of the rotation. And then there were JSP Wilson, the plastic surgeon, Harold Ellis and Professor Gerald Westbury. These people overlapped with us.[226] And there was already a multi-disciplinary team flowing between everybody there. It was a great time to be there as a junior. Because I think a lot of animosities and difficulties between specialties, if not disappeared, had almost dissolved between these people. Which was very good.

Can you tell me about how the head and neck cancer patients were managed, who did what?

---

226 See chapter 7 on how a lecture from JSP Wilson in Cork inspired a young David Vaughan towards cancer surgery.

At Westminster a lot of it was done by the oral and maxillofacial doctors, with input from plastics, and those who felt they could provide the beginnings of microvascular work. So, in reconstruction, there was a plastic input. It was pretty harmonious, actually. Neurosurgeons also could be wheeled in from Atkinson Morley.[227] A good example of that would be clivus access via the Le Fort I operation, which we'd combine with the neuros on.[228] Then of course there was oral prosthetics. In its day, it was a centre of excellence for prostheses.

John Cawood was an oral surgery registrar in Edinburgh, his chief was WD MacLennan, and relationships with the plastic surgeons were also harmonious [1973-1977].

MacLennan was a powerful man; politically, clinically, and personality-wise, he had a huge presence in Edinburgh, particularly with his connection with the Royal College in Edinburgh, being a past Dean.

There was a very convivial relationship between MacLennan and Campbell Buchan, the plastic surgeon. He had a very strong relationship, personal and professional, he was highly respected. We were fortunate in that there was such a good personal relationship between the two specialties.

One big lesson I learned from MacLennan was teamwork. He said, 'You play to strengths and you play for the team,' and that was also brought out in his own life in that he was a very good sportsman. He had played rugby for Scotland. His approach to rugby wasn't dissimilar to his approach to surgery or life in general. It was, 'Work it out laddie, do your homework, and then work hard having focussed on what you need to do. Then make sure you do it better than anybody else, then hide it and don't go out and boast. Let actions speak louder than words.' That was his ethos, and that's what I think we all benefited from.

He was a wonderful mentor. He carried the torch, and he built wonderful relationships with other specialities and I think oral surgery stood out. We had our own ward; we had our own operating theatre. MacLennan himself had a medical degree, but we always had a senior

---

227 Atkinson Morley was a specialist neurology and neurosurgery hospital in Wimbledon. It was closed and its services moved to St George's Hospital in 2003.
228 Surgical access through the base of the skull into the brain via a maxillary osteotomy at Le Fort I level.

house officer from the medical firm permanently in the department, so we had medical backup and access to support. He always built this wonderful team round about him and people worked for him because he was admired so much.

Every month he had what was called the Greeting Meeting. So all the staff would assemble, that was fellow consultant John Gould, senior registrar, registrars, senior house officers, any students that were around, nursing staff, porters, and then the most important of the lot, the tea ladies, and the orderlies. And he sat and held court, and he went round everybody and said, 'Do you have any beefs?' And he gave everybody an opportunity to say what they wanted to say, for good or bad, and invariably it got back down to the tea ladies. They were the ones that really could cut loose, they had nothing to lose, and complained about this, that, and the next thing. Everything was discussed, so if there were problems within the department they were ironed out and people had an opportunity to talk.

He just moulded our unit, which was the firm, and people would work their butts off because he set such a good example. And I think that's what I learned most from MacLennan was the team approach. Don't go out looking for trouble. Make friends, don't make enemies, you gain nothing. So that was a huge lesson and stood me well I think in my career. And he was modest, a very important quality.

So he was an inspiration to you ?

Absolutely. Not just to me, to many. To Scotland. He was the Norman Rowe of Scotland.[229]

Mike Awty:

MacLennan was a nice entertaining chap to deal with. 'Make sure you do it better than anybody else, then hide it and don't go out and boast, action speak louder than words'. That's exactly it, that was my philosophy, they were wise words and that paid dividends for me. At East Grinstead we couldn't boast because that would have brought house down, and I said we must look after our patients to the very best of our ability. The plastic surgeons were ganging up on me. Terry was not there much because he was politicking most of the time and the

---

229 See obituary: Professor William Donald MacLennan HDD, FDSRCS (Ed), FRCS (Ed) 1921–2002. British Journal of Oral and Maxillofacial Surgery 2003 41, 1–2

shit used to come my way.

I had a whisper from the chief theatre technician, he said 'I support you because you do it better than they do, you look after your patients better than they do.' The plastic surgeons were pretty casual about just about everything. This chap was very loyal to the plastic surgeons but he was a bit cheesed off by some of their senior registrars. If you don't have the theatre staff and a very powerful theatre technician supporting you then you are lost. That helped with my philosophy of taking control of our field. That was my thesis. I was chuffed that he's noticed that we were much more careful in looking after the patients.

Brian Avery was senior registrar at Canniesburn, where it was not rosy [1978-1983].

There was quite a lot of hostility between the max-fax surgeons and the plastic surgeons, particularly over oncology. I can remember doing a superficial parotidectomy with my boss Amir El-Attar, doing it with him, and it took a long time because I wasn't experienced but I did it; I think the whole operation took about four hours. The patient was fine, and we got the tumour out and no facial nerve damage. A couple of weeks later, bearing in mind I was a senior registrar, a plastic surgeon stopped me in the corridor and he shouted at me at the top of his voice that I was not to do these sorts of operations and it was outrageous that max-fax surgeons were doing things like superficial parotidectomies.

I have to say I stood my ground and said, 'You know, I do what my bosses tell me and my boss said I could do it and he was there throughout the operation and in fact you shouldn't be talking to me about this, you should be talking to my boss because I do what I'm told.' Amir El-Attar was away, and I got no support and I was near to applying for jobs for a consultant post and I was very worried because the plastic surgeon was a very influential person; he was head of the unit and he was very famous. He was the president of the Royal College of Surgeons and Physicians of Glasgow, and I thought my career was over.

Amir El-Attar came back from holiday, and he was a tough guy, was Amir when he needed to be, and he went round and told the plastic surgeon exactly what he thought. I have to give the plastic surgeon his due; he came up to me a few days later and apologised to me and said he should never have shouted at me in the corridor like that and he appreciated it was something that he should've sorted out with my consultant boss. So that ended happily, I'm pleased to say.

Khursheed Moos, consultant at Canniesburn.

Some of my senior registrars, notably Brian Avery, had done parotidectomies and had been taught that prior to coming to us. He wanted to do a case and I saw no objections to it as he had been trained. There was a huge row with plastic surgery over that and a lot of unpleasant things were said about him, but fortunately the result was good and it was done competently without complications. But those were some headaches we had at Canniesburn over the years, and they continued when Amir El-Attar retired and Graham Wood was appointed.

Rob Hensher's senior registrar rotated to University College Hospital [1985].

This job was senior registrar in the 'Plastics and Maxillofacial Unit', so there were two consultant oral and maxillofacial surgeons and two consultant plastic surgeons, and I worked for them both.

I think I'd been in the right place at the right time. I just got to do everything I wanted. And I got really properly taught about wounds, and how to close them, plastic procedures, management of burns. It was invaluable to have that kind of input. Participation in management of patients from other specialties. All that plastic input was wonderful, private and National Health Service. I was scooped into the whole thing. Maxillofacial varied from taking out a wisdom tooth to craniotomies for the children at Great Ormond Street.

The consultants were David James, and Raymund O'Neil, then replaced by Malcolm Harris when I was there. I couldn't have asked for anything better. And Mike Brough and Brian Morgan on the plastics side. So, all I had to do was turn up. It was very busy, and by now I had a lot of responsibility of managing all the juniors, because they kind of reported to me.

So, was there was no evidence of animosity in the unit?

Not between the plastics and the oral and maxillofacial surgeons. We had our run-ins occasionally with other specialties. ENT, for example, used to get very grumpy with us. I don't know why. It must have been something the grown-ups had fought about, but I didn't really get mixed up in it. I didn't really see very much animosity at all. I used to do osteotomies with the plastics registrar; we would operate together.

The theory was that it was important to let each other see each other's specialty, and it was better to work with each other. I didn't want to do plastics or cosmetic boob lifts and everything but it was great seeing it and helping the boss do the breast reductions, and implants, and so on, because it gives you the other person's flavour. I don't believe in fighting with colleagues; I think it spoils everything, not only for the patients, it spoils everything for you as well. And, if you behave like a prat, you probably are being one.

Rob was appointed as a consultant in Cheltenham in 1986.

We covered Cheltenham, Gloucester, and Cirencester hospitals. The two consultants who were there before had been singly qualified and were from that era when a lot of stuff had been scooped up by the plastic surgery service. When we then replaced these guys was the only time I've really ever come across the historic animosity between the specialties.

I'd been there about four days and I was having dinner with a few of the other consultants in order to welcome me there. A plastic surgeon who worked at another hospital not far away made it plain to me he didn't like the look of me, and, he said, and I'll quote him, 'If you want a fight, you can have one.' I said, well, I don't want any fights I suggest we all treat what we get sent, don't you? It gave me food for thought, really. Over the years, I think things settled down a little bit really, when he got more than enough work to keep him occupied. We were too busy to argue with one another. But I found that profoundly disappointing. You could say I'd been naïve, because I'd never come across such behaviour before.

Tony Markus started as senior registrar at Mount Vernon [1979].

That was about the time that John Langdon wrote his famous leader in the Annals of the Royal College of Surgeons, about the management of head and neck cancer.[230] And I remember a plastic consultant came in to the theatre complex and was absolutely explosive, saying, 'Have you read this editorial in the Annals by this dentist, Langdon, saying that the maxillofacial surgeons should be doing the head and neck

---

230 See: Team Approach in the management of oral cancer. Annals of the Royal College of Surgeons of England. Rapidis A. Angelopolous A. Langdon J. 1980 62 116 - 119.

cancer?' I can still remember the look on his face. But it was onwards and upwards, and that was very much the starter's gun for our specialty in head and neck cancer.

This very reasonable paper on the team approach paper caused some controversy. John Langdon:

Yes, that caused a lot of flak even letters in the British Medical Journal.[231] I thought it was perfectly innocuous, but that's what the atmosphere was like in those days. Well, water off a duck's back, really. It's been my role in life, actually, to say the unsayable.

Andy Brown was a senior registrar at East Grinstead from 1976 and consultant from 1981.

There's a lot of facial trauma, and increasingly soft tissue trauma which has come into our specialty. In those days, when I was appointed, we wouldn't have stitched up a single laceration on the face. That would have gone to the plastic surgeons. By the time I was appointed at East Grinstead in 1981, we hadn't won the battle as to who did soft tissue facial trauma.

John Williams was a senior registrar at Roehampton. By this stage, Norman Rowe had really established himself with the plastic surgeons? [1970].

Oh, yes, there wasn't a battle in that respect. There were battles, but not serious ones. I can remember when I went there as an honorary supernumerary registrar[232] that I was working with Dickie Battle and I carefully sewed up something one day and he said, 'Very good, my boy.' Took some scissors, cut the lot out and said, 'Now do it properly.'

Although there was mild friction, the battles over us doing the zygomas was over. There wasn't a question of them being done by the plastic surgeons and us alternately, they were ours. It wasn't all that long before that the plastic surgeons were doing zygomas. At places like Mount Vernon, the dentally qualified people could not put a knife to skin, which was far removed from anything that I had had the experience of. I mean, removing submandibular salivary glands was

---

231 See malicious letter in the British Medical Journal: dental surgeons without a medical qualification. Davis P BMJ 12th July 1980 and a nice reply from Beggs. F in BMJ 26th July 1980. Also in later edition of the Annals from Poole M. Annals 1980 62(4):309–310. and Davis P. in same issue and reply by John Langdon.
232 When he was on an elective as a medical student.

something I was doing as a senior house officer with Paul Bramley, and that was soft tissue work totally. We were already taking over those soft tissue things that were in our patch.

Russell Hopkins became a consultant in Cardiff in 1968. The plastic surgeons were nearby in Chepstow; their unit was to close and they wanted to move to Cardiff.

Later on, I became chairman of the medical staff committee, for the whole of South Glamorgan, and the move was to take place to come into Cardiff, and the plastic surgeons accused me of being fundamental in them not moving into Cardiff. But, in all honesty, it had nothing to do with me, I just did nothing to help them. It was a decision taken entirely by the Welsh office, nothing to do with South Glamorgan, and they went to Swansea in the end, to be near the oil refinery, which is the obvious place, and the steel works where the burns are. But they never forgave for me something which I'd had nothing to do with.

Adrian Sugar spent two years as a senior registrar in Chepstow. How were relations with plastic surgeons there [1978-79]?

It probably took me the best part of a year to realise. I was naïve, but I'd never worked as closely with plastic surgeons before, and I had never appreciated before, the serious animosity that was clearly there.

The initial hostility that I experienced in the Chepstow unit upset me enormously. Just to give you one example, that I had nowhere even to hang my coat when I arrived. I didn't have an office, of course. All the plastic surgery juniors did, and there was a lot of negotiation going on about finding somewhere for me. And eventually they agreed that I could have somewhere, and I shared a room in an outlying, remote building with no external lights on the walkways with live rats. They had a rat house which they used for practising micro-surgery for the registrars, and that was where they put me.

It was not a nice atmosphere in the unit; it was horrendous, and plastic surgeons were always trying to interfere right the way through my senior registrar training. The senior plastic surgeon could be one of the most venomous towards our specialty.

We often used to run a quiz for the medical staff, for the surgeons at Christmas time. And the tradition was that the senior registrars would organise it, and that was me and Martin Milling. And so, Martin and I wrote a quiz with multi-choice answers etc, and all the doctors working in plastic surgery including visiting students and all the max-fax department including visiting students, went into the quiz. The consultants all came as well. And on this first time that we did it, the person who won the quiz was a dental student who subsequently became, some years later, my registrar and is now a consultant in Gloucester and Cheltenham, Jerry Farrier. The senior plastic surgeon who had entered the quiz was disgusted that this dental student had won, and he made his views not too quietly. But it tells you something about his knowledge, doesn't it?

In the early days of the Cardiff Dental Hospital and School there were only two National Health Service consultants, Derek Seel, orthodontics and Russell Hopkins, oral surgery. Derek Seel has previously told me he and Russell had opposed, at committee, some senior academics being given honorary consultant contracts as they did not meet the training criteria for consultant status. But this was before Adrian Sugar had been appointed as senior registrar. Adrian:

Yes, there were some terrible rows between the senior academics on the one hand and Derek and Russell that they told me about. The rows got so bad at one stage, before my time, that they made some sort of peace treaty with Brian Cooke and others to allocate areas of responsibility that were academic and areas that were hospital.

When I was an undergraduate dental student in Cardiff, I went to some of Brian Cooke's oral medicine clinics. My memory is that there were only ever three patients. I remember a patient coming with a mouth cancer, and Cooke referred it to ENT. I was surprised because Russell Hopkins was working in the building and was doing cancer. Adrian Sugar:

That was very characteristic of what he did. I recall when the move of the plastic unit from Chepstow was being discussed, and when I say discussed, discussed behind closed doors and also discussed in the press, and Mike Green was by then the equivalent of clinical director of the plastic surgery department, he was having meetings behind closed doors with Brian Cooke. How do I know that? Because I was in the dental hospital when Mike Green walked through the door and said, 'Hello, Adrian,' and I said, 'What brings you here?' 'Oh,' he said, 'I've got a meeting with the Dean.'

And after that meeting with the Dean, I got summoned by the Dean to be told in graphic details the nature of the discussions that he'd been having with Mike Green, which included carving up facial trauma and bringing it under the thumb of the plastic surgeons with the max-fax surgeons being invited to treat cases when the plastic surgeons thought it was appropriate. And he asked me whether I thought this was a good idea, and I said, 'Professor Cooke, have you discussed this with Mr Hopkins or Mr Wolfle?' 'Oh, no,' he said.

So, I think he was being incredibly mischievous and of course, he must have known that I would tell Russell about this, which I did of course, and of course he and John Wolfle and Cooke got together and they gave him hell and told him to mind his own business.

But why would he would send a cancer case to ENT?

He liked playing games.

Adrian was appointed as a consultant in Chepstow in 1985. How did you get on with the plastic surgeons then?

Michael Earley had been appointed in the previous year, so he was a new boy already in Chepstow as a plastic surgeon. And Michael and I decided in the month or two before I took up post we wanted to work together, and so we decided we wanted to set up a cranio-facial clinic.

It started in September '85 and went on every month and continued after we moved to Morriston in '94. It was a wonderful learning experience because, to be honest, neither of us knew much about congenital syndromes, and especially when it came to hemifacial microsomia, Treacher Collins, Crouzon's, etc, but we were determined to learn, and we weren't going to learn by experimenting on patients. We were going to learn by seeing patients, by working out from the literature. The two of us drove to Oxford one evening, to hear Tessier[233] speak and have a private meeting with him and asked him some questions etc, and it was very valuable. So it was great to have somebody amongst the plastic surgeons that wanted to work with me, and I wanted to work with them. We also did cancer cases together with free flaps. It was a nice collaborative experience, the like of which you don't get often.

Not all opposition was from plastic surgeons. Adrian had been to Middleborough long after he had worked there as a registrar to do a locum for one of the consultants.

---

233 Paul Tessier, French plastic surgeon widely acclaimed pioneer of cranio-facial surgery as known as the 'Father of Cranio-facial Surgery'.

It was before Brian Avery was appointed. I was on call one weekend and a patient was referred to me by one of the senior orthopaedic surgeons. The patient had what he thought might be osteomyelitis of mandible and he was right; he had that. I had a little chat with him after I'd confirmed the diagnosis and he asked me if I'd take over his care, and I booked him to do a decortication and get rid of any dead bone etc, under general anaesthesia on a Saturday morning.

The anaesthetist was a guy I'd encountered before when I'd worked up there as a registrar and he refused to do it. He said, 'Tell Mr Sugar to ring me.' So, I rang him and I said, 'I understand that there's a problem,' and he said, 'Yes, I don't think you should be doing this patient.' I said, 'What do you mean?' He said, 'Well, osteomyelitis, that's a matter for the orthopaedic surgeons.' I said, 'Yes, but this patient has been referred to me specifically by the senior orthopaedic surgeon who has seen him and who has made a diagnosis of mandibular osteomyelitis, and asked my opinion, and I've told him I thought he was quite right. He's asked me to treat the patient.' He said, 'Yes, but the patient has also not been seen by the doctor on the ward.' I said, 'What's the doctor on the ward?' 'Oh,' he said, 'we have an agreement that patients must be seen by the doctor on the ward.' I said, 'We have our beds on a general surgery ward and I've never heard of anything such as that. I'll make enquiries if you like.'

And I did. I spoke to the general surgeon on call and he said, 'Who is it who's talked all this shit,' he said. And I told him, and he said, 'Not him again.' He said, 'Don't concede at all Adrian, not a word,' he said, 'there's no such agreement. If he wants my senior house officer to examine your patient, I will refuse, and in fact I'll tell him now not to do that. Your patient has been seen by our house officer and registrar, and that is perfectly satisfactory for me and should be for him. If he wants to look at the guy medically himself, he's welcome to do it, isn't he?' And he also assured me of his complete and total support on this matter. Well, I was in a quandary quite what to do about that.

So, anyway, this anaesthetist did in the end come in, and he did the case, and I treated the patient, and afterwards I consulted the hospital chief medical officer and I told him about the case. And I said I thought it was very serious because he just seemed to make excuses to not treat the patient and not treat the patient with me, and it wasn't his job to do that.

Chapter 27

The Early Greats, Terence Ward and Norman Rowe

'Sir Terence was respected, admired and even liked but Norman Rowe was loved.'

After WWII and throughout the 1950s, 60s and 70s there were two outstanding figures advancing the evolution of the specialty of oral and maxillofacial surgery from hospital dentistry. These were Terence Ward, whose clinical work was based at the Queen Victoria Hospital East Grinstead, and Norman Rowe at Rooksdown House Basingstoke and after 1959 at Roehampton Hospital.

Terence Ward started his career in dentistry as a dental mechanic before qualifying as a dentist and in medicine in 1928. It was not unusual for dentists to start as mechanics.

Mike Awty explained.

In those days in the dental undergraduate course there was a great deal of technical mechanical work, metalwork, gold work, porcelain work, so your manual dexterity was quite taxed, really. And I understood you could do your mechanics before you went to dental school. But I think that had finished before the war or at the war.

Terence Ward spent nine years working in dental practice and when WWII started he joined the RAF dental branch where he became involved in the treatment of facial injuries sustained by RAF crew at Cosford Hospital. He was influenced by William Kelsey Fry, who had worked with Harold Gillies at Queen Mary's Hospital, Sidcup in treating facial injuries in WWI and with Archibald McIndoe at the Queen Victoria Hospital East Grinstead during WWII. Kelsey Fry was a man of considerable influence, and Ward subsequently inherited Kelsey Fry's position as consultant at East Grinstead, where he continued clinical work for the rest of his life.

He became involved in all the administrative evolutions of the specialty. He was a founding Fellow of the Faculty of Dental Surgery of the Royal College of Surgeons of England, and later Dean, he was the first President of the British Association of Oral Surgeons and later was President of the International Association of Oral and Maxillofacial

Surgeons.[234]

Mike Awty knew him well as a senior house officer, senior registrar, and finally as consultant colleague at East Grinstead.

He was a very strong personality; he had very strong feelings for the profession and he was a good networker. He played golf with the Secretary of the College; he was chums with Chief Dental Officer, there wasn't anything he didn't know that was going on, and if he thought somebody deserved a job somewhere, he would pull as hard as he could to get it for them. He was very generous. He was an absolute bastard at times, but he was very generous if he thought you deserved it. Most people that have worked for him have done all right because he was very helpful, if he thought you were a genuine person and got on with him.

What did he get his knighthood for?

I think a good network, actually. He'd been largely the instigator of the International Oral Surgery Association, he'd been an early President and founder of the British Association of Oral Surgeons. He was a leading figure, and of course he had Kelsey Fry's support.

Andy Brown:

It was really burns injuries that put East Grinstead's name on the map. However, Sir William Kelsey Fry, one of the leaders and initiators of oral surgery in the UK, was appointed in the second war and he was there in the early years after the war for just a short time before going to work at Guy's. Terence Ward, later to be Sir Terence Ward, succeeded him, and he was a very interesting character. A man who was a very determined and rather difficult taskmaster at times. However, he was one of those people who worked hard and played hard. There was a mischievousness about him. He was a bit of a practical joker and loved to be surrounded by trainees as his young acolytes, particularly if they were a little bit sycophantic. He left a mark on people who worked for him.

Paul Bramley:

I worked with him only on short attachments. He used to stroll

---

234 See: Plarr's Lives of the Fellows. Royal College of Surgeons of England. and An appreciation of the late Sir Terence Ward. Awty M. British Journal of Oral and Maxillofacial Surgery 1993 32. 128 - 129.

about with his sweatband on and theatre things, conducting everybody in the theatre in what they were doing and generally being an impressive figure. I must have actually scrubbed with him, but I can't remember that.

Ward had an immense personality; he was an Edinburgh double qualification. He was the genuine front-of-house man. He could get up and speak and persuade, and he was very persuasive. Many Australians and New Zealanders, as well as British, passed through his hands.

Terry Ward retired in 1981 and died in 1993.

Norman Rowe was born in 1915 and qualified in dentistry at Guy's in 1937. He was in the Royal Army Dental Corps during the war and afterwards qualified in medicine from Guy's. After a registrar job at Hill End Hospital he became a consultant at Rooksdown House Basingstoke where he worked with Harold Gillies, the famous plastic surgeon, who had opened the unit in WWII to treat facial injuries. He transferred to Roehampton Hospital in 1959 when Rooksdown House closed. He was a founding member of the British Association of Oral Surgeons and became the first Secretary and later President. He later became the Secretary General of the International Association of Oral and Maxillofacial Surgeons and Vice President of the European Association for Maxillo-facial Surgery.[235] He was never Dean of the Faculty of Dental Surgery of the Royal College of Surgeons of England.

Despite these offices and his participation in the administrative and political advancement of oral and maxillofacial surgery, it was for his clinical work, teaching and inspiration of generations of young aspiring surgeons that he is best admired and remembered for.

Paul Bramley worked as a registrar at Rooksdown House with Norman Rowe.

It was about '52, '53 or '54. He must have been a consultant for about two years. Norman Rowe and Homer Killey had been trainees together, and they went to medical school and boxed and coxed in relation to their duties as trainees. They both got their Licentiate in the Society of Apothecaries.

John Bradley was a registrar and subsequently senior registrar at the

---

235 Obituary: Norman Lester Rowe CBE. British Journal of Oral and Maxillofacial Surgery. 1992. 30. 199.

Westminster and Roehampton.

That was an incredible experience really, working under Norman Rowe out at Roehampton. The other consultant there was Ian Heslop, and Rupert Sutton Taylor was also on the staff at this point and he was the senior consultant.

Plastic and oral surgery had been set up to treat facial injuries in WWII, with Harold Gillies as the chief at Rooksdown House, a former mental hospital at Basingstoke. It moved to Roehampton in 1959. Roehampton House was opened as a Hospital in the first world war for soldiers with limb injuries. Rowe worked at Rooksdown and eventually moved to Roehampton.

The other man there was of course Homer Killey. When the department moved up to Roehampton, Killey got the Chair at the Eastman. These two were called Auntie and Uncle.

What was it about Norman Rowe that made him so great? Was it his interpersonal skills, was it that he was a very good surgeon, was innovative, or was he a good politician? John:

He wasn't a good politician. He was the other three. But he was not a good politician. Norman Rowe was extremely innovative, a superb surgeon and a very brave surgeon. He was always very questioning. He taught me to take on board the very important question: why? And if you ask yourself the question why, you have a fair chance that you might solve a problem, but it also brings an enormous amount of fun as a result with it. Norman Rowe was too much of a gentleman to be a politician; you've got to be a bit of a bastard for that.

One of his great sadnesses, to be frank, was not being elected Dean of the Faculty. And it was because he was too nice. He didn't do it. And it was envy, because he was damn good at his job and this is what he was, which was a shame. Not a good politician, but as a man, brilliant.

Rob Hensher was a senior registrar on the Roehampton rotation. One year was spent working in Münster, West Germany. He gave me insight into the nickname 'uncle' [1984].

He was my boss but this this was more personal. When I worked in Germany he wrote to me regularly, semi-clinical but also on social matters. His letters were enjoyable and amusing. He kept that up for the whole year I was in Germany. I thought that was unique. The social and intellectual and generous nature took me aback; it was indeed like reading letters from an uncle.

John Williams became an honorary supernumerary registrar at Roehampton as his medical student elective. He subsequently became registrar and senior registrar. His former chief Paul Bramley had advised him to contact Norman Rowe.

Paul Bramley was very keen that I worked with Norman Rowe.

Almost everyone I spoke to regarded Norman Rowe as a saint and there were people queuing up to be trained by him but when they were being trained by him, they were holding a retractor and they weren't actually doing much cutting themselves? John:

That was perfectly true until John Bowerman came online. John Bowerman changed all that when he was a senior registrar. John was a bit older than the average and he told them, 'Look, I'm not learning anything by sitting on the end of a retractor. I need to do these procedures with you assisting me.' And that was the moment that both Norman and Ian Heslop in particular, who was even more anxious to do the thing himself, began to recognise that.

Peter Leopard and I were senior registrars together, and we both had a lot of clinical experience in what we'd done before we went there. We were able to apply that because Norman Rowe from the very first day that I went there took me through the very first procedure I did, which was a genioplasty. Now I knew about genioplasties but I hadn't done one and he said, 'No, no, you'll do that,' and I did the operation; he assisted me. That was the start of it and from there on in we did a lot.

I was one of the first of the senior registrars there who genuinely got a lot of hands-on experience, and I really did. I think we were the first unit to do bi-maxillary osteotomies in the same procedure, because it had always been done in two stages before.

I was told that Norman Rowe won over because of his intellect, his analysis of the situation, and that he was just such a polite, nice chap. He won people over; he didn't push for things, but they came to him because of that?

Exactly right. He really was the most polite individual you could think about. Even when he was cross with somebody, he was still remarkably polite. Those of us who knew him well, knew when he was cross because he had a midline vein on his forehead which would then stand out like a beacon. You knew then that he was a little disappointed, shall we say?

Russell Hopkins was a registrar at St Peter's Hospital Chertsey and Holy Cross Hospital Haslemere before he went to medical school. They were outreach departments of the Roehampton unit.

Norman Rowe differed greatly from some people subsequently. Norman wanted to come in for everything. For any facial injury that was out of hours, I had to ring Norman to tell him and he would come in. So I was actually getting less operating as a registrar than I had as a senior house officer. So I got fed up with this, and after a bit I got so fed up that I started to lift the cheekbones and show Norman the next day. He got quite angry at this, but he got used to it and ultimately he left me alone do to the stuff that I thought I was competent at and I called him in for the middle thirds and the big stuff.

Norman Rowe also did some work at the Eastman Dental Hospital. David Vaughan was a locum registrar at the Eastman Dental Hospital while he was a medical student. He was not so impressed.

I was doing my time at the Eastman; we treated inpatients there in Burkhardt Ward. Anyway, this young girl came in with a parotid tumour and the great Rowe had decided to operate on her at the Eastman. And there was a big bluff anaesthetist, Tom McEwan who adored Norman Rowe, because Norman Rowe was a gentleman. He was very polite to everybody.

I watched him doing the parotidectomy and did essentially what one would describe as a Millin's prostatectomy on it. He stuck his finger in, wriggled it around, it burst, the jelly flew everywhere and a piece was given to the pathologist who ran off as if he had the sacred host in his hands. And of course the facial nerve was never found, and it was sewn up, and this was considered to be a fantastic success. That's when I realised that dentists cannot teach individuals to do soft tissue surgery; you've got to be taught by other people who can do soft tissue surgery.

I asked John Williams if he thought that the Roehampton/Westminster department really led the way before East Grinstead in terms of the advancement of the specialty.

I don't think there's any doubt about that. I mean for example, it was when I was a consultant in Chichester that I went and talked to the people at East Grinstead about doing parotidectomies and the plastic people were in there too and they said, 'Well, what about a nerve stimulator?' And I said, 'I think if you need a nerve stimulator you're not doing the right operation because you must be able to see the nerve.' Well, you can't always see the nerve,' and I said, 'Yes, you can, you have to,' and so I reflect on that inasmuch as saying that's how much ahead we were in the broader aspects of the specialty that were developing.

I have been told that the reason was that Sir Terence Ward why he was so influential in medicine and dentistry was because he played golf with all the right people.

Yes, it was contacts, definitely contacts.

But he must have had a lot of ability as well?

Well, don't forget, the specialty was in those days very much more oral surgery. The max-fax element was only just coming in and at East Grinstead the plastic people did a lot of the trauma, whereas with the Roehampton crowd, Norman Rowe and Ian Heslop, all that crowd had got a lot more surgical experience as a result of this rather quieter approach than the Terry Ward type approach, and I think that was why there was a difference.

But he was competent in doing what he was doing, which was the oral surgery side of things. And it would be quite wrong to say he wasn't competent doing the max-fax side. He was, but it was a different kind of competence.

Paul Bramley was looking for a job in the early 1950s after he came back from Africa. He took a registrar job with Norman Rowe rather than a senior registrar with Terence Ward. He explained why.

There was an opportunity to go to two places, which I thought would be useful. One was East Grinstead, with Terry Ward, and the other one was with 'Uncle' Norman Rowe. I thought about it. I had met Norman before, and I'd met Ward before. I didn't apply for East Grinstead because my estimate of Ward was he was a pirate in a minor sort of way, and really not the best influence, which was really cut first and think later, if at all. Whereas Norman had an analytical mind; he saw a problem, he thought it out, and he worked off the literature and delivered the goods in a most caring manner. Also, he was a very nice man, so I went there.

Ward's lectures inferred that bigger is better and his slides showed material he never touched himself. This was the piracy bit! It was so upsetting to see that and know the real truth of Ward. But he had a very influential personality. He engineered his knighthood and tried to make the House of Lords on the same basis, but didn't receive the support that he might have had.

John Williams.

Terry Ward was so blunt and rude. Norman Rowe just would not get on with such people very easily because he was polite. He didn't have a good relationship with Terry Ward. Terry Ward was Dean of Faculty,[236] and Norman was never was, and this is the sort of issue that went between them. Terry Ward was the hail fellow, well-met sort of person, and Norman was the concerned, discerning, quiet person, but a very shrewd clinician and a very good one.

Norman was wonderful. He gradually increased his field and depth of knowledge, and they produced the book. That was a big fillip for them.[237] And he then moved Rooksdown into Roehampton.

Mark Cutler was a maxillofacial technologist working with Derek Henderson at St Thomas' Hospital when Brian Conroy offered him a job in the laboratory at Roehampton.

Norman Rowe retired a couple of years before I started at Roehampton, but he used to come back and visit and his presence was still very much felt there. He was still the main man, even though he'd gone.

When Mr Rowe was visiting, we would know a few days before when he was coming. It was almost like Captain's rounds on a ship. The place would be tidied up, I've been nowhere else like it. He must have had a terrific influence on the place when he was there.

I never met Sir Terence Ward or Norman Rowe but have listened to people who have spoken about them and I formed the impression that Sir Terence was highly respected, admired and even liked, but that Norman Rowe was loved. I put this to Mike Awty.

That's exactly right. There had been much animosity between the units but that had largely ceased. I had enormous respect for Norman

---

236 Faculty of Dental Surgery of the Royal College of Surgeons of England.
237 Fractures of the Facial Skeleton was published in 1955.

and in his quiet way I felt that I had his support.

Two years after I had interviewed him for this book my former colleague and friend Richard Thornton told me that he had anaesthetised for Norman Rowe when he was a senior house officer in anaesthetics at the Westminster Hospital. I asked him for his recollection. Richard:

There can hardly be any chapters in this book which do not include some reference to Norman Rowe. The chapter on anaesthetics is one, but even here there is a sense of omission which should be corrected.

Many of the modern anaesthesia techniques developed alongside the needs of maxillofacial surgery; the abandonment of nitrous oxide and introduction of total intravenous anaesthesia being one example. The junior anaesthetists such as myself, lucky enough to train at the Westminster group hospitals, benefitted from the experience of working in the oral and maxillofacial theatres, and especially when Norman Rowe was the surgeon. The surgical voices in this book all witness to his calm and utterly supportive care of those in the training stages of their careers. I would like to add my voice (as an outsider as it were) to these contributions.

Quite often I would be giving the anaesthetics for a Norman Rowe list which could include some complex cases. There were many consultant surgeons, and I don't blame them, who would have made it clear that they were not happy at having to work with a senior house officer gasman. Such lists would be a fraught experience, very stressful.

In contrast, Norman Rowe was without exception the most supportive consultant, not just to the anaesthetist but to the whole theatre team. His calmness was legendary. His skill as a surgeon took away many anaesthetic worries. And when problems did arise, his polite and good-humoured support allowed one to work as a valued team member to resolve the issue. His support was there wherever and whenever needed. Anaesthetic room to recovery and back to the ward. This was the setting for an environment in which one could learn and develop as an anaesthetist; and more importantly to the huge benefit of his patients. Norman Rowe was one of the greatest, if not 'the' greatest, of role models for anyone aspiring to reach the pinnacle of their profession.

John Langdon first met Norman Rowe when he was a senior house officer at the Eastman in 1966, but really got to know him when he became a consultant colleague at Roehampton in 1977.

He was delightful, very cultured. When you're two consultants in the unit, you don't actually work together very much because your sessions are on interlocking days. But Wednesdays at Roehampton was a big teaching day, so all of us would be there on a Wednesday.

There'd be a grand round where visitors from all over the world would turn up and we'd do a teaching round. And then there was a big clinic, nominally Norman Rowe's clinic. But we were all there. Then the rest of the week we didn't really overlap, except that we would all have lunch together in the consultant's office, which was when I really got to know Norman. He was a very cultured man, he could talk with a depth of knowledge on many interesting topics.

But he was also a bitter man. He felt very hurt that Terence Ward had a knighthood and Norman didn't and that really wrangled him. It came up more than once in conversations.

Norman Rowe travelled widely throughout the world giving talks and demonstrating operations and things and he'd met many people on his travels and therefore he knew many people. There was always an open invitation, if they were ever in the UK, to turn up on the Wednesday and meet everybody. And these people would pitch up from the States, from South America, from India, all sorts of places. And the impressive thing was, Norman would always know their names, the names of their wives, how many kids they had and precisely when and where they'd met. Wonderful ability; he was so good with people that way.

The other extraordinary thing about him was that he wasn't somebody who was always showing off, quoting papers. But if you were talking about a particular subject, he'd say, 'Ooh, so and so wrote a paper. It was in whatever journal in 1963.' And he was always correct; he had a phenomenal memory.

His nickname, when I first came across him at the Eastman, was Uncle. Which he was; an avuncular figure. You always felt you were part of his family, his coterie. I never heard him criticise a colleague, as a personality or as a surgeon, ever. And I never met anyone who didn't respect him and hold him in regard. Somebody else who I had huge respect for and knew as a colleague was Gerald Westbury, who was a surgeon at the Westminster and the Royal Marsden who made his reputation as a sarcoma surgeon. Occasionally, when I was a consultant, I would take a difficult case to Gerald Westbury at the Marsden for an opinion. I'd pitch up with the patient and ask his advice. And he always asked after Norman. So there was somebody in a totally different specialty who had regard and respect for him.

So were you somebody who loved Norman Rowe?

Yeah, absolutely, absolutely.

Sir Paul Bramley gave the eulogy to Norman Rowe at his memorial service at St Clement Danes Church on November the 29th 1991. When I interviewed him in 2014, he read it to me in his study at Hathersage. His love for the man was apparent not just in the words but in his voice, which broke with emotion several times. I don't believe it was published, so here it is as Sir Paul read it to me.

He was a special person.

When he left Malvern College in 1932 his housemaster did not think much to his prospects and his school report reads, 'I am sorry he is leaving so young as his medical attainments are naturally far short of hospital requirements. I only hope that this premature end to his schoolwork will not handicap him later on.'

After qualification at Guy's and marriage to Cynthia, he worked for several years in general dental practice in the west country, take-home pay three guineas a week, an important background to his later work triggered an interest in prosthetics and orthodontics. Later he used to run an orthodontic clinic on Saturday morning at Rooksdown House. From what we remember, it was mainly removable appliance expansion of the upper arch with the retraction of the incisors. You must realise this was long before orthodontics expressed any pretensions to being anything other than a black art.

Five years' war service culminating in the Normandy landings and experience with the 86th General Hospital directed his ambitions towards maxillofacial surgery. His symbolic relationship with Paddy Killey began when they were trainee specialists at Hill End under Mr Ben Fickling and Mr Rainsford Mowlem. By some subtle boxing and coxing, they both ended up with a Higher Dental Diploma Edinburgh and medical qualifications, and in 1948 were two of the first three to gain the FDS exam by examination; the third was the late Tom Battersby.

In September 1948, he was appointed consultant at Rooksdown

House, soon to be joined again by Killey. As a medical student, Norman distinguished himself when clerking for the eminent physician and cardiologist, Sir John Coneybeare, Norman presented the patient, noting a diastolic murmur. Sir John said, rather testily, 'There is no murmur, the heart sounds are perfectly normal.' Our hero, not one bit abashed, said, 'Sir, if you place your stethoscope just here and listen very carefully you can just hear it.' You can imagine the tension.

The book 'Fractures of the Facial Skeleton' was published in 1955. The run-up to this was an infuriating time for his juniors. Notes, X-rays and photographs often went missing. Only after exhaustive searches were they found stacked under Killey's bed. He was the magpie for the first edition.

Norman fell under the innovative, imaginative and somewhat eccentric spell of Harold Gillies. Together they made substantial advances in the surgery of facial deformity. At the beginning, he was only allowed to drill holes in the bone and pass the stainless steel wire. Norman, and this was absolutely characteristic of him, took the problems back to first principles, applied analytical thought, burnt the midnight oil and became such a fount of wisdom and competence that bit-by-bit total management of these cases naturally and unobtrusively came his way.

With the aid of his Francis Barnett motorbike, he developed and ran an oral surgery service in Southwest Thames, Lambeth, Mayday, Croydon, Epsom, Dorking, Chertsey, Aldershot, Haslemere, Woking and St Richard's Chichester. There was nothing before that. Just what do you owe to him in Southwest Thames? The Rooksdown unit closed in 1959 and transferred to Queen Mary's Roehampton and his contract changed to that hospital and to the Westminster and also to the Eastman Hospital. At the Westminster, he played a valued part in the team approach to cancer management and at the Eastman provided new horizons. And I could tell you they needed it.

Norman Rowe was at the frontiers of oral surgery. Roehampton, his main base, became a place of pilgrimage for trainees and consultants alike. There were always large numbers of visitors, and the theatre superintendent was forced to complain that the laundry could not provide any more than 25 extra gowns per day. His care of patients, his bedside and outpatient teaching, his lecturing and publications proceeded on an ever deepening and ever widening scale. He maintained a huge professional personal correspondence, much with his former trainees and also as a consultant's consultant. Eponymous lectures rolled in, and he became increasingly held in worldwide regard. He lectured and operated in at least 40 countries and was made an honorary member of 20 national oral and maxillofacial societies.

We all remember with amazement the tours de force he put on in public lectures. However, sometimes his juniors were not that delighted when they were kept late at night while he, Uncle, having got into the subject, dotted the 'i's and crossed the 't's in an encyclopaedic manner, when all they could think of was the sort of reception they were going to get from their young wives being late home yet again.

He had great pleasure in the fact that his own father, himself and his son David, belonged to the Most Excellent Order of the British Empire. Medals, fellowships, prizes all came his way in liberal profusion, and yet, he did not change. He remained a man of true humility, always approachable, always listening to you, always interested, always courteous and a sense of fun very near the surface. Right throughout his life, he maintained a striking sense of integrity and honour.

There's another side of Norman's work, which must be mentioned because it illuminates aspects of his character, and that is in the organisation and administration of his profession. We have the formation of the British Association of Oral Surgeons due to a small group of men, but mainly to him. He saw the problems and was prepared to do the hard work in resolving them. He did painstaking research to create the constitution, conducted the endless negotiations with the Charity Commissioners and planned with the College of Heralds the Coat of Arms, resulting in the stunning gold, pink and apple green crest.

As the first secretary, for five years, he got the Association up and running. He was entrusted with high office in both international and European associations. Self-control and quiet dignity and logical persistence bore fruit in the long negotiations to win pay parity for oral surgeons and indeed all dental consultants in the National Health Service. His courage was put to the test over several other issues affecting the development of the specialty and he was not found wanting.

In a letter to the Times you could read the following: 'I was a pretty young woman and involved in a disastrous accident converting me from that into a hideous, disordered facial wreck. I eventually went to see Norman Rowe. I knew at once this man could help me. His courtesy, his humility, was apparent. When he had to do the second operation for me, it happened to be my birthday. He bought me 12 red roses.'

Chapter 28

The Influence of the British Association of Oral and Maxillofacial Surgeons.

'It was an exciting time, and it brought people together'

The British Association of Oral Surgeons, subsequently called the British Association of Oral and Maxillofacial Surgeons, was formed in 1962. What has been its impact on the development of the specialty over the years?

John Langdon:

It gave us a corporate pride, a corporate voice. It put us on an equal footing, in the Royal College of Surgeons in London, with all the other specialty societies, which were all housed in the same building. We had the same status with our own Specialist Advisory Committee.

It brought together, the big names who as big personalities wouldn't naturally work together. I mean, Russell Hopkins, Norman Rowe, Gordon Hardman, so many of them, latterly David Vaughan, people who wouldn't necessarily naturally gel together were dragged together for the corporate good. It was a period of time when there was a lot of innovation. We had some very enthusiastic senior registrars, like David Vaughan and Bob Ord, young consultants like myself, who had fought to get salivary glands and cancer in the first place. And others doing cleft work. It was an exciting time, and it brought people together. We had a journal that was reasonably well respected. It was an essential part of our development.

Ian Martin:

I think the fundamental thing was the vote that was held around 1981, which said that within ten years you're going to have to have dual qualification because we think we should go with the predominantly northern European model of dental, oral, and maxillofacial surgery. Which means you've got to have the registerable qualification of medicine and dentistry to progress.

That was probably the most important thing that the specialty did. The Speciality Advisory Committee was predominantly six members elected from the specialty Association. And the Specialist Advisory

Committee became a member of the Joint Committee for Higher Surgical Training, as it was, as well as being a member of the Joint Committee for Specialist Training in Dentistry. So they still kept a foot in both camps. I think it was Peter Banks when President of the British Association of Oral and Maxillofacial Surgeons that took the Specialist Advisory Committee into the joint committee.

By the time the British Association of Oral Surgeons decided that everyone should have a medical qualification, it was already impossible for a trainee to advance to senior registrar status without medicine, so did it really make any difference at all? John Langdon:

It made a difference because dentally qualified applicants to medical school often found it difficult to get a place. The appointment committees would say, 'Well, why should we give you a place to do medicine, you're already qualified professionally. Whereas if we appoint a school leaver, we've got another doctor. You're not going to be a doctor.' But once it was mandatory, that made a big difference to their argument, their bargaining power, if you like.

After the British Association of Oral Surgeons became the British Association of Oral and Maxillofacial Surgeons in 1982/3, another British Association of Oral Surgeons was created for the dentally qualified oral surgeons.

Ian Martin:

The British Association of Oral and Maxillofacial Surgery has had a chequered career. My own view was always that it ought to have learnt the lesson of what happened in 1962. Until 1962 oral surgery was a second-class citizen within the Association of Plastic Surgery, and then those people like Terry Ward and others got fed up with being second class citizens; they weren't allowed to have full voting rights.[238] So they went and set up the British Association of Oral Surgeons to give them their own autonomous voice as a specialty.

I was strongly of the view, as both the chairman of the Specialist Advisory Committee, and later on as the chairman of the Association, that we ought to have learnt the lesson from that and created a home within the British Association of Oral and Maxillofacial Surgeons for singly qualified oral surgeons, and surgical dentists. I was never of the

---

238 They were admitted to the British Association of Plastic Surgeons as 'Associate Members'.

view that they were likely to take the Association over by revolution and change its whole character and disenfranchise us in terms of in our surgical credentials. That just didn't seem to me to be likely, and it was much more dangerous for them to go off and do their own thing.

We had a fairly widespread programme of putting forward four options for the membership to vote on, ranging from full inclusion of all oral surgeons as full fellows of the Association with voting rights and eligibility to be council and President, ranging to get rid of the need for a dental qualification and have just maxillofacial surgery like in southern Europe. We had various people doing video clips, and I travelled up and down the country presenting that and leading the debate in many units. Unfortunately, we didn't get the result I would have preferred, which was a fully inclusive specialty.

And surprise, surprise, the oral surgeons said, right, well we're going to set up our own association then. We now know what then happened was the Association realised with some embarrassment that the previous name, the British Association of Oral Surgeons, was not in any way protected under patent or anything else. So this new association, which was naturally antipathetic toward us as a specialty, was set up and was the British Association of Oral Surgeons. I think that was a big diplomatic error and we should have created a home where they felt they were part of a wider specialty.

The consequences are two different specialties now, and one's dental, and they're still pretty antipathetic. The only good thing is because there was no money behind that there are still very few training programmes in oral surgery, and so it's not really taken off in the way that some people would have hoped it would have done.

John Cawood commented [1991/92].

In 1991 the General Dental Council proposed the establishment of an 'Oral Surgery' specialist list based in the primary care sector. At the time I was on the council of the British Association of Oral and Maxillofacial Surgeons and the council of the Royal College of Surgeons of Edinburgh and I voiced my objections to the hijacking of the title Oral Surgeon in both chambers. My concern was they would take a title that they were not entitled to.

I raised my objections both in Edinburgh and at the British Association of Oral and Maxillofacial Surgeons, but in the beginning I felt very much on my own; there was very little support from my colleagues. I really had to bang on a lot to get this issue addressed.

I sent a letter to key individuals including the Dean in Edinburgh, the presidents of the British Association of Oral and Maxillofacial Surgeons and the European Association who had received copies of the document and were very concerned. Anyway, there was lots of discussion and we managed to change the name of this new specialist from Oral Surgeon to Surgical Dentist. I was happier with that solution because it continued to link the title Oral Surgeon with Maxillofacial and confined the new specialist to the high street and not into secondary care, which was my main concern.

John Langdon:

There was all the unnecessary and unpleasant split going on between maxillofacial surgery and oral surgery. A lot of us in the British Association of Oral and Maxillofacial Surgeons, including me when I was President and David James before me and Peter Leopard before that, were fighting to keep the oral surgeons on board.

All they wanted was a bit of recognition and a bit of status, respect for what they were doing. We argued that there was a place for singly qualified oral surgeons to do the routine dental alveolar surgery. It became apparent that if your personal practice was maxillofacial surgery, you didn't have the operating capacity, let alone the time, to be doing routine dento-alveolar surgery, and to an extent, it was a different skill set. Because of intransigence, there was this horrible split which has done none of us any good and has led to the destruction of academic maxillofacial surgery.

Chapter 29

Brian Conroy and the Evolution of Maxillofacial Technology

'It's become much more science based, it was a craft in the 1960s'

Mark Cutler is a consultant maxillofacial prosthetist and manager of the maxillofacial laboratory and prosthetics clinic at the Queen Victoria Hospital, East Grinstead. He told me of how the discipline has changed since the days of the 'dental mechanic'. Mark had decided at school that he wanted to become a maxillofacial technician. His initial training was at the Brooklands College in Surrey [1980-83].

I think I came in as the word 'mechanic' was being dropped, just. I remember picking up the careers leaflet that said 'dental technician'. I only became a dental technician because I knew that was the way you became a maxillofacial technician.

In those days, the qualification was changing from City and Guilds over to the National Diploma in Dental Technology. The course changed dramatically in the late '70s and it became more science based in the early 1980s with the National Diploma. The only college in the south offering a National Diploma in those days was Brooklands. I got a place there on the full time dental technology course. That was for three years, plus a final fourth year which was vocational training out in the laboratory before we could then get our Dental Technician Advisory and Educational Board accreditation.

The Dental Technician Advisory and Educational Board is defunct now. In those days to work in the National Health Service or in a halfway decent laboratory you had to have Dental Technician Advisory and Educational Board accreditation, especially for us who had been full-time students who most of the old dental mechanics didn't rate at all.

When I was on my full-time course, I went to a few maxillofacial units; I came here to East Grinstead when I was 18. I had been on the course for a couple of years and then one guy here looked me up and down and said, 'Who are you then?' as if I was some long-haired yobbo and I said, 'Hello, my name's Mark, I'm interested in becoming a maxillofacial technician.' 'Where are you studying?' 'Dental

Technology, Brooklands', 'You're not a full-time student are you?' 'Yes I am.' 'As long as you have a hole in your backside, you'll never be a maxillofacial technician, you won't have the skills.' So, okay thanks for that, so I kind of left it at that and, well actually here I am now running the lab at East Grinstead, so that one came out nicely.

Mark is also running the clinical service.

Yes, the prosthetic clinic as well. Obviously things have changed since those days. But what he said annoyed me, I thought, well that's rude. All the dental mechanics up to that point had trained part time and worked in either a hospital laboratory or a commercial laboratory. They didn't rate us full-time students highly at all. Leap forward 20 years and the dental technology basic qualification is the Honours Degree at Manchester or Cardiff, or wherever, and it's really all full time now. They do their three or four years and they come out with a BSc.

I suppose they thought you were lacking the practical experience if you're in college?

Of course, you passed the prosthetics module having only made three sets of dentures, whereas these guys had made three hundred sets in their old City and Guilds course. I'd probably have felt the same.

But even as a teenager, I recognised that the industry was changing, particularly the materials that were being used. These guys had never heard of cross linked polymers or silicones. They were aware of cobalt-chrome because that was a dental material and also gold. But they were unaware of materials like tantalum, titanium and palladium and all of those things that can be used for not only dental technology also any technology around the head and neck.

At Brooklands College we used to have four sessions a week of practical experience, two days in the training laboratory. Then we used to have six sessions a week of either theory or in the materials laboratory. We used to have an anatomical and pathological laboratory at the college as well. The college used to bring in experts in metallurgy and polymers, and other material scientists, and we had anatomy and physiology lessons. We did some organ dissections and head dissections; it was terrific training.

I did my final, fourth year, at Guy's Hospital as a dental technology student in the prosthetics laboratory. The Chief Dental Technician was Ken Jordan, and he was a super guy, he had a heart of gold. He was just about to retire and he could see how the industry was changing and needed people like us to come in and take it forward with new materials and techniques, all the things we do now.

When I finished my four years I looked around for a maxillofacial trainee job. In those days there were no formally recognised maxillofacial trainee posts; it was more of an apprenticeship with somebody in a maxillofacial lab. In the mid-1980s you needed to become a member of the Institute of Maxillofacial Technology, so you then had to sit the Certificate for Maxillofacial Technology to become a full member. You couldn't get a job in a maxillofacial laboratory unless you had full membership. It was almost impossible, and it's still almost impossible.

In those days, they wouldn't accept anybody that didn't have at least two years' experience plus another advanced certificate in a dental technology specialty. So I had to either do orthodontics, prosthodontics, or crown and bridge restoration technology. I did the advanced prosthodontics certificate and that took me two years [1984-86] and then when I'd completed that; I signed on to do the maxillofacial course.

In reality, even in those days, it was an eight-year career path, four years of dental technology, two years advanced dental and then two years of a maxillofacial course. And it's the same today. The students do four years for the BSc; they do three years for the MSc and they have about a year vocational training before they can apply for full membership. So the names of the qualifications have changed, but apart from that nothing else has.

Mark went to work at the London Hospital [1986-88].

The London had a very good oral surgery laboratory. I was introduced to making cap splints, as we still did in those days, arch bars, osteotomy planning, acrylic cranial implants, and also some simple facial prostheses. We also made some very simple intraoral splint devices, one piece obturators and things like jaw exercisers. Richard Lory was my vocational tutor, and I studied at the South London College part time to do the National Certificate of Maxillofacial Technology.

Mark became a full member of the Institute of Maxillofacial Technology in 1988.

I wanted to get to work in a bona fide maxillofacial unit, which the

London wasn't really to my mind. So when a job came up at St Thomas' Hospital working for Derek Henderson, I applied and was appointed. That was terrific because all they did was trauma and orthognathic surgery and I made lots of cap splints and arch bars, a few facial prostheses and some quite complex intraoral devices that Derek wanted.

Derek used cap splints for everything. I mean, he used them for fractures and orthognathic planning and we had the Levant face frames;[239] we used to make those up and arch bars. We made a lot of wrought arch bars using nickel silver half round wire and the odd intraoral appliance for people that had trauma, gunshot wounds, or industrial accidents. But the best thing about working at St Thomas' was that you were on call. They provided a maxillofacial trauma service, so one week in every two I was on call for 24 hours a day, seven days a week. And that got me into the pattern of working, which I still do now here at Queen Victoria Hospital. Of course, we don't make cap splints when we're called anymore; we make suck down splints and arch bars, and we still do the odd gunning splint.

My boss there was a chap called Jim Briggs. He was an ex-Royal Army Dental Corps mechanic, as was, and was just coming up to retirement. He'd become an oral surgery technician and then a few years before I went there, he went and did the maxillofacial course, joined the Institute and became a Maxillofacial Technician.

Derek Henderson and Jim would discuss orthognathic cases. Mr Henderson would come into the laboratory and they would sit and discuss them. Sometimes Jim and I used to go to the clinic and then we'd sit with the patient with Derek. Derek Henderson also used to take us junior staff into theatre and show what a bi-maxillary orthognathic procedure was all about. He used to get us to hold the clamps and see how difficult it is to free off the maxilla, and also Derek used to get his housemen to make a set of cap splints.

That was great because in the laboratory we could see how difficult their life was and the housemen would come into the laboratory and

---

239 The Levant frame was used to stabilise a fractured maxilla by attaching a silver cap splint to a plaster head cap or supra-orbital bone pins. See: Experience with the Levant frame for cranio-maxillary fixation. Levant BA, Cook RM, & Macfarlane WI. British Journal of Oral Surgery 1973. 11. 30-35.

see just see how long it took to make some of the things we had to make, and how involved the process was. We didn't just open a packet and pull them out.

How long did it take to make silver cap splints?

To start with, it took me about ten hours. But by the time I'd starting working here at Queen Victoria Hospital 15 years later, it took me about two; if I had all the furnace timings right and the materials at exactly the right temperature. The first thing you had to was get the impressions, pour them up and then section the model so the occlusion was spot on. Then you had to make the device in wax, then you had to invest and then cast that in silver and then trim the silver up and solder on any locking plates, etc.

Cap splints allowed people to have orthognathic surgery before modern orthodontics and allowed difficult trauma cases to be done before mini plates came in?

That's right, it was a closed reduction, wasn't it? With large and difficult fractures such as gunshot wounds where you had bits of the mandible missing, it was good to put an extension bar across and just glue on a couple of cap splints.

You mentioned that you used to make jaw exercisers. What was that about?

Well, back in the day a very simple jaw exerciser would be a trismus screw. It would be a plastic device with a thread on it that the patient wound between the teeth that literally prised their jaws apart. We still make those. And then later on we would make devices that would bolt onto the cap splints with a piece of elastic in between, just so they could get used to opening and closing their mouths. Almost like some sort of physiotherapy appliance. Of course these days you can buy them ready to go out of pack, but in those days it was high-tech stuff.

And what other devices you mentioned did he get you to make?

Well, we used to get patients who had lost teeth and significant amounts of alveolar bone and maybe sections of hard and soft palate. So we would make intraoral prostheses that were a bit weird. They'd be sectional devices, or they'd be obturators, to make good the damage that had been caused by an industrial injury, a road traffic accident or a gunshot wound.

Was there any skin grafting done in the mouth? Because at one point skin grafting was done in the mouth, wasn't it, and prostheses were made with gutta percha to hold them in?

Yes, the epithelial inlay trays. I made a few of those for Derek. He would make good the soft tissue damage. I remember making a few lower cap splints that would have a rod and tube on the front and a metal plate. Then we would use gutta percha, warm it up in hot water in theatre, prise it onto the plate and then prise it down into the defect, do the screws up and it would hold a gutta percha pack in position for a few days or weeks. That wasn't very often.

We didn't do cancer cases; they'd be all trauma of some description. I remember, for example, we had a chap once who fell off some scaffolding, and he landed face first on something quite sharp and awkward, and he'd literally given himself a hemimaxillectomy. He lost that part of his face and his eye, and I made a sectional obturator for him in hard acrylic.

Mark applied to work at Roehampton with Brian Conroy in 1989. Norman Rowe had recently retired.

I just trotted along to Roehampton one day to speak to Brian Conroy just out of casual interest, and he offered me a job on the spot. I think in those days there just weren't many of us around doing these sorts of things, so there were always plenty of jobs to be had.

The department was in temporary type buildings, single level, and the maxillofacial surgery clinics were at the front of Roehampton House and the laboratory was at the far side of the huts. We had our own prosthetics clinic, which was the first time I'd come across a designated maxillofacial prosthetics clinic.

We had four dental technicians, two doing denture prosthetics and two doing orthodontics. And we had five maxillofacial prosthetists who saw patients, went to theatre and worked in the laboratory. That was the first time that we made domiciliary visits; we used to pop out to patients in their homes and in the hospice. I used to go with Brian to Kingston somewhere. That was the first proper head and neck maxillofacial prosthetics unit I worked in.

The first thing that hit me at Roehampton was how much time we spent in the operating theatre. We were taking facial impressions, intraoral sectional impressions, and of head and neck resection cases. The thing I was particularly interested in was burns.

It was in the late '80s and the early '90s that I realised that the referrals to the maxillofacial laboratory were not just from maxillofacial surgeons. We had neurosurgeons, ENT surgeons, plastic surgeons, and general surgeons refer patients. Also, we made some little devices for anaesthetists. Some referrals came from GPs or general dental practices for various little bits and bobs. So it was then that I became aware that the maxillofacial laboratory was the place to go if you wanted something made.

I had to grow up a bit quickly at Roehampton and learn how to work in the operating theatre, as well as the clinic and the laboratory, helped by John Bowerman and Brian Conroy. We had a prosthetics clinic which was run by us maxillofacial prosthetists, and we were the clinicians, the technicians, the support staff, the laboratory aid and everything else.

Was there a problem with the General Dental Council with this about non-dentists taking impressions?

The simple fact was that a general dentist wouldn't want to do what we were doing. And if somebody has half their face missing and their insides are exposed to the rest of the world, what's an intraoral impression and what is just an impression?

A few years ago when statutory registration of dental technicians came in, I went to a meeting at the General Dental Council and we had a discussion around exactly what the maxillofacial prosthetists did. Well, we take intraoral impressions, but not really of teeth, of just the big holes where their jaws used to be. And sometimes those impressions involve the rest of the face because they have an oro-antral or oro-facial fistula that we need to record somehow and then make a device for. But there's been no real problem, not in my experience.

Brian Conroy had a terrific reputation within oral maxillofacial surgery for the work that he did, mostly in co-operation with Norman Rowe. What was the man himself like? What was he like to work with and for?

Brian was an enthusiast. Brian studied for his MPhil. and then PhD. at Surrey University. I remember Brian saying, 'I've been so lucky in my life because my job has been my hobby.' And it really was with Brian. He really ate, slept, dreamt, worked maxillofacial technology, he did nothing else. He didn't even get married until he was 40. I didn't think he knew what the fairer sex was until later on in life.

He was a Yorkshireman, and he didn't suffer fools, a Yorkshireman with a Scotsman's business acumen. He hated waste, and waste meant anybody sitting around doing nothing. Not that we have a chance at Roehampton. But if he saw something not being done properly or in the most efficient or effective way, he would let you know straightaway, so he was a difficult man to work with.

In physical appearance he was very short, just under five foot tall; he had a mop of bright white hair. When I met him he was in his late fifties and he was like a bulldog. He was a very squat, powerful little guy and his patients worshipped him. Before people like Brian came along, I'm not quite sure what happened to these patients, whether they were left in a side room to wither away or just stayed indoors for the rest of their lives. Brian had hundreds of patients that were seen at Roehampton and he'd given them new faces, new jaws, and in those days, skull plates even.

He reconstructed large sections of the skull for the neurosurgeons at Atkinson Morley[240] using the tantalum and titanium plates or polymer implants that we made in the laboratory. In those days we used to go along to Atkinson Morley and help the surgeons fit them, because we didn't have the 3D technology and the scanning technology we have now. The implants were very difficult to fit, mechanically and technically difficult, so we'd be there in theatre, bending the plates, drilling the bone, providing instruments for neurosurgeons to rebuild some of these quite large cranial reconstructions.

The guys at Atkinson Morley worshipped Brian, they thought he was the best thing since sliced bread. I remember the first day I went down to the burns unit to talk to the two plastic surgeons. I introduced myself, and suddenly, 'You must work with Brian Conroy then,' 'Err, yes, I do' and straightaway it was, 'What can we do for you?' They absolutely worshipped Brian Conroy; they thought he was terrific.

I met the Chief Executive of Roehampton Hospital a couple of times and I think before he used to make any big key decisions about staff, he would come and ask Brian first. That was the impression I got, anyway. He ruled the roost at Roehampton with a rod of iron. He was

---

240 Atkinson Morley was a specialist neurology and neurosurgery hospital in Wimbledon. It was closed and its services moved to St George's Hospital in 2003.

a difficult man; today it wouldn't be allowed, in these politically correct times, to say half the stuff he said to people, or treat them in the way he did; he fell out with a lot of people because, if he didn't perceive that you met his standards, he was your enemy for life. There was no grey area with Brian; you were his best friend or his mortal enemy. There was nothing in between. I became Brian's deputy and half of the time I was pouring oil on troubled waters.

Brian Conroy was the key player in the Institute of Maxillofacial Prosthetics and Technology; he started it. Just after WWII you had chaps working in the Emergency Medical Service hospitals such as Canniesburn,[241] Mount Vernon[242], Roehampton[243] and East Grinstead. After the war they came together to talk about oral surgery technology and Brian was quite young in those days, and he had the wherewithal to say, 'Well, let's make a list of all these chaps who are working in these oral surgery laboratories and we'll formalise this; we'll make a list and we'll start a contact database.'

Perhaps he wouldn't have used those words, but Brian Conroy was really the first one to get everyone together in the oral surgery laboratories. They all met for the first time together in 1957 in a pub in the Charing Cross Road. Jim Briggs, who I worked for at St Thomas' was one of the chaps who attended that first meeting. It was Brian Conroy, Alan Roberts, Professor Roberts and he's just retired as Vice Chancellor of Leeds University, Harry Lockwood from Mount Vernon, Walter Smith from Canniesburn, Stanley Brasier from Chepstow, Reg Eden from Charing Cross. There were about 12 or 13 and they came together from far and wide in the UK to form the Association of Maxillofacial Technicians.

Their first job was really to formalise the qualification because in those days there was no formal qualification. They approached City and Guilds, who were the craft examiners and said, 'Can we devise a qualification in maxillofacial technology and use you as the

---

241 The Canniesburn unit was descended from the Ballochmyle EMS hospital.

242 Mount Vernon wasn't an EMS hospital for plastics and jaw injuries during the war, that was at Hill End but the unit did move to Mount Vernon in 1953.

243 Roehampton was designated as an EMS hospital for facial injuries in WWII but it was quickly moved to Stoke Mandeville as it was considered too close to London and was at risk from bombing. The department Mark was in evolved from the EMS hospital at Rooksdown House, Park Prewitt, Basingstoke which moved to Roehampton in 1959.

examiners?' And City and Guilds said, 'Fine, we'll have you on board.' So, I think in 1956, that's when the City and Guilds course in maxillofacial technology started. Then coming forward in the history, in 1963 the first scientific congress was organised, here at the Queen Victoria Hospital, East Grinstead, organised by the Association of Maxillofacial Technicians. It was March 1963.

Brian was quite a political animal. He didn't want to be seen to be all things to all men, so he made Ralph Sharpe the Chairman and Terence Ward was the President; they asked an oral and maxillofacial surgeon to become our first President of the Association of Maxillofacial Technicians.

That first meeting and every two years since we have had the scientific congress. We have them all over the place now; we've been to Utrecht, France, Ireland and Scotland.

John Langdon became a consultant at Roehampton, where he worked with Brian Conroy as a colleague [1987-1993]. Later after retirement he was a friend.

Brian Conroy was an extraordinary guy. He had a wonderful mind, an excellent pair of hands, but not very good interpersonal skills. The technical laboratory at Roehampton was quite big, but it was always unhappy because of his interpersonal skills. However I always got on with him very well.

Brian would get frustrated with his colleagues if they couldn't see what he was getting at or couldn't achieve what he thought they should achieve or what he wanted to happen, whether they were surgical or technical colleagues. He would come to theatre and scrub up and take over if you weren't careful.

But he had a wonderful mind, was very inventive and technically very talented. We were quite close after he retired, living nearby we saw quite a lot of each other socially and, after Norman Rowe died, through the educational foundation we started. [244]

What was his legacy to technology or to the specialty overall?

I guess his major contribution was three dimensional planning. This was in the pre-computer days, when full faced models were made

---

244 See obituary by John Langdon: Brian Francis Conroy MBE M. Univ FIMPT LCGI 1932–2010 British Journal of Oral and Maxillofacial Surgery 2010 58 (5) 402-403.

out of radiographs and complicated jigs and things. He had these very complicated jigs that would hold the skull and orientate it in the appropriate plane, on which you could do your model surgery. And he did most of the model surgery. When I was at the London, Gordon Seward would carve up all his own models for orthognathic surgery. At Roehampton they were all carved up in the lab by Brian and presented to you as a fait accompli with precise measurements. 'You want three millimetres forwards and rotation upwards of twenty degrees' and all the rest. But I think he was the first person in the UK who came to grips with changes in all three dimensions.

He drove the Institute of Maxillofacial Technicians forwards; he professionalised it. I think prior to that it was largely a lot of dental technicians who ended up in hospitals doing oral surgery technical work.

I understand he was very much involved in making new instruments.

Yeah, Norman Rowe would come up with the concepts, such as his orbital retractors, maxillary disimpaction forceps, or his spreaders, and Brian would come up with a prototype in the lab.

Mark Cutler was at Roehampton for six years [1990-96].

After a couple of years Colin Haylock, who was Brian's deputy, left to work at another hospital and I applied for the Deputy Head of Department and I got the job. But that was as Brian was retiring, so as Brian came in later each day and did less operational stuff, so by the time I left Roehampton, I was kind of running the place really and Brian had almost retired. And as I left to come to East Grinstead, Brian retired from Roehampton and of course Roehampton closed.

Mark went to East Grinstead.

My official title in those days was Manager of the Maxillofacial Laboratory and Prosthetics Clinic.

I applied for the job in 1995 and I had to work out three months' notice at Roehampton. Brian was very upset; well, he didn't speak to me for a year after I left. I went from being his First Lieutenant to being his mortal enemy for a while. Obviously East Grinstead was the main competitor for Roehampton, and I agonised over applying for the job. I went and spoke to Colin Haylock who'd left Roehampton by then; he had been the lecturer on my maxillofacial course at South London. Colin said 'Oh don't worry about it, you have to cut your own path in life and not what other people want you to do.'

And what did you find?

A lot of the staff had been here for a long time and they were very good oral surgery mechanics, very good dental technicians. You could give them something to make and they would make it. But when I came here we weren't using modern up-to-date silicone materials for facial prostheses. We were still a bit stuck in the cap splint age; cranioplasty implants were still being made using acrylic, not titanium or any other material; they'd never heard of lasers or Labcam or anything like that. It was very much an oral surgery laboratory from the 1970s. I don't think any of the guys had ever done a paper, or had stood up and given a lecture at one of the Institute conferences.

By the 1980s the Association had become the Institute of Maxillofacial Prosthetics, rather than the Association of Maxillofacial Technicians. And that was to reflect the fact that a lot of the guys working then were being referred patients directly, were seeing patients, and were completely accountable and responsible for the patient care they were providing. They weren't subservient or responsible to any other clinician; they were their own men, and the Institute had to represent those people and the name change was just a consequence of that representation. That was 1988 and of course the Institute became a registered charity in 1995.

What have been the main changes in maxillofacial technology on the national scene throughout your career so far?

In the 1970s, the maxillofacial oral surgery technicians were just making cap splints and doing osteotomy planning, perhaps. Since then it has been moving more towards health care science and away from dentistry.

In the late '80s, early '90s, I did an audit of the 20 biggest maxillofacial laboratory services in the UK. It was quite a simple one, but the key thing we found was that most of our referrals didn't come from dentally qualified surgeons. Most of what we were now doing came from neuro, ENT, burns, plastics, GPs even. So what's happened nationally in the last 30 years is that the oral surgery technician has gone from making cap splints and arch bars, to making deep buried cranio-facial implants and facial prostheses, and oro-facial prostheses, using things like osseo-integrated implants as well.

We've come to a point now where I'll have a prosthetics clinic and

350

I'll ask one of the surgeons to come along to it, to see a patient. I'll ask them if they can put an osseo-integrated implant into there so we can put a facial prosthesis in, and they go, 'Yeah, sure, that's no problem.' They kind of go away now and they make a joke, 'Oh, I had to go across to Mark's clinic and see a patient for him.'

Nationally over the last 30 years it's become much more science based, it was a craft in the 1960s. A lot of the work I do now is planned using computers. We use computerised tomography and surface scanning to plan virtually all the cranio-facial implants, the deep buried ones, even the osseo-integrated implants, and mandibular tray implants. Now we have lasers; I have two lasers in the laboratory for welding materials like pure titanium. We have an inert gas environment casting machine for casting pure titanium which is a very difficult material to process. There are few places outside maxillofacial work that can do that.

What regulation and legislation has affected practice of maxillofacial technology?

The biggest thing that's hit us in the last 20 years is the Medical Devices Directive from Europe. In 1994 the European Community decided that those who placed medical devices on the market must be held accountable and responsible for their work and their practice. From 1996 anybody providing a patient with a medical device, in our case a custom made medical device, has had certain hoops to jump through. Now you have to use appropriately qualified staff, have an auditing process, a paper trail from where the silicone was dug out of the desert to where it was processed into polydimethylsiloxane, to being turned into a facial prosthesis or obturator. Also, the machinery that's being used in a laboratory and the appropriateness of the laboratory practice that you are carrying out.

I know Medical Devices Directive impacted on dental technology a bit, but the devices that are made in a dental laboratory are nowhere near as risky as the devices made by us. For example, you don't need to cut somebody's scalp open and screw it onto their skull. In the 1990s that really shook up maxillofacial laboratories significantly; some laboratories just couldn't maintain the standards that were required.

In recent years we've had the statutory regulation of dental professions, including dental technology. Some of us working in maxillofacial technology now have to register as dental technicians with the General Dental Council to make intraoral appliances, and that was another cost in time and money to comply with. Then in July 2008 the Department of Health stipulated by a directive that if you want to practise as a maxillofacial prosthetist, you have to be a full member of the Institute of Maxillofacial Prosthetics. That was quite easy because about 99 percent of us already were, so it wasn't a problem.

In effect, in the last 20 years we've had three significant pieces of legislation that have stopped corners being cut, helped quality to stay high and evidence good training for maxillofacial prosthetics for the next generation.

What about registration with the General Dental Council? Clearly you don't need registration with the General Dental Council to fit extraoral appliances?

No, you don't. At first, that piece of red tape confused and slightly annoyed me. But then to work in maxillofacial prosthetics you have to train first as a dental technician. You don't know how to use or process the materials in the right way unless you've had the experience in a dental laboratory to start with. And of course you need to know about occlusion, how to make an obturator, how to make a large oro-facial prosthesis with a face, a jaw and teeth replacing alveolus and hard palate. You can't do that if you don't even know how the teeth are supposed to come together, and of course you have to have some form of dental qualification to do that.

Appendix 1
The Interviewees

Professor Sir Paul Bramley Qualified 1944

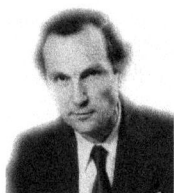

Paul Bramley was born in 1923 and trained in dentistry in Birmingham, qualifying in 1944. He started his career as Resident House Surgeon to the inspirational Harold Round (the first person in the UK to qualify as a dentist with a degree), at the Queen Elizabeth Hospital Birmingham for a year before being called up for War Service. Sir Paul spent two-and-a-half years mostly in the Middle East, during which time he qualified as a parachutist in Palestine and was blown up by Irgun Zvai Leumi, a terrorist group while he was Officer in Charge of a troop train.

Back in Birmingham, Sir Paul was flattered to be offered a position in Harold Round's dental practice but declined as he wanted to do medical training, which he started in Birmingham in 1948, qualifying in 1952. He then spent a year as a volunteer medical officer in a Church of Scotland Mission Hospital in Kenya where he practised mostly general surgery and tropical medicine.

On return to England he worked part time in the Schools Dental Service and Maternity and Child Welfare Services while waiting for a suitable career post to materialise, which it did in the form of a registrar job at Rooksdown House in Basingstoke, where he worked for Norman Rowe and Homer Killey, who at the time was operating with Sir Harold Gillies.

After two years, Sir Paul unsuccessfully applied for a senior registrar job between The Westminster and St Thomas' Hospital. When the job was later offered to him he turned it down as by then he had accepted a Consultant appointment with the South Western Regional Hospital Board based at Plymouth. He started in 1954 and continued until 1969 when he accepted the post of Professor of Dental Surgery at the University of Sheffield, where he remained until 1988. For three years, he was Dean of the dental school.

Sir Paul has held many professional positions within academia and dentistry, including being a member of the General Dental Council, Chairman of Dental Protection and Dean of the Faculty of Dental Surgery of the Royal College of Surgeons of England. He was a former president of the Oral Surgery Club of Great Britain and British Association of Oral Surgeons. He was a Royal College of Surgeons Faculty of Dental Surgery Colyer Gold Medal winner and was knighted in 1984.

I interviewed Sir Paul at his home in Hathersage over two days in September 2014. He died in 2020.

Gordon Fordyce Qualified 1946

Gordon Fordyce was born in 1925. He started his undergraduate training at the dental school in Dundee, which was part of St Andrew's University, at 16 and qualified four years later in 1946.

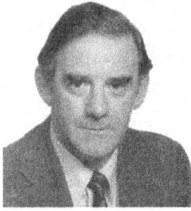

After qualification, he worked for a few months in general dental practice before being called up into the Army for National Service. He provided dental treatment for Army recruits at Chester and Carlisle before being posted to Klagenfurt in Austria, where he worked initially as a dental officer and later as a senior dental officer. Here he had his first experience in the management of jaw injuries.

After National Service he returned to Dundee where he took advice from a professor of anatomy who told him that the newly introduced Fellowship in Dental Surgery of the Royal College of Surgeons of Edinburgh would be the route to an appointment as a consultant dental surgeon in the new National Health Service.

In 1949 Gordon became a demonstrator in anatomy at Dundee while he studied for the primary Fellowship examination. Later that year, at 24, he was appointed as a registrar to the Jaw Injuries Unit at Hill End Hospital near St Albans in Hertfordshire.

Gordon was soon promoted to senior registrar and still held this position when the unit moved to Mount Vernon Hospital in Northwood in 1953. When he finished his training time he was promoted to senior hospital dental officer at Mount Vernon before being appointed a consultant dental surgeon for two sessions (half days) per week at the Royal Free Hospital and subsequently part-time consultant at St Albans and Mount Vernon. Gordon retired from clinical practice in 1988.

Gordon became an elected member of the General Dental Council but his biggest achievement was as Post Graduate Dental Dean of the British Postgraduate Medical Federation, where he was responsible for introducing vocational training for dentists in the National Health Service, which was started in 1988.

Gordon was awarded the Tomes Medal, the Queen's Silver Jubilee Medal in 1977, and was appointed an Officer of the Order of the British Empire in 1988. He is a past President of the British Association of Oral Surgeons.

I interviewed Gordon at his home in Hampshire in April 2012. He died in 2018.

Michael Awty   Qualified 1953

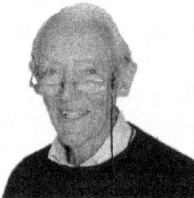

Michael Awty was born in 1930 and went to Guy's Hospital to study dentistry in 1948. He opted to go early to the 'Pre-Med' year for sciences in order to ensure he started his undergraduate training before he was called up for National Service. Mike graduated in 1953 and, after a house job at Guy's, went to East Grinstead for a second job working for Sir Terence Ward in what became a long relationship. During this second job he was called up for National Service, and Sir Terence, who was a Consultant to the Royal Air Force, could use his influence to secure Mike a place in the RAF and an overseas posting to his liking.

After basic RAF training Mike was posted to Kuala Lumpur where he provided dental treatment to all three services at base for two years, and where, in his free time, he could join helicopters supplying SAS patrols fighting communist terrorists in the jungle.

Mike started the medical course at Guy's in 1956, qualifying in 1961. After Medicine and house jobs in Lewisham and the Metropolitan ENT Hospital in Kensington, he went to the Eastman Dental Hospital in 1963, and spent a few months in periodontology before being appointed as a registrar in oral surgery. There he worked with Professor Homer Killey, Norman Rowe and Professor Robert Bradlaw and passed his Fellowship. He then moved back to East Grinstead as senior registrar and was appointed there as a consultant in 1965.

In 1968 on information from Sir Terence the Government seconded Mike to Kaduna in Northern Nigeria to set up a maxillofacial surgery service in conjunction with the Nigerian Army, to cope with a large build-up of maxillofacial injuries from the ongoing civil war. This gave a unique exposure to major facial injuries, mostly gunshot wounds, later providing excellent experience to senior registrars, who followed on for six-month secondments for many years.

Mike retired from National Health Service practice in 1992 and private practice in 2000. He is a past Treasurer and President of the British Association of Oral Surgeons. I interviewed him at his home near East Grinstead in 2014.

Laurence Oldham Qualified 1955

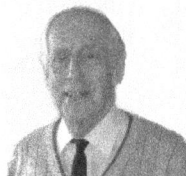

Laurence Oldham was born in 1931 and entered Dental School in Birmingham in 1950, qualifying in 1955. He took up a non-resident house job at the Birmingham Dental Hospital involving being on call at the General Hospital for three evenings a week and alternate week ends resident. After six months Laurence became the resident house surgeon at the General Hospital which provided his first real exposure to surgery.

After two years of house jobs, Laurence was called to his National Service in the RAF. After four weeks initial training at RAF Halton near Aylesbury which was the headquarters of the RAF Medical and Dental Branches, he was posted to the Air Ministry Dental Centre in London which was at 114 Harley Street, London where he provided general dental services to RAF personal. Later he was posted to Oakington near Cambridge and later was back in London to complete his two years of National Service.

After National Service he spent four months in National Health Service dental practice in Wimpole Street, which confirmed to him that he wanted to pursue a career in surgery. After attending the primary fellowship course at the Royal College of Surgeons and spending several months as a locum registrar, firstly at the Royal Dental Hospital and later back in Birmingham, he set off to the United States on a Rotary Foundation Scholarship to Philadelphia where he attended a preparatory course for oral surgery residents at the University of Pennsylvania.

On returning to the United Kingdom in 1960 Laurence became an assistant lecturer in the oral surgery department of the Manchester dental school, which lasted for five years until he became bored. In 1965 he went to Uganda to the New Mulago Hospital at Makerere University. Here he was to be fired with enthusiasm from his general surgery colleagues and gained experience which was lacking from his dental hospital time.

In 1968 Laurence returned to the oral surgery department at Manchester and later that year took a consultant post in Taunton until he retired in 1991.

Laurence was a member of the council of the British Association of Oral Surgeons.

Laurence's Memoir, One Man's Foray into Oral and Maxillofacial Surgery, was published in 2012

I interviewed Laurence at his home in Taunton in July 2012. He died in 2019.

Russell Hopkins Qualified 1956

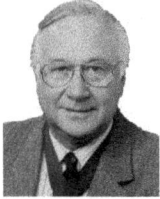

Russell Hopkins was born in 1932. Russell wanted to become a doctor but failed one part of his Higher School Certificate examinations. A year later he was one of the first to take the new 'A level' examinations and applied to do dentistry as well as medicine. He was offered a place in both courses and took the first offer he received and started the dental course in Newcastle in 1951, qualifying in 1956.

After working in Hartlepool and Cambridge in dental practice, Russell moved to Rhodesia, where he worked in Salisbury for a year. Bored with two years in dental practice Russell applied for a hospital post back in the UK in 1958.

In Nottingham, as a resident senior house officer, Russell was inspired into a hospital career by consultant Tom Battersby and decided this was the way of life for him. He went on the Primary FDS course at the Royal College of Surgeons and then became registrar at Chertsey, which was a satellite of the department at Roehampton. The consultant was Norman Rowe.

Russell entered the Royal Free Medical School in 1961 and qualified in 1964; he worked as a house physician in Croydon and a house surgeon in Wandsworth before working a for a while as a ship's surgeon, a role to which he was to return to several times during his career.

In 1966 Russell became a senior registrar in Newcastle attracted, by the prospect of working for Professor Geoffrey Howe, the first oral surgery professor in the country. After finding that much of the maxillofacial surgery was being done by the plastic surgeons and realised the limited surgical horizon of his chief, Russell decided to waste no more time and applied for and was appointed as a consultant at the new University Hospital of Wales in 1968. In 1985 he became General Manager of the University Hospital of Wales for six years while retaining one day a week of clinical work.

After six years of being General Manager, Russell declined to apply for the new post of Chief Executive and spent two years in charge of medical audit for Glamorgan, which he describes as the most unrewarding years of his career.

Russell retired at 63 but within weeks has was asked to apply for, and was accepted, as Chairman of the Glan-y-Môr and subsequently Bro Morgannwg NHS Trusts, roles he carried out until he was 73.

Russell was a President of the British Association of Oral and Maxillofacial Surgeons and was appointed an Officer of the Order of the British Empire for his service to medicine. His memoir 'A Journey Through a Life' was published in 2014.

I interviewed Russell at his home near Newport in West Wales in August 2012. He died in 2020.

Khursheed Moos Qualified 1957

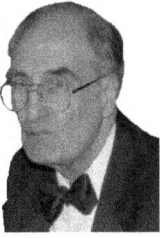

Khursheed Moos was born in 1934 and entered dental training at Guy's Hospital in 1953. After qualifying in 1957, he was appointed as house surgeon at the Royal Sussex County Hospital in Brighton for 9 months before starting medical training at University College Hospital. In 1959, after his 2nd MB exams, he was called up for National Service, and after basic training at Aldershot he was stationed at the Royal Herbert Hospital in Woolwich.

After National Service, Khursheed restarted his medical training, now at the Westminster Hospital Medical School. When he qualified in 1964, he became house surgeon to Professor Harold Ellis, which was followed by a house physician post in Warwick.

In 1966 he became registrar in dental and oral surgery at Mount Vernon where he worked under Gordon Fordyce, Paul Toller and Ben Fickling. He became senior registrar at Cardiff and was in this post when Russell Hopkins came as the consultant.

Khursheed was appointed as a consultant in Coventry in 1969 but moved to Canniesburn Hospital Glasgow in 1974, where he undertook a major clinical role in cranio-facial deformity and trauma. Khursheed has trained generations of oral and maxillofacial surgeons in the unit at Canniesburn, not only from the UK but many visiting from overseas. He has researched, taught, lectured and written widely about his subject.

After retiring from clinical practice in 1999, he has taken an honorary academic position at the Glasgow dental school as well as lecturing and teaching abroad.

Khursheed Moos is a past president of the Oral Surgery Club of Great Britain and the British Association of Oral & Maxillofacial Surgeons. He is a Frank Colyer Prize winner and is an Officer of the Order of the British Empire. I interviewed him at his home in Helensburgh, Dunbartonshire in 2013.

John Bradley Qualified 1958

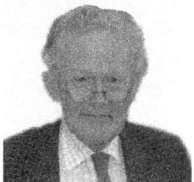

John Bradley was born in 1935 and went to Guy's dental school in 1954. Qualifying in 1958, John was rejected for National Service on health grounds and applied for hospital posts to have two years of hospital experience before a career in general practice. Having failed to secure a house job at Guy's, John was appointed house surgeon at St Thomas' Hospital. Here he worked for John Hovell, who fired his enthusiasm for surgery.

John then spent three months in general dental practice before starting work at the Westminster Hospital as a senior house officer in 1959. Here he worked for Rupert Sutton Taylor for one year before going to Salisbury for a year as a registrar. In 1962 he returned to the Westminster as a registrar which had now combined with Roehampton Hospital so he could work for Norman Rowe. John moved seamlessly to become the last singly qualified senior registrar at the Roehampton/Westminster unit in 1964 before becoming a consultant in Burnley and Bury in 1968.

As a consultant in Lancashire, John expanded the remit of the specialty locally and was instrumental in the merger of the Lancashire units to form a cohesive department known as The Four Bs (Blackburn, Bolton, Bury and Burnley).

At the end of his clinical career John became Chairman of the Bury NHS Trust. He was an editor of the British Journal of Oral and Maxillofacial Surgery and a past President of the Oral Surgery Club of Great Britain.

John was interviewed at my home in Lincoln in December 2011. His memoir Hot Spots and Hot Seats was published in 2012.

Michael Bromige Qualified 1958

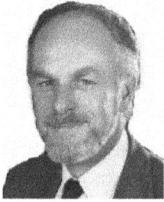

Michael Bromige was born in 1935. He started at the Birmingham dental school in 1954. After qualification in 1958, he took a house surgeon post at Selly Oak Hospital, which after six months converted to a senior house officer at slightly higher pay. After this year he worked for three months in the school dental service and then nine months in general dental practice which confirmed that this was not the career he wanted.

During a locum registrar post at the Birmingham dental hospital he was persuaded that a career in surgery would be more suitable for him than orthodontics. He became a registrar for about four years at the General Hospital. After passing his Fellowship examinations he became a senior registrar in 1964 at the Queen Elizabeth Hospital Birmingham and the Plastic and Jaw Injury Unit at Wordsley Hospital Stourbridge with trauma duties at the Birmingham Accident Hospital.

In 1968 Mike had a choice of consultant jobs to apply for and he was appointed to a part-time job at Nottingham with duties at Mansfield, where he remained until retirement in 1996.

Mike has had many management roles within the hospital service and is a past secretary of the British Association of Oral Surgeons. I interviewed him at his home in Lincolnshire in 2013.

John Williams Qualified 1961

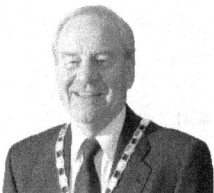

John Williams was born in 1938 and entered Guy's Hospital dental school in 1956, qualifying in 1961. He spent six months as a house surgeon at Guy's before becoming senior house officer to Paul Bramley in Plymouth for just over a year. There his leaning towards surgery as a career was confirmed, so he returned to Guy's to study medicine in 1962.

After qualifying in medicine in 1967 he worked at Guy's as a house surgeon in ENT and after his six months as a house physician he returned to Plymouth as a senior house officer in casualty and subsequently orthopaedics. In 1969 he spent some time as a registrar in general surgery before becoming the registrar in oral surgery there.

John, following advice given by Paul Bramley, had spent some time as an honorary registrar at Roehampton while a medical student. Thus in 1969 he returned to Roehampton as registrar after his time as a registrar in Plymouth and worked for Norman Rowe, John Bowerman and Ian Heslop. The following year he was appointed to senior registrar there, which involved duties at both Roehampton and the Westminster Hospital.

John Williams has held many offices within oral and maxillofacial surgery and the professions of medicine and dentistry. Among the posts he has held are President of the British Association of Oral and Maxillofacial Surgeons, the European Association and was the only UK surgeon to also have been President of the International Association of Oral and Maxillofacial Surgeons. He was Dean of the Faculty of Dental Surgery of the Royal College of Surgeons of England and Senior Vice President of the College, Editor of the British Journal of Oral and Maxillofacial Surgery and Chairman of the Confidential Enquiry into Post-operative Deaths. He established the Committee on Safety of Devices for the Medicine and Healthcare Products Regulatory Agency and subsequently became a Director.

He was awarded the Down Surgical prize by the British Association of Oral and Maxillofacial Surgeons for his outstanding contribution to the development of the specialty. He was awarded the John Tomes Medal of the British Dental Association and the Colyer Gold Medal of the Faculty of Dental Surgery of the Royal College of Surgeons of England. He has been appointed as a Commander of the Most Excellent Order of the British Empire.

I interviewed John Williams at his home near Chichester in November 2014.

John Langdon Qualified 1964

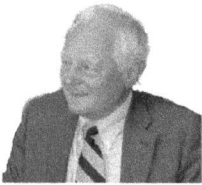

John Langdon's career evolved from failure in four of his GCE O level examinations (he was dyslexic) to becoming one of a handful of academics who made a significant impact on the practice of cancer surgery within the discipline of oral and maxillofacial surgery.

After retaking O levels John studied science subjects in senior school, which his headmaster considered the appropriate direction for his less able pupils, and started dentistry in 1960 at the London Hospital Dental School. John enjoyed clinical dentistry and won four prizes for his performance. He qualified in December 1964.

After dental house jobs at the London and a senior house officer job at St George's and the Royal Dental Hospital, he sought career advice from Sir Robert Bradlaw, the Dean at the Eastman Dental Hospital. Sir Robert appointed him on the spot to work under Professor Homer Killey, Lester Kay and Norman Rowe. A registrar job followed back at the London and its satellite department in Honey Lane Hospital, Waltham Abbey.

After medical studies at the London he eschewed the teaching hospital for house jobs at Harold Wood Hospital where he gained general surgery experience which would be the envy of a present day specialist registrar.

Immediately after his house jobs John became a senior registrar at the London where he observed the meticulous cancer and salivary gland surgery of Professor Gordon Seward.

After two years he resigned from the London as it was becoming increasingly unpleasant for him because of homophobia. However, he was quickly appointed to a senior registrar post at King's College Hospital and a few months after that as a consultant at

Roehampton and Ashford Hospitals. Both applications and appointments were encouraged, and in some part facilitated, by the kindly Malcolm Harris, who was a senior lecturer at King's at that time.

At Roehampton John became a colleague of the inspirational Norman Rowe who encouraged him in expanding their remit to include cancer surgery which had hitherto been exported to other specialties. This development was made against considerable opposition.

After six years at Roehampton, John became senior lecturer and subsequently professor of oral and maxillofacial surgery at King's College London and combined a head and neck cancer surgery practice with undergraduate and postgraduate teaching.

John Langdon wrote many journal articles, especially on cancer, and many chapters and books, several of which became standard texts for oral and maxillofacial surgery. He took on many roles in external bodies and health working parties, always promoting the contribution that oral and maxillofacial surgeons could offer.

John was awarded the Down Surgical Prize by the British Association of Oral and Maxillofacial Surgeons for his outstanding contribution to the development of the specialty. He was awarded the Sir Stanford Cade Memorial Medal and lecture. He was the first maxillofacial surgeon to be elected President of the British Association of Head and Neck Oncologists and is a former President of the Institute of Maxillofacial Prosthetists and Technologists, the Section of Odontology at the Royal Society of Medicine and the British Association of Oral and Maxillofacial Surgeons He was elected a fellow of the Royal Academy of Medical Sciences in 1998 and a Fellow of King's College London in 2002.

John told me the inspirational story of his career in oral and maxillofacial surgery at his home in Somerset in September 2020.

Andrew Brown Qualified 1968

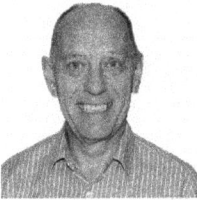

Andrew Brown went up to Guy's Hospital dental school in 1963 and qualified with LDS in 1968 and BDS in 1969. After qualification he became the resident house surgeon at Guy's. By this time Andy had realised that the top people in the dental profession, i.e. the consultant dental surgeons, at least at Guy's, were both medically and dentally qualified. He applied to Guy's medical school and after a few months break following his house job; he started the medical course, qualifying in 1973.

After medical school Andy was inspired by the cancer surgery of Omar Shaheen, the ENT Surgeon whose house surgeon he became at Guy's; afterwards he was a house physician at Greenwich Hospital.

Uncertain of the future direction of his career, he was advised at Guy's to get the advice of Professor Killey at the Eastman Dental Hospital. When Andy went to see Professor Killey, he offered him a job as registrar at the Eastman where he remained for just under two years before following a previously trodden path to senior registrar at East Grinstead which he started in 1976.

He was appointed as a consultant at East Grinstead in 1981 where he started a head and neck oncology practice and subsequently taught many trainees, wrote and lectured on his main subject.

Andy is a former President and Chairman of Council of the British Association of Oral and Maxillofacial Surgeons and a recipient of the Down Surgical Prize for his outstanding contribution to the development of the specialty. .

I interviewed Andy at his home in East Grinstead in December 2012

John Cawood Qualified 1969

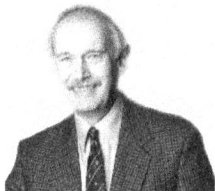

At school John Cawood applied for dental school because his friend Graham Wood (who also became an oral and maxillofacial surgeon) had decided to. He studied in Dundee, where the University of St Andrews students were located, and qualified in 1969.

At dental school he was alerted to the opportunity for interesting clinical work in oral and maxillofacial surgery when some dental school staff were involved in a road accident and suffered facial injuries. They were treated by Derek Henderson, who had lectured to the students about his specialty.

After graduation John went into a general dental practice in Glasgow which failed to inspire him, so he became a senior house officer in oral and maxillofacial surgery in Southend.

A registrar job in Edinburgh followed, where he worked under the inspirational William MacLennan, and the major clinical work was facial injuries. A senior registrar job in Liverpool followed, at the end of which he went, as part of a recognised exchange programme, to Miami.

But he was at the end of his training time, and there was a glut of senior registrars applying for very few consultant jobs, so he took time out to go to Seattle as a resident. In Seattle the main clinical interest was facial deformity and the resident job he took was more of a structured training post rather than a service job in the manner of an apprenticeship in the UK. John then went for a short period to Arnhem where he was inspired by their clinical work in pre-prosthetic surgery.

John was appointed as a consultant in Chester in 1983. He developed a special interest in rehabilitation after cancer surgery as part of the emerging Liverpool consortium. He has lectured, written and published widely, particularly in his special interests of implantology, pre-prosthetic surgery, rehabilitation and osteosynthesis of facial fractures. He has also been an editor of the International Journal of Oral and Maxillofacial Surgery and has contributed to national and international committees.

John was the King James IVth Professor awarded by the Royal College of Surgeons of Edinburgh, he won the British Association of Oral and Maxillofacial Surgeons Presidents Prize and was a founding member of the Strasbourg Osteosynthesis Research Group.

I interviewed John in November 2020 during the Covid pandemic via Zoom.

David Vaughan Qualified 1969

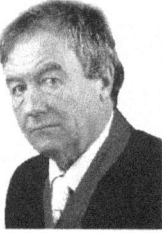

David Vaughan was born in 1944 and went to Dental School in Cork in 1962, qualifying in 1969. He worked in dental practice for a few months before deciding he didn't like it and then entered the medical school in Cork qualifying in 1974.

After house jobs at St Finbarr's Hospital Cork and the university teaching hospital, he undertook four years of general surgery training there with a view to becoming a head and neck oncology surgeon. This was followed by six months of plastic surgery, which failed to impress him.

David had spent some time in London doing locum work when he was a medical student so he then migrated to the Royal Marsden Hospital in London where he worked as a senior house officer/registrar before becoming a registrar at the Eastman Dental Hospital in 1979 where he remained for five months. David gained a senior registrar post at East Grinstead where his senior registrar colleague was Andy Brown, who helped him with his first encounters with orthognathic and trauma surgery. At King's College Hospital, he was helped by Professor Sowray, who gave him full support in expanding the surgical repertoire.

In 1982 David was appointed as consultant oral surgeon in Liverpool, initially based at Walton Hospital. There he established a head and neck oncology practice, which he subsequently expanded to include all the oral units in Liverpool except for one. By his efforts, this became the major head and neck cancer treatment and training unit in the United Kingdom.

David Vaughan was awarded the Down Surgical Prize by the British Association of Oral and Maxillofacial Surgeons for his outstanding contribution to the development of the specialty. He is a past president of the British Association of Oral and Maxillofacial Surgeons and the British Association of Head and Neck Oncologists. I interviewed him at his home near Liverpool in January 2014.

Adrian Sugar Qualified 1970.

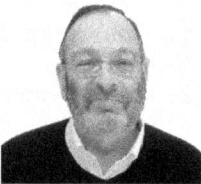

Adrian decided he wanted to pursue either medicine or dentistry at an early age and applied for both medical and dental school. However, he was put off medicine at an interview and chose dentistry. He went to the Leeds dental school, where he developed a keen interest in politics and graduated in 1970. He spent a year there as a dental house officer and then six months in general dental practice.

After six months he went to Teesside as a registrar in oral surgery. As a registrar he became heavily involved in a large workload of facial trauma. He stayed for four years but was yet to be inspired into a career in oral and maxillofacial surgery. He had never been to a national meeting or met anyone who was dually qualified and was considering giving up dentistry.

Adrian worked for another six months in dental practice, before returning to Leeds for another registrar job in oral surgery. Here he was inspired to continue in the specialty, partly by being involved with the neurosurgeons and the cranio-facial trauma. However, he felt that he needed to leave Leeds to gain adequate surgical experience so he declined to apply for a senior registrar job there and was appointed in South Wales.

Adrian started his senior registrar rotation between Cardiff and Chepstow in 1979. He was appointed as a consultant at Chepstow in 1985. As a consultant, Adrian gradually built up a practice in cleft and cranio-facial deformity while modernising the management of the routine oral surgery, moving it to local anaesthetic outpatient surgery.

In 1994, the Chepstow unit moved to Morriston Hospital in Swansea. There, with colleagues, he built up a department of eight oral and maxillofacial surgeons together with maxillofacial prosthetists, orthodontists, and restorative dentists. He continued to work on cleft and cranio-facial deformity and was clinical director of the Welsh cleft lip and palate service. Adrian has taught and lectured widely on this special interest in the UK and abroad.

He retired from full time clinical practice in 2019.

Adrian has held many administrative positions, particularly related to his clinical special interests such as President of the Cranio-facial Society of Great Britain and Ireland, Chair of the National Health Service Cleft Development Group and the British Facial and Audiological Implant Group. He had won several prizes for his work including the British Association of Oral and Maxillofacial Surgeons President's Prize and the Down Surgical Prize for his outstanding contribution to the development of the specialty.

I interviewed Adrian at his home in Caswell near Swansea in 2019.

Brian Avery   Qualified 1971

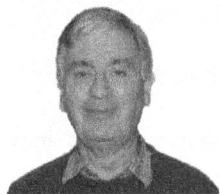

Brian Avery was born in 1947. He was accepted by four dental schools and accepted a place at Guy's which he started in 1965. After his second BDS examinations, he took a year out of dental training to do the second MB exams. He qualified in dentistry in 1971 and, after a six-month house job at Guy's and a short break, he started his medical clinical training in 1971, qualifying in 1974.

Brian spent six months as ENT house surgeon at Guy's which gave him his first exposure to head and neck oncology which was to dominate his clinical work later in his career. A house physician job at New Cross Hospital followed.

In 1975 Brian spent a year as registrar at the Eastman Dental Hospital before moving to the Westminster and Roehampton unit where he worked for John Bowerman and Norman Rowe. Brian did his senior registrar training at the Plastic and Jaw Injuries unit at Canniesburn Hospital Glasgow with Khursheed Moos and Amir El-Attar which lasted four and a half years.

Brian was a Consultant in Middlesbrough in 1983 where he practised for 26 years. There he developed cranio-facial surgery with one of the neurosurgeons but his main clinical interest became head and neck oncology.

Brian won the British Association of Oral and Maxillofacial Surgeons Surgical Prize, the Down Surgical Prize for his outstanding contribution to the development of the specialty and the Colyer Gold Medal. He was a member of the council of the Royal College of Surgeons of England and spent three years as Dean of the Faculty of Dental Surgery of the Royal College of Surgeons of England and during this time a year as President of the British Association of Oral and Maxillofacial Surgeons. I interviewed him at his home in Mordon, County Durham in 2013.

Richard Thornton Qualified 1971

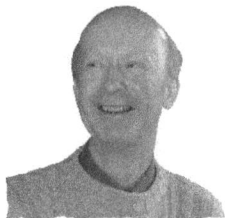

Richard Thornton was born 1946 and went to St. Thomas' Hospital medical school in 1965, qualifying in 1971. After surgical and medical house jobs at Portsmouth and Carshalton he started training in anaesthesia at the Westminster and Roehampton hospitals, where he gave anaesthetics for Norman Rowe's cases and went to the London Hospital to learn the art of outpatient dental general anaesthesia.

He was a registrar in anaesthetics at Southampton and subsequently senior registrar at University College and Great Ormond Street Hospitals and the National Hospital for Neurology and Neurosurgery, Queens Square.

In 1979 Richard became a consultant anaesthetist in Lincoln retiring in 2011. In Lincoln Richard's main interest was anaesthesia for oral and maxillofacial surgery, particularly head and neck cancer and dental anaesthesia. He became a supervisor for the dental non-consultant anaesthetists before dental anaesthesia outside of hospitals was effectively banned by the General Dental Council. For many years he taught on our Dentist on the Ward courses in Lincoln. As a friend and former colleague with whom I had worked closely, he was the natural choice to interview on the changes in anaesthesia for oral and maxillofacial surgery. I interviewed him in my home in Lincoln in 2012.

Tony Markus Qualified 1972

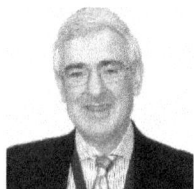

Tony Markus went to Newcastle dental school in 1968 and qualified in 1972. After a six months resident house job at the Newcastle Royal Infirmary, he did some locum work in general dental practice before going to Barts Hospital as senior house officer for a year in 1974. He then worked part time in dental practice and, after going on the Primary FDS course at the Royal College of Surgeons, he became a registrar in oral surgery at Guy's Hospital in 1975.

After a couple of years at Guy's, Tony was appointed as senior registrar by North West Thames Health Authority and started at University College and Great Ormond Street hospitals in 1977 before rotating to Mount Vernon Hospital. Later Tony had the opportunity to work at St George's Hospital.

Tony was appointed as a consultant at Poole in 1985, where he set up a multi-disciplinary team for the management of cleft lip and palate as his main surgical interest.

Tony has participated in the politics of the management of clefts and has written and taught widely on the subject. He is a former council member of the British Association of Oral and Maxillofacial Surgeons and President of the Oral Surgery Club of Great Britain. He has been awarded an FRCS 'ad eundem' and in 1993 he was awarded the

DePuy Surgical Prize by the British Association of Oral and Maxillofacial Surgeons for his outstanding contribution to the development of the specialty. I interviewed him at his home in Dorset in 2012.

Robert Hensher Qualified 1972

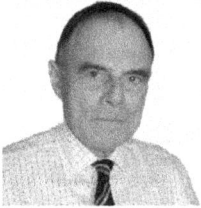

Rob Hensher went to dental school in Liverpool in 1968, qualifying in 1972. He made an early decision to make his career in music after dental school. However after his exposure to medicine as a dental undergraduate he decided upon oral and maxillofacial surgery. After just six months as a dental house officer, he entered medical school in Liverpool after which he did pre-registration house jobs in medicine and surgery followed by a surgical rotation in Liverpool.

In 1980 he moved to London and spent six months as an oral and maxillofacial senior house officer at Whipps Cross in Leytonstone before moving to the Westminster Hospital as a registrar later the same year. He also worked at Roehampton and then had the opportunity to go to New Orleans where he worked with Jack Kent, who fired his enthusiasm for temporomandibular joint disease and joint replacement.

On returning home he was immediately appointed as a senior registrar rotating between the Westminster Hospital, Roehampton, University College Hospital and Great Ormond Street Hospital. The rotation also included a year at Munster in West Germany.

In 1986 he was appointed as a consultant at Cheltenham and Gloucester where he developed a temporomandibular joint replacement practice. He regenerated prosthetic temporo-mandibular joint replacement in 1986, helping in the development of and introducing the Concepts bespoke prosthesis to The UK and Europe. Currently regarded as the gold standard.

In 2000 he moved to London to engage in full-time private practice. I interviewed Rob at my home in London in 2019.

Michael Davidson Qualified 1976.

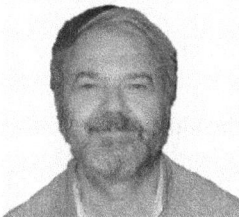

Mike Davidson was born in 1952. He went to the London Hospital dental school where he was stimulated by inspirational teachers in oral medicine, public health, one in particular in oral surgery, and academically gifted fellow students. He graduated in 1976, unsure of which aspect of dentistry he wanted to pursue, but spent six months as a resident house officer in oral surgery at the London.

After the Primary FDS course at the Royal College of Surgeons of England he became a resident senior house officer in oral surgery at the Royal Sussex County Hospital in Brighton, during his time there he decided that this was the career for him. After a short period in general dental practice he returned to the London for medical training, graduating in 1984, returning to Brighton for medical and surgical house jobs.

He gained further surgical experience as a senior house officer in Chichester in accident and emergency medicine and orthopaedics before becoming a registrar in oral and maxillofacial surgery there from 1986 to 1988. His time in Chichester was his most rewarding training experience in surgery in general as well as oral and maxillofacial surgery. After followed a senior registrar job in Leeds, after which he was appointed as a consultant in oral and maxillofacial surgery in Taunton from 1991.

Mike has been heavily involved in local and national medical politics with the British Medical Association, Royal College of Surgeons of England and British Association of Oral and Maxillofacial Surgeons, where he has served as a council member and Chairman of Council. I interviewed Mike at his home near Taunton in 2019.

Ian Martin Qualified 1979.

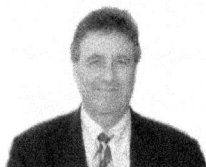

Ian Martin decided on dentistry as a career after he had visited the Manchester dental school on a school's open day. He was also swayed by seeing that the local doctor lived in a semi-detached house and had a Rover car while the dentist lived in a mansion and had a Mercedes.

Ian went to King's College London to study dentistry, where he enjoyed the congenial atmosphere and the work. He was also inspired by the oral surgery teaching; he was allowed to surgically remove a wisdom tooth right at the start of his clinical course. He won the Wallis prize and the British Dental Association-Dentsply national prize for a research project he did on halothane contamination of operating theatre air. He had decided upon a career in oral surgery by the time he qualified.

Qualifying from King's in 1979, he was appointed as a house surgeon in the dental hospital, rotating through three departments for a year. He was then appointed as a senior house officer in oral surgery. He started medical training there in 1982.

On qualifying in medicine in 1986 he did his medical and surgical house jobs at King's before going to Plymouth for two years for a rotating surgical senior house officer jobs in orthopaedics, plastic surgery and general surgery.

After his surgical experience, Ian became one of the few in oral and maxillofacial surgery to get a general FRCS before taking the Edinburgh oral and maxillofacial FRCS. In 1989 Ian was appointed as a registrar in oral and maxillofacial surgery on Merseyside before becoming a senior registrar at East Grinstead and consultant in Sunderland in 1993. His main clinical interest has been in head and neck cancer and reconstruction.

Ian has held several administrative and political positions within oral and maxillofacial surgery and medicine in general. He has been President and Chairman of Council of the British Association of Oral and Maxillofacial Surgeons, President of the British Association of Head and Neck Oncologists and the European Association for Cranio-Maxillofacial Surgery. He has been chair of the trustees and steering group for the National Confidential Enquiry into Patient Outcome and Death. He was awarded the Down Surgical Prize by the British Association of Oral and Maxillofacial surgeons for his outstanding contribution to the development of the specialty.

I interviewed Ian at his home in London in 2019.

Mark Cutler Qualified 1984

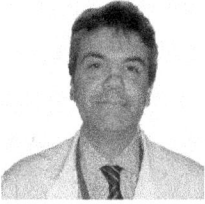

Mark entered training at the Brooklands College in 1980 to study for the National Diploma in Dental Technology, which he obtained in 1988. His course involved three years at the college with a further year of vocational training, which he undertook in the prosthetic laboratory at Guy's Hospital, before gaining accreditation with the then, Dental Technician Advisory Board.

After accreditation, Mark remained at Guy's while he prepared for the Advanced Prosthetics Certificate at the South London College from 1984 to 1986. He then worked in the laboratory at the Royal London while he studied at the South London College for the National Certificate in Maxillofacial technology from 1986 until 1988. He could then become a member of the Institute of Maxillofacial Technology.

After becoming a member, Mark very quickly found a job working in the laboratory at St Thomas' Hospital where he worked with Derek Henderson for nearly a year. He then moved to Roehampton where he worked for seven years, five of them as deputy to Brian Conroy, the chief technician. In 1996 he moved to East Grinstead as consultant maxillofacial prosthetist and manager of the maxillofacial laboratory and prosthetics clinic.

Mark was awarded an MBE for services to maxillofacial prosthetics in 2011, I interviewed him at the Queen Victoria Hospital, East Grinstead in February 2013.

Appendix 2
Some Hospitals Mentioned in the Text

The development of oral and maxillofacial surgery took place in many hospitals throughout the UK, but dental surgeons (as they were then called) from departments descended from the EMS (Emergency Medical Services) hospitals, which were set up to manage facial injuries in WWII, had a disproportionate influence on the specialty.

In 1932, the political situation in Europe suggested that another war might come, and so the Army Council set up a committee on the setting up of special emergency hospitals to treat facial injuries in any future war. On the committee was plastic surgeon Harold Gillies and also dental surgeon William Kelsey Fry who had worked together at Frognal House, Sidcup in treating facial injuries in WWI. Also involved was prominent medically qualified dental surgeon William Warwick James, who had worked on facial injuries in south London at the Royal Victoria Patriotic Asylum, which had been requisitioned for war work and became the 3rd London General Hospital until 1920.

The committee made recommendations which were reported in 1935.[245] They recommended that there be special hospitals of 200 beds each which could expand to 500 beds to treat patients with fractures needing the attention of dental surgeons and injuries to hard and soft tissues needing the help of plastic or other specialised surgeons.

In 1938, the Emergency Medical Service was established to organise hospitals in anticipation of injuries resulting from possible enemy bombing. When war came several were set up around the United Kingdom, four around London. In 1939 the committee sent Gillies and Kelsey Fry to look at prospective sites for the hospitals which they did between April and September that year. They decided that Hill End near St Albans, Rooksdown House at Basingstoke, the Queen Victoria Hospital at East Grinstead and Queen Mary Hospital, Roehampton were suitable. However, the Roehampton unit was soon moved to Stoke Mandeville.

It is no coincidence that it was from two of these that many of the original movers and shakers of the specialty originated and by the 1960s and 1970s they were taking their pick of the bright young medically qualified dentists who wanted to come into the specialty and these are thus overrepresented in among those I have interviewed.

Rooksdown House, Park Prewitt Hospital, Basingstoke (moved to Roehampton in 1959)

Gillies and Kelsey Fry decided that Rooksdown House would be the premier site for taking soldiers with facial injuries and would be modelled on Queen's Hospital in Frognal House, Sidcup, where they had treated WWI facial injuries. Park Prewett Hospital at Basingstoke was a large psychiatric hospital which was taken over by the Emergency Medical Service during WWII. Rooksdown House was a large house in the grounds which housed the private psychiatric patients.

When Gillies arrived to work there in 1940, the psychiatric patients had already

---

245 Report to the Army Council of the Standing Committee on Maxillo-Facial Injuries. (1935) HMSO.

been displaced and Rooksdown was being occupied as a home for nurses from St Mary's and Westminster Hospitals. Gillies was in charge of Rooksdown House, but there were other plastic surgeons who worked there as well, and other medical staff.

Kelsey Fry decided that he would not go there with Gillies but work with plastic surgeon Archibald McIndoe, who was Gillies cousin, at East Grinstead. There were other dental surgeons. One was Martin Rushton who eventually became the Dean of the Faculty of Dental Surgery of the Royal College of Surgeons of England and of Guy's dental school.

After the war finished, the Emergency Medical Service moved out of Park Prewitt and psychiatric patients returned. However, there were still many patients still needing facial surgery and Rooksdown House continued treating them. In 1948 when the National Health Service started it was taken over and became the Regional Centre for Plastic Surgery and Jaw Surgery for the South West Metropolitan Region, which it remained until 1959 when the unit was moved to Queen Mary Hospital, Roehampton. The psychiatric patients returned to Rooksdown House in 1961.

Norman Rowe arrived at Rooksdown House in 1948, having been a registrar at Hill End Hospital, St Albans, and was joined within a year by Homer Killey who had been a registrar at Hill End with him. Sir Paul Bramley worked as a registrar at Rooksdown House under Norman Rowe and described in his interview the relationship between them and how Rowe took on some of the surgery.[246]

Queen Mary Hospital, Roehampton

Queen Mary Hospital, Roehampton, was based on what was a country house and had been requisitioned in WWI to treat war injured soldiers much as Frognal House in Sidcup had.

Roehampton became the premier centre for orthopaedics and particularly the treatment of those with limb injuries and rehabilitation of amputees and had a large prosthetic limb producing facility. At the outbreak of WWII Roehampton already had a plastic surgery department, the chief being Thomas Pomfret Kilner who was another of the four original British plastic surgeons who had been trained by and had worked with Gillies at Sidcup. Subsequently they had fallen out. At the time Queen Mary Hospital, Roehampton was run by the Ministry of Pensions and so did not become one of the major sites for the management of facial injuries, although there was discussion that it would take some. However, it was soon decided that Roehampton was too close to London for such a facility and the unit was moved to Stoke Mandeville Hospital.

The Rooksdown House unit moved to Roehampton in 1959.

Queen Victoria Hospital, East Grinstead

The Queen Victoria Hospital was opened as a cottage hospital in 1863. During WWII it was taken over for the management of facial injuries sustained by RAF crew.

---

246 For an in depth description of Rooksdown House in WWII see: Millar, Simon 2015 Rooksdown House and the Rooksdown Club: A Study Into the Rehabilitation of Facially Disfigured Servicemen and Civilians Following the Second World War. Doctoral thesis, University of London. Available to download at: https://sas-space.sas.ac.uk/6264/

In 1939 it was extended by the erection of huts in adjacent land purchased for that purpose, and from 1941 Archibald McIndoe was in charge of the hospital as the plastic surgeon. There were other surgeons there and William Kelsey Fry was the consulting dental surgeon supported by resident dental surgeons Alan McLeod, Rae Shepherd and Gilbert Parfitt. Early on they were joined by Alex MacGregor, who went on to work with Rainsford Mowlem at Hill End, Martin Rushton, who subsequently worked with Gillies at Rooksdown House, and Wilfred Fish. There were 4 dental surgeons and five technicians.

Although the hospital was given over to treat RAF crew, Archibald McIndoe, who was in charge, remained a civilian. Terence Ward was in the RAF and in 1940 he was seconded to East Grinstead by the RAF dental service and in 1941 left to be in charge of the maxillofacial unit as Cosford.

At the end of the war Kelsey Fry left to return to Guy's, McLeod and Shepherd to their dental practices, Parfitt to the Eastman Dental Hospital to do research, and Terence Ward was appointed as consultant in oral surgery. He was heavily involved in the formation of the British Association of Oral Surgeons, and the first scientific meeting of the association was held there in October 1962.

The Queen Victoria Hospital is the only one of the special hospital units from WWII which remains on the same site and is one of the few, if not the only hospital, which retains a doctors' mess with a bar! The hospital does not provide full hospital services but is rather a specialist surgical hospital for plastic surgery, oral and maxillofacial and corneo and oculoplastic surgery as well as sleep medicine.[247]

Hill End Hospital, (moved to Mount Vernon in 1952)

Hill End Hospital was a psychiatric hospital close to St Albans in Hertfordshire and was also commandeered by the Emergency Medical Services for use in WWII. It was linked to St Barthomew's Hospital and many of the staff came from there. Rainsford Mowlem was in charge of the plastic surgery unit, which was set up in 1939 in facilities vacated by the psychiatric patients. There were two large 33 bedded wards. Two dental surgeons were appointed; these were Alex McGregor, who later became Dean of the Birmingham Dental School, and Ben Fickling. Later they were joined by Paul Toller.

Just like at Rooksdown House and East Grinstead, at the end of the war there remained many patients who still needed rehabilitation. The unit provided a plastic surgery and oral surgery service to a wide geographical area north of the Thames stretching from the east coast to Oxford, so it remained in service. However, it became necessary for the hospital to be returned to its original function as a psychiatric hospital and a new home was needed for the unit.

Mount Vernon Hospital had originally been the country branch of The North London Hospital for Consumption and Diseases of the Chest, a hospital in Hampstead. Artificial pneumothorax had reduced the need for hospitalisation, and so Mount Vernon principally became a radium institute to treat malignant disease. At the onset of WWII,

---

247 For detail see: The Maxillofacial Unit. Sir Terence Ward. Annals of the Royal College of Surgeons of England 1975 57. 68 - 73 and A History of the Queen Victoria Hospital, East Grinstead. Bennett J. British Journal of Plastic Surgery 1988 41. 422 - 440.

huts were erected in the grounds to take hospital patients from various hospitals from within London, and after the war these huts were vacant and were offered to the Hill End team who moved to Mount Vernon in 1953.[248]

The plastic surgery department at Mount Vernon Hospital was a major centre which attracted ambitious trainees from within the UK and overseas and made a major contribution to plastic surgery in treatment, training and research. For many years, Mount Vernon and Canniesburn were the two major plastic surgery units in the UK. But oral surgery never attained the achievements or reputation of the units at Roehampton or East Grinstead until it eventually divorced from the plastic surgery unit and moved to Northwick Park Hospital with a new generation of enthusiastic surgeons.

Ballochmyle (moved to Glasgow Royal Infirmary in 1960 and to Canniesburn in 1967)

The Emergency Medical Service decided that there should be two special hospitals in Scotland to take injuries from WWII. They were at Bangor in West Lothian and Ballochmyle in Ayrshire.

The site at Ballochmyle was chosen as it was some distance away from populated areas and therefore less likely to be affected by bombing raids but it was also a great distance from enemy action, so its intended purpose was primarily the management of civilians injured in bombing raids. The base was Ballochmyle House, a large historic mansion which was used for accommodation of staff while the hospital was built in the grounds, and comprised two blocks of eight wards each and other buildings for support services.

The plastic surgeons were led by Jack Tough and there were three dental surgeons led by consultant A Wilson who attended frequently while working in his dental practice, which was the pattern at the time. Harold Gillies attended intermittently to give moral support, occasionally to operate and play golf.

After the war, the plastic and dental surgery continued and took referrals from other hospitals and from general practitioners but it was deemed too far away from the major population areas so in 1960 it moved to the Glasgow Royal Infirmary. There was insufficient space there, so in 1967 it moved to a specially built 130 bed hospital at Canniesburn.

Plastic Surgery in Glasgow progressed but dental surgery did not until 1969 when Derek Henderson was appointed as a consultant oral surgeon and he co-operated with the plastic surgeons in the surgical management of facial deformity. He worked with Ian Jackson, who was a progressive plastic surgeon. Khursheed Moos was appointed as an oral surgeon in 1974.

It later became apparent that a specialist plastic and maxillofacial hospital working without intensive care facilities and the sophisticated imaging and laboratory support of a major general hospital was becoming untenable for medicine and surgery of the 21st Century. So in 2003 the plastic surgeons moved back to the Glasgow Royal

248 The history, antecedents and progress of the Mount Vernon Centre for Plastic Surgery and Jaw Injuries, Northwood, Middlesex, 1939-1983. Dawson R 1988 British Journal of Plastic Surgery 41. 83 - 91

Infirmary. The oral and maxillofacial surgeons divorced from the plastic surgeons and moved to the Southern General Hospital in Glasgow where they could work with the neurosurgeons on major deformity cases and also undertake head and neck cancer surgery unhindered. The oral and maxillofacial surgery service is now in the Queen Elizabeth University Hospital, built on the site of the Southern General Hospital.[249]

Gloucester City Hospital (moved to Chepstow and Frenchay Hospital Bristol in 1950. The Chepstow unit moved again to Morriston Hospital Swansea in 1994).

The Gloucester Plastic Surgery, Burns and Jaw Surgery Unit was set up under the auspices of the Emergency Medical Service between August 1943 and May 1944, later than the other special plastics units. The purpose was to treat soldiers wounded in the land war after the D-day landings. Gloucester was chosen as the site as it was expected the wounded would be brought by boat into the Bristol Channel.

The surgeon chosen to be in charge was Emlyn Lewis, who was an experienced general surgeon at St Mary's Hospital. He had prepared for the role by attending Rooksdown House once a week with Sir Harold Gillies. He went to Sunday morning rounds at East Grinstead with McIndoe and had also visited Mowlem at Hill End and Kilner at Stoke Mandeville. The unit was set up at the City Hospital in Gloucester; there were huts in the grounds that had been erected in the 1914 - 18 war.

The main work arrived four days after June 4th 1944, D day. The patients arrived not by boat but flown into RAF Wroughton. Injured soldiers were taken on alternate days to Gloucester and Rooksdown House.

As with the other special units, it continued after the war, carrying out surgery for rehabilitation and providing a service to the civilian population and for new referrals. There were a considerable number of patients from Wales so it was decided that the work should be carried out at Frenchay Hospital at Bristol providing for the southwest England and the main unit would move to Chepstow in Monmouthshire where there was a former military hospital used for prisoners of war.

The unit moved to Chepstow between May and September 1950. The dental surgeon was John Gibson, who was appointed to Gloucester with a view to moving to Chepstow. The Chepstow unit moved to Morriston Hospital Swansea in 1994.[250]

Wordsley Hospital

Wordsley Hospital, north of Stourbridge, was located in what had been a Victorian workhouse and military hospital in WWI. It was used by the Emergency Medical Services during WWII, with additional buildings added. After the National Health

---

249 A Short History of Oral and Maxillofacial Surgery in Scotland. Khursheed Moos. Dental History Magazine Vol 3 No 1. 7 - 12 and History of the West of Scotland Plastic Surgery Unit: 1940-1986. McGregor I, Watson R. British Journal of Plastic Surgery 1998 51. 333 - 342.
250 The information for this account is largely based on: Personal memories of the Gloucester unit 1943-1950. Edwards L. British Journal of Plastic Surgery 1985 38. 55 - 69. This paper as it includes a good account of how facial trauma was managed at the time and much social history particularly concerning the move to Chepstow and accommodation of staff.

Service started, the Birmingham Regional Hospital Board appointed a plastic surgeon O Mansfield who had received training at Hill End and he was supported by a dentist, J Knight. Subsequently, the Plastic Surgery Unit grew as did the oral surgery support and provided a service to a large area of the West Midlands extending as far west as Hereford.[251]

The hospital finally closed in 2005.

---

251 The development of Plastic Surgery in the West Midlands Region. North J. British Journal of Plastic Surgery 1987 40. 317 - 322.

Appendix 3
Timeline

Of some significant dates and others of relevance or interest in the evolution of medicine, dentistry, surgery and particularly British oral and maxillofacial surgery

12th Century.

St Bartholomew's Hospital London was formed in Smithfield.

13th Century.

Practitioners of surgery in England became associated with barbers.

St Thomas' Hospital London founded.

15th Century.

1460 The Barber-Surgeons were incorporated as one of the livery companies of the City of London.

16th Century.

Girolamo Fracastoro in Italy claimed that particles in the air could be transferred and cause disease.

1505 The Seal of Cause of the Royal College of Surgeons of Edinburgh was confirmed by Royal Charter by King James IVth of Scotland.[252]

1518 The Royal College of Physicians of London was founded by Henry VIII.

1540 The scattered guilds of barber-surgeons within England united to form a united Company of Barber-Surgeons.

1563 Queen Elizabeth's Statute of Artificers gave the Guilds and Companies powers that allowed the Company of Barber-

Surgeons to have full control of deciding who was fit to practise surgery. It later became widely disregarded by the courts.

17th Century.

1618 The physicians published a Pharmacopoeia in London, but there was no restriction on who could take or administer the medications.

1675 Antonie von Leeuwenhoel reported to the Royal Society that he had identified 'little animals' in rainwater using a microscope he had developed. This was initially regarded with scepticism.

18th century.

1711 William Cheselden (1688-1752), who was qualified with the Grand Diploma of the Barber-Surgeons, started lecturing and became Surgeon to St Thomas' and St George's Hospitals. He developed the lateral lithotomy operation.

1715 Westminster Hospital founded.

1721 Guy's Hospital founded.

1728 John Hunter (1728-1793) widely regarded as the founder of modern scientific surgery was born.

1729 Cheselden published: 'Atlas of the Human Bones or Osteographia'.

1733 St George's Hospital founded.

---

252 The Seal of Cause gave exclusive rights to perform surgery within Edinburgh and imposed the duty to ensure all apprentices were tested.

1736 Percival Pott (1714-1788) took the Diploma of the Barber-Surgeons. He became Surgeon at St Bartholomew's Hospital where he lectured and described Pott's fracture of the fibula.

1740 the London Hospital founded.

1745 The surgeons parted from the barbers to form their own 'Surgeons Company' with its own premises in the Old Bailey.

1745 The Middlesex Hospital was founded.

1746 William Hunter started his anatomy school in London. It was the first medical school in the city.

1748 John Hunter came to London and worked as an assistant to his brother William. They started a collection of diseased organs from cadavers and described them.

1749 John Hunter started training at the Royal Hospital, Chelsea with William Cheselden.

18th century (second half) private medical schools opened around London.

1760 John Hunter was commissioned as an army surgeon, having trained at Barts with Percival Pott after Cheselden died.

1763 John Hunter, in partnership with dentist James Spence, experimented with tooth transplants.

1764 John Hunter started his own anatomy school.

1768 John Hunter was elected as surgeon to St George's Hospital. He started his museum of anatomical specimens.

1773 The Medical Society of London formed, where physicians, surgeons and apothecaries met.

1785 The Middlesex Hospital took on a teaching role.

1793 Matthew Baillie (John and William Hunter's nephew) produced 'The Morbid Anatomy of some of the most Important Parts of the Human Body' and in 1799 'Atlas of Human Diseases'.

1793 John Hunter died. His collection of pathological and anatomical specimens was purchased by the government in 1799 and presented to the Royal College of Surgeons; it became the basis of the Hunterian Museum.

1799 The first dental surgeon was appointed at a London hospital at Guy's.

19th Century.

1800 The Surgeons' Company became the Royal College of Surgeons in London. The Surgeon's Hall in Old Bailey was in a 'ruinous state' so they moved to new premises in Lincoln's Inn Fields.

1805 The Medical and Chirurgical Society of London was formed. It eventually became the Royal Society of Medicine.

1814 The Apothecaries Act empowered apothecaries to examine all persons who could practise as apothecaries. Educational standards included an apprenticeship of 5 years, a course of lectures in anatomy and physiology and lectures on the theory and practice of medicine. They also needed to have attended the wards of a hospital for 6 months. Apothecaries were also entitled to practise surgery and act as 'general practitioners' but they could only charge for drugs dispensed.

1818 The Hunterian Society was formed in 1818 by Sir William Blizard of the London Hospital.

1819 The stethoscope was introduced.

1821 The Charing Cross Hospital was the first hospital to open with a specific teaching role.

1823 The Lancet started publication by Thomas Wakley; it was published weekly for the medical profession. Wakley described the Royal College of Surgeons as 'a constitutionally rotten concern'.

1831. The Times reported that on Thursday December 1st a maxillectomy operation was scheduled at St Bartholomew's Hospital which was: 'so rare that it excited such interest in the faculty and the unprofessional public that when the patient and surgeon arrived a multitude so dense and intractable had assembled that neither patient nor surgeon could gain admittance and the operation was postponed'. On Saturday December 3rd the surgeon, Mr Earl, removed the tumour which hung from the floor of the orbit to the lower jaw in 16 minutes after securing the common carotid artery.[253]

1832 The Provincial Medical Society was formed in Worcester; it was to become the British Medical Association in 1856.

1834 University College Hospital (formerly known as the North London Hospital) was opened for teaching.

1838 Matthias Jakob Schleiden reported that different parts of plants were composed of 'cells'. Theodor Schwann in Berlin confirmed cells in humans.

1839 King's College Hospital was opened for the purpose of teaching.

1840 The Provincial Medical Society started publishing the Provincial Medical and Surgical Journal, which was to become the British Medical Journal.

1840 Samuel Cartwright was appointed as the first Professor of Dentistry, at King's College London.

1840s to 1970s. The 'germ theory' of disease developed gradually but cannot be assigned to any one person.

1842 Dr Crawford Long of Jefferson, Georgia in the USA made a patient insensible using ether while he removed a neck tumour and subsequently for eight other operations. This was probably the first recorded use of general anaesthesia. Publication and knowledge of this was not revealed until 1849, some years after the use of ether had been generally accepted. It is also possible that this had been preceded by the use of ether three months beforehand by William Clark who administered it for a dental extraction carried out by a dentist, Elijah Pope, in Rochester, New York.

1843 The Royal College of Surgeons of London became the Royal College of Surgeons of England. The first Fellows of the college were appointed by election from among the members.

1844 The first examination for the Fellowship of the Royal College of Surgeons of England. Candidates had to be 25 years of age, of good character, have studied for six years (three in a London hospital and one as a house surgeon or dresser in a recognised hospital), have written up six clinical cases and written examinations in physiology, surgery, therapeutics and pathology. 24 candidates passed the first Fellowship examination. However, practice without qualification continued.

1844 The first record of inhalation general anaesthesia. Dentist Horace Wells in Hartford, Connecticut instructed his assistant Dr Riggs to administer nitrous oxide to him and remove his painful tooth.

1846 Dentist William Morton administered ether at the Massachusetts General Hospital for removal of a neck lump. This event was widely reported and ether became widely used once it was realised what agent he had used.

The first report of a general anaesthetic in England. Dr Francis Boott administered ether for a dental extraction in Gower Street, London, and told Robert Liston, a

---

253 Reported in 'The Times' December 6th 1831. See: The Times Digital Archive online for this and other operation reports.

surgeon at the nearby University College Hospital who carried out an amputation with ether the following week. There were some reports of a possible previous administration in Dumfries, Scotland.

1847 James Simpson published 'On a New Anaesthetic Agent, More Efficient than Sulphuric Ether' in The Lancet. Chloroform displaced ether as the most popular anaesthetic agent and remained so until beyond the end of the century.

1853 John Snow, probably the first doctor in England to specialise in anaesthesia, administered 15 minims of chloroform, via a handkerchief, to Queen Victoria for the birth of Prince Leopold. News of this helped anaesthesia become more widely accepted; it had been condemned by the church.[254]

19th century (second half) The Infirmaries in towns were being opened.

1858 The UK parliament passed the Medical Act which gave recognition to 'legally qualified medical practitioners' and set up the General Medical Council to monitor professional training, register qualified persons and de-register them if necessary.

Rudolf Virchow published his book 'Cellular Pathology'. He had recognised that the cell theory could be applied to disease. He discovered leukemic cells in a lymph node and described thrombo-embolism.

The Dental Hospital of London was established. It eventually became the Royal Dental Hospital. It closed in 1985.

1859 The first Medical Register was published.

1860 The LDS diploma was established

by the Royal College of Surgeons of England.

1860 By now all the London hospitals had dental surgeons appointed to them. These were mostly medically qualified men who practised dentistry. Specialist surgeons were not appointed to the hospitals until many decades later.

1861 The National Dental Hospital opened, students were taught dentistry. It eventually became the dental school of University College Hospital.

1863 A United States congressional enquiry was set up to examine the evidence and award an honorarium to the discoverer of anaesthesia but it was unable to come to a conclusion.

1867 The clinical thermometer was introduced.

1867 Joseph Lister reported a series of 11 cases of compound fracture of the leg, with only one death from 'hospital disease' when using carbolic spray. He called this technique 'antisepsis'.

1870 Julius Cohnheim, a pupil of Virchow, reported his technique of freezing a specimen with carbon dioxide in order to examine it quickly under the microscope while the surgeon was still operating.

1872 John Morgan warned about the danger of chloroform in the British Medical Journal. He quoted mortality rates from combined British and American data. Death rate of 1:23204 for ether, 1:2873 for chloroform and 1:5588 for a mixture of both.

1875. Joseph von Gerloch developed

---

254 Another claim on the title of Britain's first anaesthetist was dentist James Robinson. See: The Life of James Robinson Britain's First Anaesthetist. Richard H Ellis. Dental Historian Oct 1985 18-20. Also see: A Treatise on the Inhalation of the Vapour of Ether for the Prevention of Pain in Surgical Operations. Robinson K. 1847. Both sourced from the British Dental Association Library.

stains for tissues and Wilhelm His had developed the microtome.

1878 The Dentists' Act was passed.

1879 The first Dentist's Register was established and kept by the General Medical Council. The act precluded the use of the description of 'dentist' or any other term suggesting registration to anyone other than registered dentists or registered doctors. It did not make practice by unregistered persons illegal.

1879 The LDS diploma was established in Edinburgh, Glasgow and Ireland.

1884 The first use of local anaesthesia. Carl Koller applied 2% cocaine to the eye of a patient having surgery for glaucoma in Germany. Later that year, William Halsted and Richard Hall in New York reported that they had injected cocaine as an infiltration to produce local anaesthesia and had numbed teeth with an inferior dental nerve block.

1886 Medical Act. New registrants had to be qualified in medicine, surgery and gynaecology.

1887 An early recorded use of histopathology was of specimens taken from the larynx of Kaiser Frederick III the Crown Prince of Prussia and Germany. Sir Morell Mackenzie, an eminent throat specialist advised that a piece of the growth be removed and examined under a microscope by an expert. Two specimens were taken and examined by Professor Rudolf Virchow, who concluded the specimens were benign so laryngectomy was avoided. The Crown Prince died of laryngeal cancer.

1890. A steam steriliser was used in Germany, antisepsis became asepsis.

1892 The Society of Extractors and Adaptors of Teeth was formed to represent the interest of unregistered dental practitioners.

1891 (about) George Washington Crile (1864-1943) noticed that removal of an isolated lymph gland containing metastatic cancer from the lip, tongue, tonsil, scalp or cheek was followed by recurrence in nearly all cases. He advocated a 'block dissection' of the glands of the neck (after clamping the carotid artery!).[255]

1894. Rubber gloves were used during surgery by Halsted in Baltimore. Cuthbert Wallace was the first surgeon in the UK to use the aseptic technique.

1895 Wilhelm Roentgen in Würzburg discovered X-rays. The first image of human tissue was of his wife's hand.

1896 The first use of X-rays in England was reported in the Lancet. It was an image of a bullet in a hand.

1896 Possibly the first use of therapeutic radiation. Emil Herman Grubbé assembled an X-ray machine in Chicago and used it to treat a woman with carcinoma of the breast. He subsequently suffered and died from multiple cancers caused by his exposure to radiation.

1890 The Lancet reported that they had received a copy of a petition signed by past and present dental surgeons to the board of management of the London Hospital with a request that it be made compulsory 'for all candidates for the post of dental surgeon to be registered on both the Dental and Medical Registers.'

1897. William Arbuthnot Lane first used a 'no touch' technique for operating at

---

255 See: Treatment of Malignancy. Crile GW. Annals of Surgery 1931; 93(1):99-108. He described his thoughts and technique in: George Crile: An Autobiography with edited sidelights by Grace Crile (2 volumes) 1947. Sourced from Royal Society of Medicine Library.

Guy's Hospital.

20th Century.

1906 The first university qualifications in dentistry were established in Birmingham and Dublin.

1909 A legal case ruled that not only was it not illegal to practise if unregistered, it was permissible to use the title 'Dentist'. The Society of Extractors and Adaptors of Teeth became the Incorporated Dental Society.

1915 Roehampton House in South London was taken over to become Queen Mary's Hospital for the rehabilitation of amputees injured in WWI.

1916 Captain Harold Gillies returned from France and reported to the Cambridge Military Hospital Aldershot where he took over two wards for the management of facial injuries.

1917 The Frognal Estate at Sidcup was taken over to become the Queen's Hospital for the treatment of facial injuries and the facility at Aldershot was moved there.

1920 Harold Gillies' book 'Plastic Surgery of the Face' was published.

1922 The Dentist Act 1922 made it illegal to practise dentistry without being registered but the register included dentists who were unqualified but already practising.

1925 Treatment of facial injuries at Queens Hospital Sidcup ceased and the remaining patients were transferred to Queen Mary's Hospital Roehampton

where they continued to be treated by Gillies and Kilner.

1928 Alexander Fleming noticed the antibacterial properties of the penicillin mould at St Mary's Hospital.

1928 Ivan Magill published his paper on endotracheal anaesthesia. He had developed the technique with Stanley Rowbotham while working at Sidcup with Gillies.[256] Magill acknowledged Charles Elsberg had previously developed an endotracheal technique in America.[257]

1930s Alexandro Vellebona, in Italy, developed the technique of tomography using a moving X-ray source and plate to image a slice of tissue. Tomography was the technique routinely used in maxillofacial surgery to visualise orbit floor fractures until computerised tomography was invented.

1935 The Report to the Army Council of the Army Advisory Standing Committee on Maxillo-Facial Injuries was published. It advised on the hospitals and facilities needed in any forthcoming war.[258]

1940s Techniques of extracting and purifying penicillin were developed and tested, initially on mice, so it was available for therapeutic use by 1945.

1940 'Injuries of the Face and Jaws, with Special Reference to War Casualties' was published. It was authored by William Warwick James and Ben Fickling and was based on their First World War experience and their records from the Third

---

256 See: Endotracheal Anaesthesia. Magill I. Proceedings of the Royal Society of Medicine. 1928;22(2):83-88.
257 See: Clinical Experiences with Intratracheal Insufflation (Meltzer), with Remarks upon the Value of the Method for Thoracic Surgery. Elsberg CA Ann Surg. 1910;52(1):23-29.
258 Authored by William Kelsey Fry, Harold Gillies and William Warwick-James the committee made recommendations on the treatment and setting up of special hospitals for facial injuries in any forthcoming war. All three had extensive experience in WWI. Sourced at the British Dental Association Library.

London General Hospital.[259]

1941 The Royal College of Surgeons in London was bombed. 2/3rd of Hunterian Museum was destroyed, including 10,000 of John Hunter's specimens.

1942 The Beveridge report formed the basis of the Welfare State and National Health Service.

The Dental Treatment of Maxillo-Facial Injuries by W Kelsey Fry, P Shepherd, A McLeod and W Parfitt was published. The authors were working on WWII facial injuries at East Grinstead.

1943 Streptomycin was first isolated in New Jersey. It became the first antibiotic capable of curing tuberculosis.

1948 The National Health Service was inaugurated on July 5th.

The Faculty of Dental Surgery of the Royal College of Surgeons of England was inaugurated. The first Fellowship in Dental Surgery of the Royal College of Surgeons of England examinations were held.

1949 The first Fellowship in Dental Surgery of the Royal College of Surgeons of Edinburgh examinations were held.

1955 The first edition of Fractures of the Facial Skeleton by Norman Rowe and Homer Killey was published and helped establish dental surgeons as predominant in facial trauma.

1956 Ian Donald first used ultrasound to monitor obstetric development in Glasgow, using a machine developed with engineer Tom Brown.

1961 The first therapeutic use of a laser. Charles Campbell and Charles Koester used a ruby laser to destroy a retinal tumour in New York.

1962 The British Association of Oral Surgeons was founded; the first President was Terence Ward.

1963 The British Journal of Oral Surgery was first published.

1964 The carbon dioxide laser was invented by Kumar Patel at the Bell laboratories

1966 The British Association of Oral Surgeons Memorandum on Post Graduate Training reported: 'Council were unanimously of the opinion that in the future development of oral surgery a registered medical qualification will tend to come to be regarded as desirable for the holder of a consultant appointment in dental surgery who aspires to have full medical charge of his beds.'

1971 Dr Geza Jako first used a carbon dioxide laser to treat a laryngeal cancer in Boston.

1976 The first computerised tomographic scanner was used. The technique was developed by Godfrey Hounsfield when working for EMI and independently by Dr Allan M. Cormack in Massachusetts. It was known as the 'EMI scanner' and was used for brain scanning.

1970s (late) The first dental panoramic X-ray machines became widely available.

1977 The first MRI body scan was performed on a human using an MRI machine developed by American doctors Raymond Damadian, Larry Minkoff and Michael Goldsmith. The first magnetic resonance scanners became available for medical use in 1981.

---

259 The Third London General Hospital operated in Wandsworth from 1914 -1920. It had been the Royal Victoria Patriotic School and was requisitioned for the duration of the war. The original Victorian building is now apartments.

1978 The council of the British Association of Oral Surgeons agreed to pursue their recommendation that new consultant dental surgeon posts dealing predominantly with oral surgery be advertised as Consultants in Oral Surgery.

1981 The British Association of Oral Surgeons endorsed the conclusion of its 1979 Working Party that future consultants in the specialty should hold both medical and dental qualifications and that this should be a mandatory requirement within 10 years.

1982/3 The British Association of Oral Surgeons became the British Association of Oral and Maxillofacial Surgeons.

1984 The British Journal of Oral Surgery was renamed the British Journal of Oral and Maxillofacial Surgery.

1985 The first specialty examination in oral and maxillofacial surgery for the FRCS diploma of the Royal College of Surgeons of Edinburgh was held.

1995 The first digital dental panoramic X-rays system became available.

The specialist register of Oral and Maxillofacial Surgery was created by the General Medical Council in accord with the European Union Specialist Medical Qualification Order (Article 8).

The John McLean Archive

John Mclean was a well-known restorative dental surgeon and materials scientist who combined a career in private dental practice with research into dental materials and teaching at Guy's and the Eastman dental hospitals. He authored dozens of research papers and was the editor of a standard book on dental ceramics. He was a president of the British Dental Association and on his death he left a legacy to the Association which was used to fund the John McLean Oral History Archive.

The archive was established to record the changes in dentistry since the inception of the National Health Service and comprises oral history interviews and witness seminars, which have been published.

Acknowledgements

I am indebted to my subjects for their time in allowing me to interview them and for reading and checking the final text for accuracy of their meaning and making suggestions. The British Association of Oral and Maxillofacial Surgeons allowed me access to the minutes of their council meetings and other documents. Rachel Bairsto, the head of museum services and archives at the British Dental Association, administered the John McLean history archive and arranged for the professional transcription of the audio recordings. The British Dental Association own the copyright of the original recordings and transcriptions and allowed me to use the material. The images on the front cover are from the slide collections of the late Gordon Hardman and Gordon Fordyce which were donated by their families to the British Dental Association archive. The libraries of the British Dental Association and Royal Society of Medicine hold a wealth of historical books and journals which I have referred to. My wife Maralyn has line edited the text and given me good council in content editing.

Also by Andrew Sadler

Dentist on the Ward: An Introduction to Oral and Maxillofacial Surgery and Medicine For Core Trainees in Dentistry – *Andrew Sadler and Leo Cheng*

Core Oral Surgery for Dental Students: Essential Knowledge for Qualifying Dental Examinations – *Andrew Sadler and Edmund Bailey*